Radiotherapy for Hodgkin Lymphoma

Lena Specht • Joachim Yahalom
(Editors)

Radiotherapy for Hodgkin Lymphoma

Springer

Prof. Lena Specht
Departments of Oncology and Haematology
Rigshospitalet
University of Copenhagen
2100 Copenhagen
Denmark

Prof. Joachim Yahalom
Department of Radiation Oncology
Memorial Sloan-Kettering Cancer
1275 York Ave
New York
10021-6094 NY
USA

ISBN 978-3-540-78455-5 ISBN 978-3-540-78944-4 (eBook)

DOI 10.1007/978-3-540-78944-4

Springer Heidelberg Dordrecht London New York

Library of Congress Control Number: 2010930080

Cover design: eStudio Calamar, Figueres/Berlin

Printed on acid-free paper

Springer is part of Springer Science+Business Media (www.springer.com)

Preface

The major goal of developing this book is to optimize radiotherapy for Hodgkin lymphoma by providing clinicians who treat patients with this disease with a comprehensive account of the background for radiotherapy for Hodgkin lymphoma, the rationale for radiotherapy in a modern combined modality setting, and the data that document its contribution to the best outcome for patients. Special emphasis is given to the changes in volume and dose that have evolved over the past 2 decades, and the use of modern advanced technologies in imaging and radiotherapy planning and delivery in order to accurately target involved sites and protect adjacent organs.

Radiotherapy was the first curative treatment modality for this previously lethal disease, and the achievements of the pioneers of curative radiotherapy for Hodgkin lymphoma represented some of the earliest success stories of the non-surgical treatment of cancer. With the advent of effective multiagent chemotherapy regimens, the role of radiotherapy changed. Radiotherapy now became part of multimodality treatment. Moreover, the long-term toxicity of the very extensive radiation fields of the past became apparent. This led to a virtual scare of radiotherapy in certain circles, and efforts were made to replace combined modality treatment with chemotherapy alone, almost no matter how intensive, with surprisingly little regard for the long-term toxicity of chemotherapy itself.

Recent evidence on the consequences of omitting radiotherapy altogether in the treatment of Hodgkin lymphoma demonstrates that such a strategy is not yielding the best possible results with regard to cure. In early-stage disease, the interim analysis of the large H10 trial of the EORTC/GELA/IIL demonstrates that in patients who were rendered PET-negative after two cycles of ABVD, the substitution of radiotherapy with more chemotherapy in favorable and unfavorable patients results in significantly higher relapse rates than standard treatment with less chemotherapy followed by involved node radiotherapy (INRT). In advanced disease, where many regarded radiotherapy as of no additional value, the recent analysis of the British LY09 trial demonstrates that the omission of radiotherapy seemed to be to the detriment of the chance of cure also in these patients. Finally, the concept of mini-chemotherapy with mini-radiotherapy has been shown to yield excellent results in patients with favorable and unfavorable early-stage disease, as demonstrated by the final analyses of the German Hodgkin Study Group HD10 and HD11 trials.

Radiotherapy remains the most effective single modality for the treatment of Hodgkin lymphoma. The modern application of this treatment modality, with lower doses and with very much reduced volumes, has proved effective and reduced the toxicity of this treatment tremendously. Highly advanced technologies within imaging, e.g., PET/CT-scanning, image co-registration, four-dimensional scanning and motion compensation, and within treatment planning and delivery, e.g., intensity-modulated radiotherapy, arc-therapy, image-guidance and motion gating or tracking, have revolutionized radiotherapy. These techniques allow highly conformal radiotherapy, sparing large volumes of normal tissues while maintaining target coverage. Such techniques can and should be employed in the treatment of Hodgkin lymphoma. We and others have developed these techniques, which are employed in the treatment of Hodgkin lymphoma in several large institutions on both sides of the Atlantic. It is our sincere hope that this book will aid radiation oncologists worldwide in implementing modern highly conformal radiotherapy in the multimodality treatment of Hodgkin lymphoma to the benefit of present and future patients.

This book could not have been written without the generous help of many colleagues who have contributed their knowledge and expertise to the different chapters of this book, and we wish to express our sincere gratitude for their contribution and support.

Finally, we want to dedicate this book to our spouses, Henrik and Judith, who have been most patient throughout and given us support and encouragement when we needed it most.

Copenhagen, July 2010 Lena Specht
New York, July 2010 Joachim Yahalom

Contents

History of Radiotherapy of Hodgkin's Disease (Now Hodgkin Lymphoma)

1

Lena Specht and Saul Rosenberg

Contents

1.1 Introduction

In December, 1895, Wilhelm Conrad Röntgen first published his discovery of X-rays in a short communication to the Medical Physics Society of Würzburg, Germany, entitled "Über eine neue Art von Strahlen" ("On a New Type of Rays") (Röntgen 1895; Lederman 1981; Dubois and Ash 1995). The biologic effects of the new rays were soon discovered, and they were almost immediately used in dermatology and to treat superficial cancers.

In Chicago, in 1902, Pusey published what appears to be the first documented case of radiotherapy of Hodgkin's disease (Pusey 1902). Figure 1.1 shows a 4-year-old boy with the diagnosis of Hodgkin's disease. The enlarged glands on the right side of the neck had been removed surgically, and in September, 1901, the boy was referred to Pusey "for exposure of the glands on the left side of the neck." "There was a mass of glands on the left side as large as a fist. Under *x*-ray exposures the swelling rapidly subsided, and in 2 months the glands were reduced to the size of an almond." In 1903, Senn, also from Chicago, published in more detail his cases of "that strange disease known as pseudoleucæmia, or Hodgkin's disease" (Senn 1903); the first case is shown in Fig. 1.2. This patient was "forty-three years of age, a saloon keeper and farmer by occupation. The glandular affection dates back a year, having commenced in the cervical region almost simultaneously on both sides, and involves now very extensively the glands of these localities as well as of the axillary and inguinal regions. The increased respiratory movements and dullness over the anterior mediastinum indicate the extension of the disease to the bronchial and mediastinal glands. Spleen considerably enlarged." The treatment started on March 29, 1902, and the patient "received thirty-four treatments as

L. Specht (✉)
Departments of Oncology and Haematology, The Finsen Centre, Rigshospitalet, University of Copenhagen, 9 Blegdamsvej, 2100, Copenhagen, Denmark
e-mail: specht@dadlnet.dk

S. Rosenberg
Division of Oncology, Stanford University, 269 Campus Dr, Rm 1115, Stanford, CA 94305, USA
e-mail: saul@stanford.edu

L. Specht and J. Yahalom (eds.), *Radiotherapy for Hodgkin Lymphoma*,
DOI: 10.1007/978-3-540-78944-4_1, © Springer-Verlag Berlin Heidelberg 2011

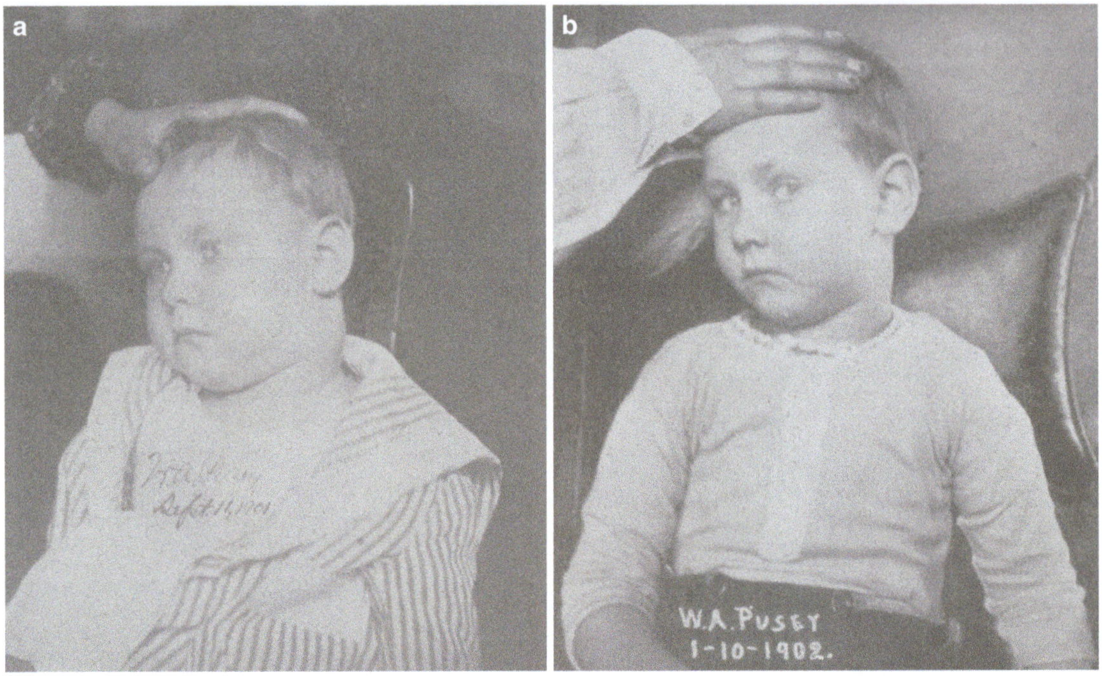

Fig. 1.1 A case of Hodgkin's disease that was treated in 1901 by W. A. Pusey, Professor of Dermatology in the Medical Department of the University of Illinois. (**a**) The patient on September 11, before the start of radiotherapy. (**b**) The condition on January 8, 1902, after the patient was treated intermittently from November 1901. This seems to be the first documented case of radiotherapy for Hodgkin's disease (from Pusey 1902)

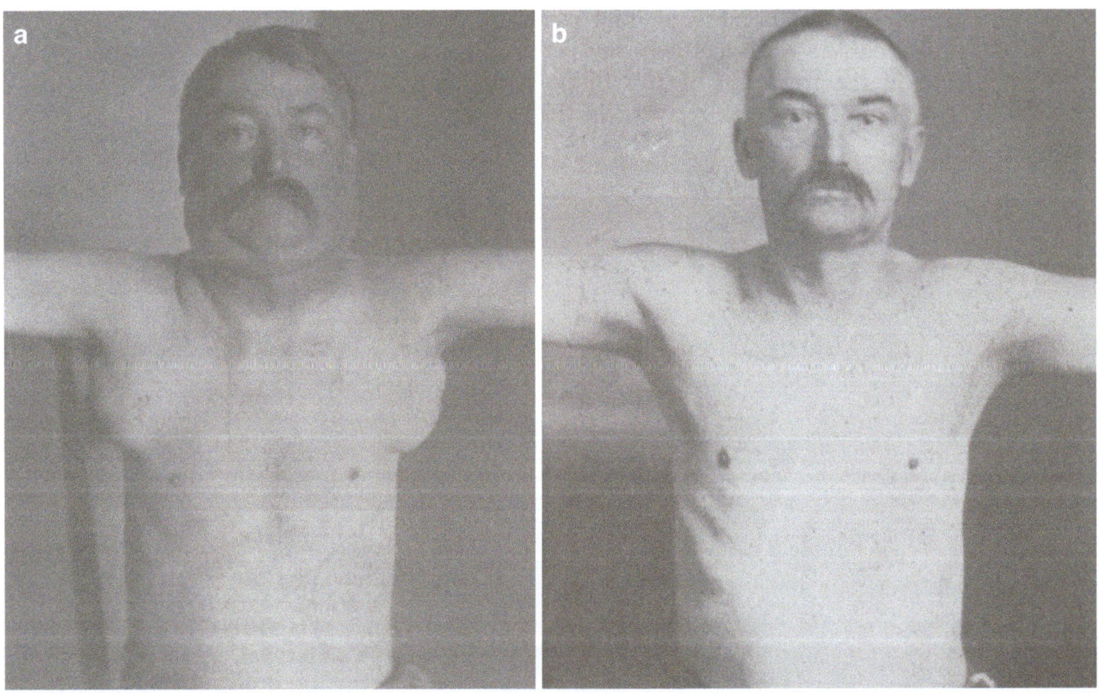

Fig. 1.2 A case of pseudoleucæmia, or Hodgkin's disease, that was treated in 1902 by N. Senn, Professor of Surgery, Rush Medical College, Chicago. (**a**) The patient before radiotherapy. (**b**) April 24, 1902, at the end of radiotherapy (from Senn 1903)

follows: right side of neck one minute, left side of neck one minute, neck from before backward one minute, neck from behind forward one minute, each axilla one minute, each groin one minute, spleen one minute. Daily sittings for the first ten days; 60 volts 8 ampères were used each day; distance of tube from surface twelve inches, a medium vacuum tube being used." At the end of treatment on April 24 "all of the glands subjected to the x ray treatment have nearly disappeared." Senn concluded that "the eminent success attained … by the use of the x ray can leave no further doubt of the curative effect of the Röntgen therapy in the treatment of pseudoleucæmia."

The optimism created by these early reports of almost miraculous responses to X-rays was soon tempered by the reports of almost inevitable recurrences (Coley 1915; Desjardins and Ford 1923; Minot 1926). For the next 40–50 years radiotherapy came to be regarded as a palliative treatment.

1.2 Radiotherapy as a Curative Treatment Modality

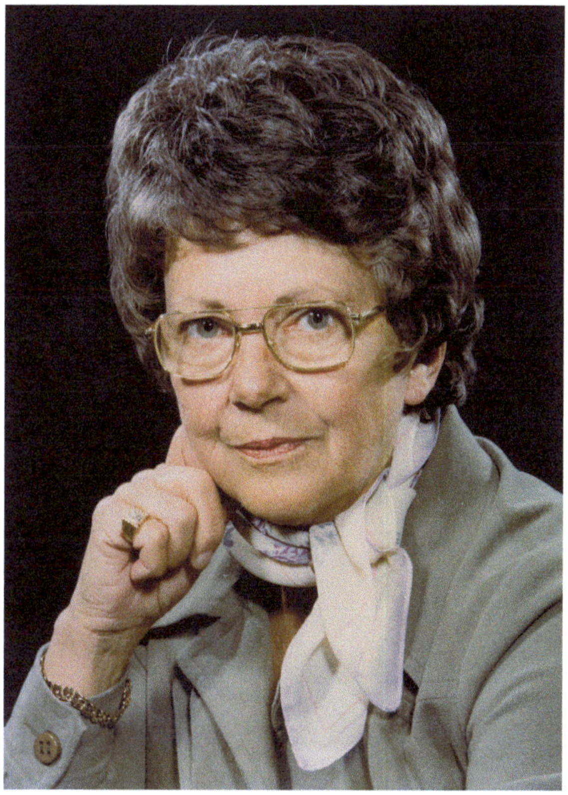

Fig. 1.3 Dr. Vera Peters, Princess Margaret Hospital, Toronto, Canada, pioneer of curative radiotherapy for Hodgkin's disease

Technical advances gradually allowed larger and deeper volumes to be irradiated with better control of dosage. Some radiotherapists began to use extended field radiation therapy for patients with Hodgkin's disease with doses as high as possible. The pioneer of this concept was René Gilbert from Geneva, Switzerland, who reported that prolonged remission could be achieved with this method (Gilbert 1925; Gilbert and Babaïantz 1931).

Vera Peters in Toronto (see Fig. 1.3) in 1950 presented the first definitive evidence that patients with early stage Hodgkin's disease could be cured with radiotherapy (Peters 1950; Peters and Middlemiss 1958). Eric Easson from Manchester, UK, in 1963 confirmed, with somewhat more convincing statistical methods, that localized Hodgkin's disease (i.e., lymphadenopathy confined to one or two contiguous anatomical sites) was probably curable with radical radiotherapy (Easson and Russell 1963; Easson 1966). These results were achieved with kilovolt radiation, and doses of more than 20–27 Gy could seldom be given.

The development at Stanford of the linear accelerator enabled Henry Kaplan in 1956 to start treating patients with Hodgkin's disease with high-dose (30–40 Gy), extended field radiotherapy including all major lymph node regions, the so-called total lymphoid radiotherapy (Rosenberg and Kaplan 1970), see Fig. 1.4. Figure 1.5 shows Henry Kaplan and Saul Rosenberg at their weekly Hodgkin's disease staging conferences at Stanford. In 1962, he published his first results with this technique in patients with localized disease (Kaplan 1962), demonstrating dramatic improvements in survival compared with patients treated palliatively. Analyses after longer follow-up of the results of radical radiotherapy with megavolt equipment (linear accelerators) compared with palliative radiotherapy and radical radiotherapy with kilovolt equipment demonstrated the highly significant improvement in the prognosis for these previously incurable patients (Kaplan 1966), see Fig. 1.6. Total or subtotal lymphoid irradiation with megavolt equipment became the standard treatment for early-stage Hodgkin's disease on both sides of the Atlantic.

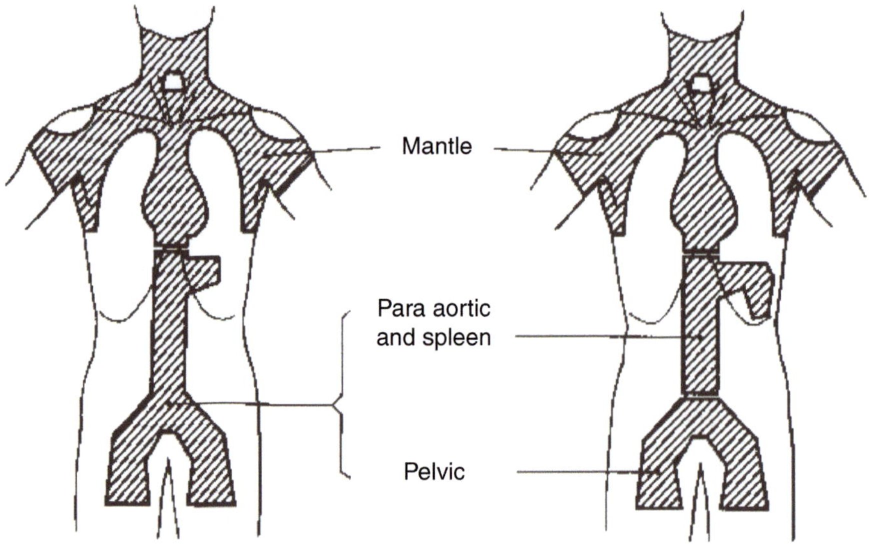

Fig. 1.4 Diagrams of the total lymphoid radiotherapy of Hodgkin's disease for splenectomized (*left*) and non-splenectomized (*right*) patients developed by Henry Kaplan at Stanford (from Rosenberg and Kaplan 1970)

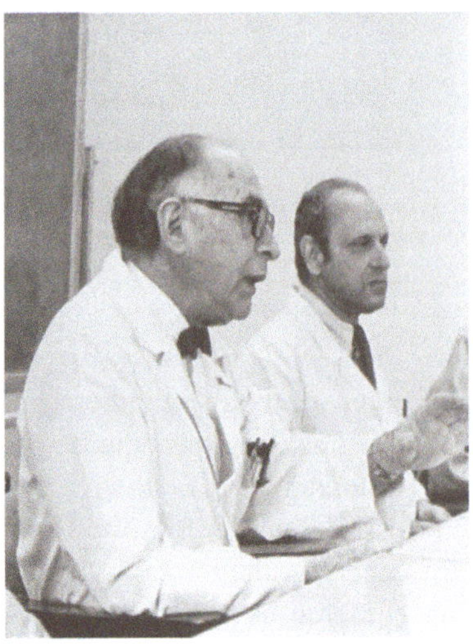

Fig. 1.5 Professor Henry Kaplan and Professor Saul Rosenberg, Stanford University, at their weekly Hodgkin's disease staging conference

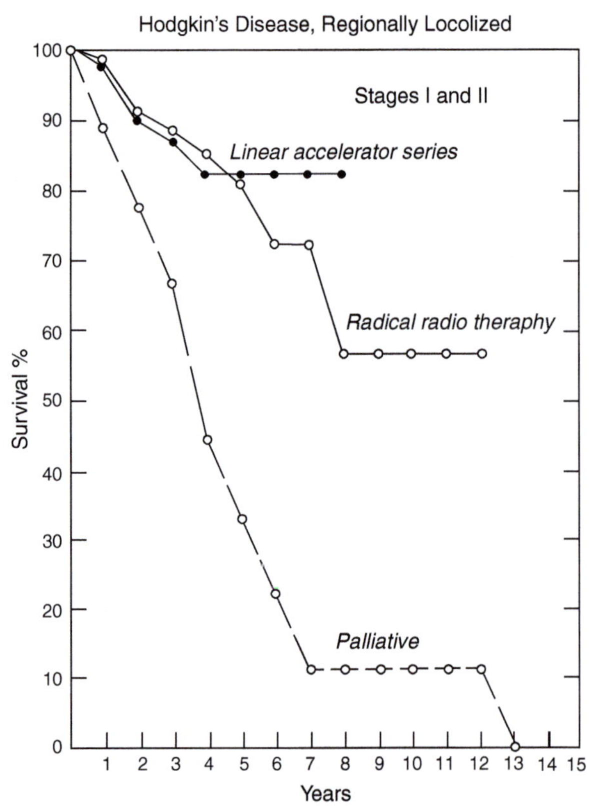

Fig. 1.6 Results of treating localized stages I and II Hodgkin's disease with different radiotherapy methods, megaVoltage with linear accelerator, radical radiotherapy with kiloVolt equipment, and palliative radiotherapy with kiloVolt equipment (from Kaplan 1966)

1.3 Radiotherapy as Part of Combined Modality Treatment

With the advent of chemotherapy for Hodgkin's disease, combining the two treatment modalities became an issue. At first, monotherapy with vinblastine in combination with extended field radiotherapy was

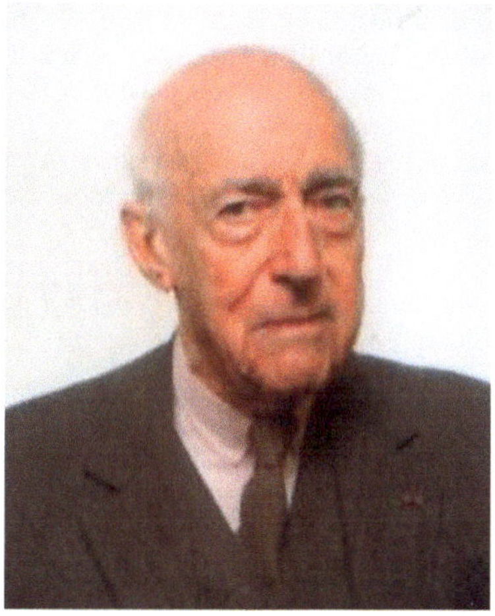

Fig. 1.7 Professor Maurice Tubiana, Institut Gustave Roussy, Paris, France, pioneer of radiotherapy for Hodgkin's disease and founder of the Lymphoma Group of the European Organization for Research and Treatment of Cancer (EORTC)

tested by Maurice Tubiana (see Fig. 1.7) from Paris, France, in the first randomized study by the European Organization for Research and Treatment of Cancer (EORTC) Lymphoma Group (Tubiana et al. 1979), demonstrating superior relapse-free survival with adjuvant monochemotherapy. Later randomized trials testing more effective chemotherapy regimens with radiotherapy, carried out first at Stanford (Hoppe et al. 1985) and later at other centers, showed superior relapse-free survival but no significant difference in overall survival (Specht et al. 1998). However, long-term follow-up of the very extensive radiotherapy demonstrated very significant long-term sequelae (Henry-Amar 1983; van Leeuwen et al. 1994; Travis et al. 1996; Hoppe 1997). Moreover, in the setting of effective chemotherapy, the extensive radiation fields were no longer needed (Specht et al. 1998). Hence, the use of radiotherapy for the treatment of Hodgkin's disease changed dramatically, from total or subtotal nodal radiotherapy to involved field radiotherapy including only the involved lymph node regions (Yahalom and Mauch 2002). With the advent of even more sophisticated techniques, including advanced imaging and highly conformal treatment planning and delivery, even smaller treatment volumes, including only the lymph nodes actually involved by lymphoma, are now being implemented (Girinsky et al. 2006).

Radiotherapy remains a highly effective treatment for Hodgkin's disease. With the implementation of the new advanced technologies in radiotherapy planning and delivery, radiotherapy can be used as a highly effective and precise tool to maximize the chance of cure while minimizing toxicity in patients with Hodgkin's disease.

References

Coley WB (1915) Primary neoplasms of the lymphatic glands including Hodgkin's disease. In: Binnie JF (ed) Transactions of the American surgical association. William J. Dornan, Philadelphia

Desjardins AU, Ford F (1923) Hodgkin's disease and lymphosarcoma; clinical and statistical study. JAMA 81:925–927

Dubois JB, Ash D (1995) The discovery of X-rays and radioactivity. In: Bernier J (ed) Radiation oncology: a century of progress and achievement. The European Society for Therapeutic Radiology and Oncology, Brussels

Easson EC (1966) Possibilities for the cure of Hodgkin's disease. Cancer 19:345–350

Easson EC, Russell MH (1963) The cure of Hodgkin's disease. BMJ 1963:1704–1707

Gilbert R (1925) La roentgenthérapie de la granulomatose maligne. J Radiol Electrol 9:509–514

Gilbert R, Babaïantz L (1931) Notre méthode de roentgenthérapie de la lymphogranulomatose (Hodgkin): résultats éloignés. Acta Radiol 12:523–529

Girinsky T, van der Maazen R, Specht L et al (2006) Involved-node radiotherapy (INRT) in patients with early Hodgkin lymphoma: concepts and guidelines. Radiother Oncol 79:270–277

Henry-Amar M (1983) Second cancers after radiotherapy and chemotherapy for early stages of Hodgkin's disease. J Natl Cancer Inst 71:911–916

Hoppe RT (1997) Hodgkin's disease: complications of therapy and excess mortality. Ann Oncol 8(Suppl 1):115–118

Hoppe RT, Horning SJ, Rosenberg SA (1985) The concept, evolution and preliminary results of the current Stanford clinical trials for Hodgkin's disease. Cancer Surv 4:459–475

Kaplan HS (1962) The radical radiotherapy of regionally localized Hodgkin's disease. Radiology 78:553–561

Kaplan HS (1966) Long-term results of palliative and radical radiotherapy of Hodgkin's disease. Cancer Res 26:1250–1252

Lederman M (1981) The early history of radiotherapy: 1895-1939. Int J Radiat Oncol Biol Phys 7:639–648

Minot GR (1926) Lymphoblastoma. Radiology 7:119–120

Peters MV (1950) A study of survivals in Hodgkin's disease treated radiologically. Am J Roentgenol 63:299–311

Peters MV, Middlemiss KCH (1958) A study of Hodgkin's disease treated by irradiation. Am J Roentgenol 79:114–121

Pusey WA (1902) Cases of sarcoma and of Hodgkin's disease treated by exposures to X-rays - a preliminary report. JAMA 38:166–169

Röntgen WC (1895) Über eine neue Art von Strahlen. Sitzungsberichte der physikalisch-medicinischen Gesellschaft zu Würzburg Sitzung 30:132–141

Rosenberg SA, Kaplan HS (1970) Hodgkin's disease and other malignant lymphomas. Calif Med 113:23–38

Senn N (1903) The therapeutical value of the Röntgen ray in the treatment of pseudoleucæmia. NY Med J 77:665–668

Specht L, Gray RG, Clarke MJ et al (1998) Influence of more extensive radiotherapy and adjuvant chemotherapy on long-term outcome of early-stage Hodgkin's disease: a meta-analysis of 23 randomized trials involving 3, 888 patients. International Hodgkin's Disease Collaborative Group. J Clin Oncol 16:830–843

Travis LB, Curtis RE, Boice JD (1996) Late effects of treatment for childhood Hodgkin's disease. N Engl J Med 335:352–353

Tubiana M, Henry-Amar M, Hayat M et al (1979) Long-term results of the E.O.R.T.C. randomized study of irradiation and vinblastine in clinical stages I and II of Hodgkin's disease. Eur J Cancer 15:645–657

van Leeuwen FE, Klokman WJ, Hagenbeek A et al (1994) Second cancer risk following Hodgkin's disease: a 20-year follow-up study. J Clin Oncol 12:312–325

Yahalom J, Mauch P (2002) The involved field is back: issues in delineating the radiation field in Hodgkin's disease. Ann Oncol 13(Suppl 1):79–83

Background and Rationale for Radiotherapy in Early-Stage Hodgkin Lymphoma

2

Lena Specht and Andrea K. Ng

Contents

L. Specht (✉)
Departments of Oncology and Haematology, The Finsen Centre, Rigshospitalet, University of Copenhagen, 9 Blegdamsvej, 2100 Copenhagen, Denmark
e-mail: specht@dadlnet.dk

A.K. Ng
Department of Radiation Oncology, Brigham & Women's Hospital and Dana-Farber Cancer Institute, Harvard Medical School, 75 Francis St, ASB1-L2, Boston, MA 02115, USA
e-mail: ang@lroc.harvard.edu

2.1 Introduction

The curative role of radiation therapy for patients with HL was first established in 1950 by Dr. Vera Peters in Toronto (Peters 1950), based on the concept of contiguous spread of HL. Based on her results and the results of other pioneers, notably Dr. Henry Kaplan at Stanford, extended-field radiotherapy was established as a curative treatment for stage I, II, and some cases of stage III disease, as detailed in Chap. 1. For a number of years, radiotherapy was the only known curative treatment for HL.

With the introduction in 1964 by Dr. Vincent DeVita at the National Cancer Institute of combination chemotherapy with mechlorethamine, vincristine, procarbazine, and prednisone (the MOPP regimen), cures could be achieved even in patients with advanced disease (DeVita, Jr. et al. 1970). The MOPP regimen also proved effective in the treatment of recurrences after extended-field radiotherapy for stage I–III disease (Horwich et al. 1997). Randomized trials were then carried out, testing if the addition of chemotherapy to radiotherapy up front could improve outcome compared to radiotherapy alone with chemotherapy reserved for recurrences. Meta-analysis of these trials showed that the risk of recurrence was significantly reduced by the addition of chemotherapy up front, but that OS was not influenced, at least in the short term (10–15 years) (Specht et al. 1998).

The need for the extended radiation fields when effective chemotherapy salvage of recurrences was available was also tested in a number of randomized trials. Meta-analysis of these trials showed that the risk of recurrence was significantly reduced by the use of

L. Specht and J. Yahalom (eds.), *Radiotherapy for Hodgkin Lymphoma*,
DOI: 10.1007/978-3-540-78944-4_2, © Springer-Verlag Berlin Heidelberg 2011

Table 2.1 Definition of favourable and unfavourable (intermediate) early-stage Hodgkin lymphoma

	GSHG	EORTC	Stanford	NCIC
Risk factors	(a) Large mediastinal mass (b) Extranodal disease (c) ESR ≥ 50 without B-symptoms or ≥30 with B-symptoms (d) ≥3 nodal areas	(a) Large mediastinal mass (b) Age ≥ 50 years (c) ESR ≥ 50 without B-symptoms or ≥30 with B-symptoms (d) ≥4 nodal areas	(a) B-symptoms (b) Large mediastinal mass	(a) Histology other than LP/NS (b) Age ≥ 40 years (c) ESR ≥ 50 (d) ≥3 nodal areas
Favourable	CS I-II without risk factors	CS I-II (supra-diaphragmatic) without risk factors	CS I-II without risk factors	CS I-II without risk factors
Unfavourable	CS I or CS IIA with ≥1 risk factors CS IIB with (c) or (d) but without (a) and (b) (which are included in advanced disease)	CS I-II (supra-diaphragmatic) with ≥1 risk factors	CS I-II with ≥1 risk factors	CS I-II with ≥1 risk factors

GHSG: German Hodgkin Lymphoma Study Group; EORTC: European Organization for Research and Treatment of Cancer; NCIC: National Cancer Institute of Canada; ESR: erythrocyte sedimentation rate; LP: lymphocyte predominance; NS: nodular sclerosis; CS: clinical stage

more extensive radiotherapy, but that overall survival was not influenced (Specht et al. 1998). Hence, in the setting of effective chemotherapy, the extended radiation fields were no longer needed.

During the era when MOPP was the standard systemic therapy for HL, radiation therapy alone was routinely given for patients with pathologically confirmed early-stage disease, sparing these patients from the toxicity of MOPP chemotherapy. In 1973, Dr. Gianni Bonadonna in Milan introduced the combination chemotherapy regimen consisting of adriamycin, bleomycin, vinblastine, and dacarbazine (the ABVD regimen) (Bonadonna et al. 1975). This regimen proved more effective and less toxic than MOPP (Canellos et al. 1992; Duggan et al. 2003; Somers et al. 1994). Gradually, combined modality therapy became the standard treatment for early-stage HL. This change was initially based solely on the superiority of combined modality treatment with regard to recurrence-free survival. However, very long-term follow-up of randomized trials has also shown a significant OS benefit of combined modality therapy over radiation therapy for patients with early-stage disease (Ferme et al. 2007; Specht 2003). This superiority seems to be based on the adverse influence of the long-term toxicity of intensive therapy for recurrences (Franklin et al. 2005; Specht 2003).

Issues around the radiation therapy component of combined modality therapy include the optimal radiation dose, radiation field size, and treatment technique, and whether it can be eliminated in selected patients based on initial clinical characteristics or response to systemic therapy. Over the years, trials have been designed and conducted to address these questions.

In the design of most clinical trials for early-stage HL, patients are frequently classified into favorable versus unfavorable groups according to the presence or absence of prognostic factors. The classification criteria can vary from group to group, but disease bulk, number of sites of disease, constitutional symptoms, and/or sedimentation rates are among factors that are typically used. Summarized in Table 2.1 are definitions of favorable and unfavorable-prognosis early-stage HL as defined by several major groups active in HL trials. A clear understanding of specific selection criteria for inclusion in various clinical trials will allow a better appreciation of the applicability of the trial results to individual patients.

2.2 Combined Modality Therapy for Early-Stage Hodgkin Lymphoma

As part of combined modality therapy, the optimal radiation doses and field sizes have been explored by a number of trials. Specifically, in an effort to reduce toxicity, investigators have addressed the question of radiation dose de-escalation and radiation field-size reduction in the context of combined modality therapy.

2.2.1 Radiation Dose and Fractionation

In the era of treating HL with radiotherapy alone, 40 Gy was for a long time considered the tumoricidal dose based on the original publication by Henry Kaplan (Kaplan 1966). Later analyses indicated that tumor control was achieved at lower doses and was dependent on tumor size at the time of irradiation (Mendenhall et al. 1999; Schewe et al. 1988; Vijayakumar and Myrianthopoulos 1992). A re-analysis of the available dose–response data from patients treated with radiotherapy alone showed no positive dose–response relationship at doses above 32.5 Gy, and because of the wide confidence limits of the estimates no appropriate dose levels for various tumor burdens could be estimated (Brincker and Bentzen 1994). Moreover, the available data did not show a major importance of overall treatment time in the range from 4 up to 6–7 weeks. The capacity of the lymphoma cells to repair sublethal damage appeared to be small suggesting that dose per fraction is not very important for the dose needed to obtain tumor control. Hence, choice of fractionation does not seem to be critical, and schedules with a low degree of damage to the normal tissues should therefore be selected. The randomized HD4 study by the German Hodgkin Study Group (GHSG) documented that for subclinical involvement 30 Gy was equally effective as 40 Gy (Duhmke et al. 2001).

The appropriate radiation dose after chemotherapy in early-stage HL was examined in two trials for patients with favorable-prognosis disease and in one trial for patients with unfavorable-prognosis disease.

The European Organization for Research and Treatment of Cancer (EORTC) H9F trial was a three-arm trial in which all patients received six cycles of epirubicin, bleomycin, vinblastine, and prednisone (EBVP) (Thomas et al. 2007). After a complete response, patients were randomized to receive no further treatment, 36 Gy, or 20 Gy of involved-field irradiation (IFRT). Patients with a partial response all received 36 Gy of IFRT with or without a 4 Gy boost. As will be discussed in a later section, the chemotherapy-alone arm was closed early due to lower than expected event-free survival. In an interim analysis of 783 enrolled patients, at a median follow-up of 33 months, the 4-year event-free survival (EFS) of patients randomized to receive 36 Gy versus 20 Gy was not significantly different (87% versus 84%) (Thomas et al. 2007).

The GHSG HD10 trial on patients with low-risk early-stage disease also explored the use of lower doses of radiation therapy as part of combined modality therapy (Eich et al. 2005). The design was a 2×2 randomization in which patients were randomized to four versus two cycles of ABVD, followed by 30 Gy versus 20 Gy of IFRT. With respect to the arms evaluating radiation doses, in the most recent interim analysis that included 1,370 patients, at a median follow-up of 41 months, the freedom from treatment failure were comparable between the two arms (94% versus 93%).

For patients with unfavorable early-stage HL, the use of lower doses of radiation therapy is being addressed by the GHSG HD11 trial (Klimm et al. 2005). Patients were randomized to ABVD versus cyclophosphamide, doxorubicin, etoposide, procarbazine, prednisolone, vincristine, and bleomycin (BEACOPP), followed by 30 Gy versus 20 Gy of IFRT radiation therapy. In the most recent interim analysis that included 1,570 patients, at a median follow-up of 3 years, there was no significant difference between the 30 and 20 Gy arms (90% versus 87%).

However, all of these trials have median follow-up time of less than 5 years, and peer-reviewed published results are not yet available. Additional follow-up is therefore needed to establish the safety of 20 Gy of radiation treatment.

2.2.2 Radiation Field Size

Among patients with favorable-prognosis early-stage HL, no randomized trials have been conducted comparing extended-field (EFRT) versus IFRT after chemotherapy. However, IFRT was adopted as the standard arm in a number of recent European trials, including EORTC H7F, H8F, H9F, and GHSG HD10. In patients with unfavorable-prognosis disease, three trials have compared EFRT versus IFRT as part of combined modality therapy, although the results should be applicable to patients with favorable-prognosis disease as well.

In the EORTC H8U trial, two of the three arms compared four cycles of MOPP/ABV followed by either EFRT or IFRT (Ferme et al. 2007). The 5-year EFS rates were 88% and 87%, respectively, at a median follow-up of 92 months.

In the GHSG HD8 trial, 1,204 patients with CS I–II HL with adverse factors were randomized to receive two cycles of cyclophosphamide, vincristine, procarbazine, and prednisone (COPP) and ABVD followed by EFRT or IFRT (Engert et al. 2003). At a median follow-up time of 54 months, the 5-year freedom from treatment failure rates of the two arms were 86% and 84%, respectively ($p=0.56$), and the 5-year overall survival rates were 91% and 92%, respectively ($p=0.24$).

In an Italian trial by Bonnadonna et al., 136 patients with CS I unfavorable and CS IIA favorable and unfavorable HL received four cycles of ABVD followed by either subtotal nodal irradiation or IFRT (Bonadonna et al. 2004). At a median follow-up of 116 months, the 12-year freedom from progression of the two arms were 93% and 94%, respectively, and the 12-year overall survival were 96% and 94%, respectively.

The definition of IFRT was never quite clear, and the term was interpreted in different ways in different studies. Many radiation oncologists used the lymph node region diagram employed in the Ann Arbor staging classification (Kaplan and Rosenberg 1966). However, this diagram was never intended for definition of radiation fields. Commonly accepted guidelines stated that IFRT is treatment of a whole region, not individual lymph nodes (Yahalom et al. 2007; Yahalom and Mauch 2002).

The concept and guidelines for IFRT were developed for use with conventional two-dimensional (2D) treatment planning. With this treatment a considerable volume of tissue which never contained lymphoma was irradiated. However, the evidence detailed above consistently indicates that, in the scenario of combined modality treatment with efficient chemotherapy, irradiation of uninvolved lymph nodes and other tissues is not necessary. This is supported by analyses of sites of relapse in early-stage patients who were for some reason treated with chemotherapy alone (Shahidi et al. 2006). Moreover, reductions in the IFRT fields to encompass only the initially involved lymph nodes with a maximum margin of 5 cm have been shown to be safe (Campbell et al. 2008). In this study, among the 102 patients treated with chemotherapy followed by reduced IFRT, at a median follow-up of 50 months, there were three relapses, all of which were at distant sites.

Modern sophisticated techniques, including better imaging, three-dimensional (3D) treatment planning, and highly conformal treatment delivery, have opened up the possibilities to further reduce the irradiated volume in patients with early-stage HL. The EORTC-GELA Lymphoma Group (GELA: Groupe d'Etudes des Lymphomes de l'Adulte) pioneered the concept of involved-node radiotherapy (INRT), using modern 3D conformal techniques and imaging, preferably including positron emission tomography with 2-[18F]fluor-2-deoxyglucose (FDG-PET) (Girinsky et al. 2006). The specifications are in accordance with the ICRU 50/62 recommendations, although no guidelines exist taking into account the post-chemotherapy planning of a pre-chemotherapy volume (ICRU 1993). With INRT the clinical target volume (CTV) includes only the volume of tissue which contained the initially involved lymph nodes. Due to the uncertainty of the exact localization on the post-chemotherapy planning CT scan of the involved nodes on the pre-chemotherapy staging CT scans, the whole area on the relevant CT slices are included in the target definition (Girinsky et al. 2008). The corresponding planning target volume (PTV) takes into account organ movement and set-up variations, which may vary in different anatomical sites, but in general a 1 cm isotropic margin is considered sufficient. For patients in complete remission (CR) or complete remission unconfirmed (CRu) after chemotherapy, no further radiotherapy is added. For patients in partial remission (PR) after chemotherapy, a boost to the residual lymphoma mass is added. Response criteria based on CT scans are employed (Cheson et al. 1999; Lister et al. 1989), as newer response criteria based on FDG-PET scans have not been validated for treatment planning (Cheson et al. 2007). The introduction of INRT represents a drastic reduction in the irradiated volume in patients with early-stage HL. No randomized trials have compared this approach with IFRT or EFRT. However, the GHSG is planning in its HD17 study in patients with early favorable disease to randomize between INRT and IFRT (Eich et al. 2008). The INRT concept is employed in the current EORTC-GELA-IIL (IIL: Intergruppo Italiano Linfomi) H10 trial, and it is also employed for routine treatment outside of protocol in most of the participating centers. Analyses of relapse frequency and localization will be extremely important for the validation of the INRT concept.

2.2.3 Association of Radiation Dose/Field Size and Late Toxicity

Complications of radiation therapy for HL will be discussed in a separate chapter. However, it is important to recognize that because of the long latency to late effects after radiation therapy for HL, most of the data on late effects, including risks of second malignancy and cardiac disease, are based on patients treated during a time period when higher radiation doses, larger treatment fields, and less conformal techniques were used, as compared to patients treated in the modern era.

Several case–control studies have shown a clear radiation dose–response relationship on the risk of breast cancer after HL. In a large international case–control study on breast cancer after HL that included 105 cases of breast cancer and 266 matched controls, radiation dose to the area of the breast where the tumor developed in the case (and a comparable area in matched controls) was estimated for each case–control set (Travis et al. 2003). Breast cancer risk increased significantly with increasing radiation dose to reach eightfold for the highest category (median dose 42 Gy) compared to the lowest dose group (< 4 Gy) (p-trend for dose < 0.001). A significant radiation dose–response relationship was similarly demonstrated in a Dutch study that included women from the international investigation (van Leeuwen et al. 2003). The Childhood Cancer Survivor Study group recently published a case–control study on 120 cases of breast cancer (65% were in survivors of HL) matched to 464 controls by age at initial cancer and time since initial cancer (Inskip et al. 2009). Again, a significant linear radiation dose–response was observed (p-trend < 0.0001), with an estimated relative risk of breast cancer of 6.4 at 20 Gy and 11.8 at 40 Gy.

In an international investigation by Travis et al., lung cancer risk increased with increasing radiation dose to the area of the lung in which cancer developed (p-trend with dose < 0.001), with the relative risk becoming significantly increased after doses of 30 Gy or higher (Travis et al. 2002). These findings support the notion that radiation dose reduction will likely result in lower second malignancy risks.

Hodgson et al. used a validated radiobiological model that takes into account cell initiation, inactivation, and proliferation after varying doses of radiation therapy to quantify the excess risk of radiation-induced second malignancy after various radiation treatment fields and doses (Hodgson et al. 2007). The risks were estimated in 37 patients with mediastinal HL treated with IFRT to 35 Gy, and hypothetical mantle radiation therapy to 35 Gy, and IFRT to 20 Gy. The estimated relative risks of cancers of the breast and lung after "historical" treatment with mantle radiation therapy to 35 Gy were in agreement with those found in epidemiological studies. With the modern treatment of IFRT to 35 Gy, the 20-year excess relative risks of breast and lung cancer were estimated to be reduced by 63% and 21%, respectively. With potential future treatment of IFRT to 20 Gy, there were further reductions in the excess relative risks by 77% and 57%, respectively.

A significant dose–response relationship for cardiovascular complications after radiation therapy for HL has also been demonstrated. Hancock et al. showed that cardiac mortality after HL was significantly increased after doses of higher than 30 Gy to the mediastinum, but the increase was not significant after 30 Gy or lower (Hancock et al. 1993). Subsequent reports from the same group on results of a prospective cardiac screening study in asymptomatic long-term HL survivors showed an increased risk of valvular disease, diastolic dysfunction, and coronary disease, although the median dose to the mediastinum in this screened cohort was 44 Gy (Heidenreich et al. 2003; Heidenreich et al. 2005; Heidenreich et al. 2007).

There are also data to support current attempts to reduce radiation treatment field size in limiting complications. In the GHSG HD8 trial, patients on the extended-field arm were significantly more likely to experience acute side effects including leukopenia, thrombocytopenia, nausea, gastrointestinal toxicity, and pharyngeal toxicity (Engert et al. 2003). A higher risk of second malignancy was also observed in the extended-field arm compared with the involved-field arm (4.5% versus 2.8%), although the difference was not statistically significant. A subsequent analysis of 89 patients age 60 or older on this trial showed that elderly patients had a significantly inferior outcome when treated with EFRT as compared with IFRT, both in terms of freedom from treatment failure (58% versus 70%, $p = 0.034$) and overall survival (59% versus 81%, $p = 0.008$) (Klimm et al. 2007). In an Italian trial, at a median follow-up of almost 10 years, three cases of second malignancies were reported, all of which were in the EFRT arm (Bonadonna et al. 2004). In a meta-analysis by Franklin et al. on second malignancy risk after HL, the second malignancy risk after

EFRT versus IFRT was compared (Franklin et al. 2006). There was a trend of increased risk of second malignancy with EFRT with an odds ratio of 1.54 ($p=0.09$). In addition, the risk of breast cancer was higher with EFRT, with an odds ratio of 3.25 ($p=0.040$). A recent cohort study from the Netherlands on 1,122 female 5-year survivors of HL also showed a lower breast cancer risk with smaller radiation volume (De Bruin et al. 2009). In their multivariate Cox regression analyses, in which time-to-event was taken into account, women treated with mantle field irradiation (including the axillary, mediastinal, and neck nodes) had an almost threefold increased risk of breast cancer compared with those treated with mediastinal irradiation alone.

A larger radiation treatment field has also been shown to be associated with increased risk of cardiac complications. Hull et al. reported on the risk of cardiac disease in 415 HL survivors (Hull et al. 2003). The only treatment-related risk factor for the development of coronary artery disease on multivariable analysis was a matched mantle and subdiaphragmatic field as opposed to a mantle field alone or subdiaphragmatic field alone (hazard ratio, 7.8, $p=0.04$).

2.3 Can Radiation Therapy Be Safely Eliminated in Early-Stage Hodgkin Lymphoma?

As trials are being conducted evaluating reducing radiation dose and field size in combined modality therapy for early-stage HL, investigators have explored the option of eliminating radiation therapy and treating patients with early-stage disease with chemotherapy alone.

2.3.1 Trials Comparing Combined Modality Therapy Versus Chemotherapy Alone

Recently, a meta-analysis of trials testing this important question has been performed by the Cochrane Haematological Malignancies Group (Herbst et al. 2010). Randomized controlled trials comparing chemotherapy alone with identical chemotherapy combined with radiotherapy in newly diagnosed patients with HL of all ages in clinical stage (CS) I or II were included (Aviles and Delgado 1998; Bloomfield et al. 1982; Eghbali et al. 2005; Noordijk et al. 2005; Pavlovsky et al. 1988; Straus et al. 2004). These trials are summarized in Table 2.2. Trials with less than 80% of patients in CS I or II (Laskar et al. 2004; Nachman et al. 2002; O'Dwyer et al. 1985; Picardi et al. 2007), and trials where the number of chemotherapy cycles varied between treatment arms (Kung et al. 2006; Meyer et al. 2005), were not included in the main analysis, but they were included in supplementary sensitivity analyses. These trials are summarized in Table 2.3. These trials varied in the study design, patient population, types of chemotherapy, and radiation fields employed. The findings and the limitations of each of the trials are discussed below.

Aviles and Delgado from the National Medical Centre, Mexico, randomized 307 patients with

Table 2.2 Randomized controlled trials comparing chemotherapy alone with identical chemotherapy combined with radiotherapy in newly diagnosed patients with Hodgkin lymphoma of all ages in clinical stage (CS) I or II

Trial	Patient population	No. patients	Treatment arms	Median follow-up	Results
Aviles et al.	CS I–II supradiaphragmatic,	99	6×ABVD	11.4 years	DFS (12 years) 48%, OS (12 years) 59%
	bulky disease	102	6×ABVD+MFRT		DFS (12 years) 76%, OS (12 years) 88%
Bloomfield et al.	"Poor prognosis" PS I or II	18	6×CVPP	1.8 years	Complete remission 61%
		19	6×CVPP+IFRT		Complete remission 95%
Eghbali et al.	CS I–II without risk factors (see Table 2.1,	130	6×EBVP	4.3 years	EFS (5 years) 69%, OS (5 years) 97%
Noordijk et al.	EORTC criteria), in CR after 6×EBVP	448	6×EBVP+IFRT (20 or 36 Gy)		EFS (5 years) 87%, OS (5 years) 99%

Table 2.2 (continued)

Trial	Patient population	No. patients	Treatment arms	Median follow-up	Results
Pavlovsky et al.	CS I–II	142	6×CVPP	4 years	DFS (7 years) 62%, OS (7 years) 82%
		135	3×CVPP+IFRT (30 Gy)+3×CVPP		DFS (7 years) 71%, OS (7 years) 89%
Straus et al.	CS I–II and CS IIIA (13% of pts.), no bulky disease	76	6×ABVD	5.6 years	FFP (5 years) 81%, OS (5 years) 90%
		76	6×ABVD+IFRT or modified EFRT (36 Gy)		FFP (5 years) 86%, OS (5 years) 97%

CS: clinical stage; PS: pathological stage; ABVD: adriamycin, bleomycin, vinblastine, dacarbazine; CVPP: cyclophosphamide, vinblastine, procarbazine, prednisone; EBVP: epirubicine, bleomycin, vinblastine, prednisone; MFRT: mantle field radiotherapy; IFRT: involved-field radiotherapy; EFRT: extended-field radiotherapy; DFS: disease-free survival; EFS: event-free survival; FFP: freedom from disease progression; OS: overall survival

Table 2.3 Randomized controlled trials comparing chemotherapy alone with chemotherapy combined with radiotherapy in newly diagnosed early-stage Hodgkin lymphoma. Trials with less than 80% of patients in CS I or II, and trials where the number of chemotherapy cycles varied between treatment arms

Trial	Patient population	No. patients	Treatment arms	Median follow-up	Results
Laskar et al.	All stages included, in CR after 6×ABVD. Here are only CS-I-II included	44	6×ABVD	5.3 years	EFS (8 years) 94%, OS (8 years) 98%
		55	6×ABVD+IFRT		EFS (8 years) 97%, OS (8 years) 100%
Nachman et al.	Children with any stage in CR after chemotherapy. Here are only CS I-II included	173	4×COPP/ABV (no adverse factors)	Not reported	EFS (3 years) 91%, OS (3 years) 100%
			6×COPP/ABV (adverse factors)		EFS (3 years) 83%, OS (3 years) 100%
		189	4×COPP/ABV+IFRT (21 Gy) (no adverse factors)		EFS (3 years) 97%, OS (3 years) 100%
			6×COPP/ABV+IFRT (21 Gy) (adverse factors)		EFS (3 years) 87%, OS (3 years) 95%
O'Dwyer et al.	CS IB-IIIA	17	6×MOPP	6 years	Four relapsed, two died
		16	EFRT+6×MOPP		Three relapsed, three died
Picardi et al.	CS I-IV with bulky disease (≥5 cm) with residual PET mass after chemotherapy	80	6×VEBEP	3.3 years	EFS (5 years) 86%, OS (5 years) 100%
		80	6×VEBEP+IFRT (32 Gy)		EFS (5 years) 96%, OS (5 years) 100%
Kung et al.	PS I–IIIA, children	78	6×MOPP/ABVD	8.3 years	EFS (8 years) 83%, OS (8 years) 94%
		81	4×MOPP/ABVD+IFRT (25.5 Gy)		EFS (8 years) 91%, OS (8 years) 97%
Meyer et al.	CS I-IIA, without bulk (≤10 cm), unfavorable (see Table 2.1, NCIC criteria)	137	4–6×ABVD	4.2 years	FFP (5 years) 88%, OS (5 years) 95%
		139	2×ABVD+STNI (35 Gy)		FFP (5 years) 95%, OS (5 years) 92%

CR: complete remission; CS: clinical stage; PS: pathological stage; ABVD: adriamycin, bleomycin, vinblastine, dacarbazine; COPP: cyclophosphamide, vincristine, procarbazine, prednisone; MOPP: mechlorethamine, vincristine, procarbazine, prednisone; VEBEP: etoposide, epirubicine, bleomycin, cyclophosphamide, prednisone; IFRT: involved-field radiotherapy; EFRT: extended-field radiotherapy; STNI: subtotal nodal radiotherapy; EFS: event-free survival; FFP: freedom from disease progression; OS: overall survival supradiaphragmatic stage I or II disease in a three-arm study to either six cycles of ABVD, or to mantle field radiotherapy (MFRT) alone, or to MFRT to 35–38 Gy preceded and followed by three cycles of ABVD (Aviles and Delgado 1998). Only the first and last of the three arms of the study are relevant here. With a median follow-up of 11.4 years the estimated 12-year disease-free survival (DFS) of patients treated with combined modality was 76% compared with 48% for patients treated with chemotherapy alone ($p<0.01$). The corresponding figures for overall survival (OS) were 88% and 59%, respectively ($p < 0.01$).

Bloomfield et al. from the Cancer and Leukemia Group B reported on a small study in progress (Bloomfield et al. 1982). A total of 37 patients were randomized to either six cycles of cyclophosphamide, vinblastine, procarbazine, and prednisone (CVPP), or to six cycles of CVPP and involved-field radiotherapy (IFRT). Complete response rate was superior with combined modality treatment (95% versus 61%, $p=0.04$), but with a median follow-up of only 22 months from diagnosis there was no survival difference. Unfortunately, no further published data from this trial have appeared.

In the EORTC-H9F trial, CS I–II, favorable-prognosis patients were randomized after a complete response to six cycles of EBVP to the following three arms: IFRT to 36 Gy, IFRT to 20 Gy, or no further treatment (Eghbali et al. 2005; Noordijk et al. 2005). The chemotherapy alone was closed due to higher than expected number of relapses. The main criticism of this study is the inadequate chemotherapy employed. However, this study was restricted to selected patients with favorable features, and the EBVP regimen was chosen since its efficacy in combination with involved-field radiation therapy had been proven in the earlier EORTC H7F trial.

Pavlovsky et al. from the Grupo Argentino de Tratamiento de la Leucemia Aguda (GATLA) randomized 277 patients with CS I–II HL to receive six monthly cycles of CVPP followed by IFRT to 30 Gy, versus six cycles of CVPP alone (Pavlovsky et al. 1988). At 84 months, the DFS of the combined modality therapy arm was significantly higher than that of the chemotherapy-alone arm (71% versus 62%, $p=0.01$). On subgroup analysis, the difference between the two arms were highly significant among patients with unfavorable features (age >45, >2 sites, or bulky disease), with DFS of 75% in the combined modality therapy arm versus 34% in the chemotherapy-alone arm ($p=0.001$). Among favorable patients, the difference in DFS was not significant (77% versus 70%). The main limitation of this study is the inferior chemotherapy regimen used, which likely explained the poor treatment outcome especially for the unfavorable patients treated with chemotherapy alone. In addition, 45% of patients in this trial were children aged under 16. The results therefore may not be entirely applicable to the adult population.

In a Memorial Sloan Kettering Cancer Center trial, patients with non-bulky CS IA-IIB and CS IIIA were randomized to six cycles of ABVD with or without radiation therapy (Straus et al. 2004). The target accrual was 90 patients per arm. After 152 patients were accrued at 10 years, the trial was closed due to slow accrual. No significant differences in freedom from progression (FFP) (86% versus 81%) and overall survival (97% versus 90%) were found at a median follow-up of 60 months. Seven of the eight relapses in the chemotherapy-alone arm were in initially involved nodal sites. This trial, however, was underpowered to determine if the two treatment approaches are truly equivalent. Furthermore, care should be taken in the interpretation of long-term toxicity data when they become available since the majority of patients randomized to receive radiation therapy were treated with EFRT.

The meta-analysis of these five unconfounded trials in (almost exclusively) early-stage HL showed not only a highly significant advantage for combined modality treatment with regard to tumor control, but the meta-analysis also showed a highly significant ($p<0.00001$) advantage with regard to OS with a hazard ratio of 0.40 (95% confidence interval 0.27–0.59) (Herbst et al. 2010). The meta-analysis of OS is shown in Fig. 2.1.

The remaining six trials testing chemotherapy alone versus combined modality either included more than 20% of patients with advanced disease or they were confounded in the sense that more cycles of chemotherapy were given in the chemotherapy-only arm than in the combined modality arm, see Table 2.3.

Laskar et al. reported results of a randomized trial from Tata Memorial Hospital in India comparing six cycles of ABVD with or without IFRT (Laskar et al. 2004). Only patients who achieved a complete response to the chemotherapy were randomized. Patients of all stages were included, and 55% had CS I–II disease.

Study	Weight	Hazard Ratio Random, 95% CI
CALGB 7751	5.1%	0.63 [0.11, 3.65]
EORTC-GELA H9-F	4.6%	0.27 [0.04, 1.74]
GATLA 9-H-77	30.7%	0.68 [0.33, 1.40]
Mexico B2H031	50.4%	0.29 [0.17, 0.51]
MSKCC trial #90-44	9.2%	0.31 [0.08, 1.14]
Total (95% CI)	**100.0%**	**0.40 [0.27, 0.59]**

Heterogeneity: Tau^2= 0.00; Chi^2 = 3.89, df = 4 (P = 0.42): I^2 = 0%
Test for overall effect: Z = 4.57 (P < 0.00001)

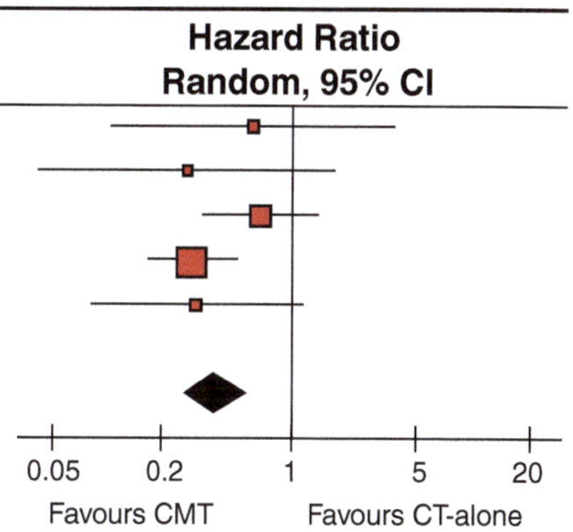

Fig. 2.1 Meta-analysis of overall survival (OS) in patients with early-stage Hodgkin lymphoma who were treated with chemotherapy alone (CT) or chemotherapy and radiotherapy (CMT). Solid squares represent effect estimates for the single trials, the size of the squares represent the weight of the individual studies in the meta-analysis. Horizontal lines indicate the 95% confidence intervals (CI). The width of the diamond shows the 95% confidence interval for the pooled hazard ratios. (Reprinted with permission from Herbst et al. 2010)

Significant differences in 6-year EFS (88% versus 76%, $p=0.01$) and OS (100% versus 89%, $p=0.002$) were observed, favoring the combined modality therapy arm. However, no significant difference was found in stages I and II with regard to neither EFS nor OS, whereas, surprisingly, significant differences were found for stages III and IV. This study is limited by the high proportion of pediatric patients, with 46% age under 15. Also, the generalizability of the results to cases seen in the western world is unclear, as 71% of cases were of mixed cellularity histology, reflecting the high proportion of Epstein Barr Virus-related cases in developing countries.

The Children's Cancer Group (CCG) conducted a randomized trial on patients under the age of 21 comparing low-dose IFRT and noradiation therapy after a complete response to chemotherapy (Nachman et al. 2002). Sixty-eight percent had CS I–II disease. Patients were stratified into three risk groups based on clinical stage and presence of adverse factors. On an as-treated analysis, the 3-year EFS of the chemotherapy-alone arm was 85%, which was significantly lower than that of the combined modality therapy arm of 93% ($p=0.0024$). The randomization was stopped on the recommendation of the Data Monitoring Committee because of a significantly higher number of relapses on the no-radiation therapy arm. Of note, among the 34 relapses with known sites of relapse in the chemotherapy-alone arm, 29 were exclusively in the original sites of disease, three were in both previously involved and new sites, and only two were exclusively in new sites. However, as in the previous study, the relevance of the results of this pediatric trial to adult patients is not clear. Moreover, the follow-up is relatively short in this study.

An early and very small trial carried out at the Montefiori Medical Center, New York, included only 33 patients and was never fully reported (O'Dwyer et al. 1985). Patients in stages IB–IIIA were randomized between EFRT followed by six cycles of MOPP or six cycles of MOPP alone. This trial did not indicate any difference between the two treatments, but it was of course far too small.

Picardi et al. conducted a randomized trial designed to evaluate whether radiation therapy can be safely eliminated if a complete response by PET scan is achieved after chemotherapy (Picardi et al. 2007). A total of 260 patients were included in the study. One hundred and sixty patients became PET-negative and had>75% reduction in the tumor mass at the completion of six cycles of etoposide, epirubicin, bleomycin, cyclophosphamide, and prednisone (VEBEP). These patients were randomized to 32 Gy of IFRT versus no further treatment. At a median follow-up of 40 months, there was a significant DFS benefit favoring the addition of consolidative radiation therapy (96% versus 86%, $p=0.03$), suggesting that even in carefully selected patients based on optimal functional imaging response to chemotherapy, the omission of radiation therapy is associated with a higher relapse rate.

The Pediatric Oncology Group carried out a study in children in pathological stage (PS) I–IIIA (Kung et al. 2006). A total of 159 patients were randomized to either six cycles of MOPP/ABVD or four cycles of MOPP/ABVD followed by IFRT to 25.5 Gy. With a median follow-up time of over 8 years no significant difference was demonstrated either in EFS or OS.

In a randomized trial conducted by the National Cancer Institute of Canada (NCIC) and Eastern Cooperative Oncology Group, patients with non-bulky CS I–II disease were stratified into low-risk (LP/NS, age <40, ESR <50, and <3 sites of disease) and high-risk groups (Meyer et al. 2005). Low-risk patients were randomized to EFRT versus four to six cycles of ABVD, and high-risk patients were randomized to two cycles of ABVD followed by radiation therapy versus four to six cycles of ABVD. At a median follow-up of 4.2 years, patients treated with chemotherapy alone had a significantly inferior 5-year progression-free survival of 87% versus 93% in patients treated with either EFRT or combined modality therapy ($p=0.006$). There were no significant differences in OS. In examining the results of this trial, it needs to be taken into consideration that the "standard arm" in the low-risk group was EFRT, which had been shown to be inferior to combined modality therapy in several randomized trials even among favorable patients, and is currently no longer viewed as standard treatment. Furthermore, as in the Memorial Sloan Kettering trial, the majority of patients assigned to receive radiation therapy were treated with EFRT, which will likely have significant contribution to late effects.

In the meta-analysis mentioned previously, analyses were made including the six trials mentioned above that did not fulfill the inclusion criteria for the reasons mentioned above. These analyses confirmed the significant improvement in tumor control and OS with combined modality treatment (Herbst et al. 2010).

There are short-term non-randomized data suggesting that radiation therapy can be omitted in patients with advanced-stage HL based on PET response at the end of chemotherapy (Kobe et al. 2008). However, it is not clear whether the results are applicable to patients with early-stage HL. The results of the study by Picardi et al. mentioned above do not point in that direction (Picardi et al. 2007).

One of the key criticisms of trials that showed a significantly inferior outcome in the chemotherapy-alone arm was the inadequate chemotherapy used in some of the trials. These include the CVPP regimen used in the study from Argentina (Pavlovsky et al. 1988), the EBVP regimen used in the EORTC H9F trial (Eghbali et al. 2005; Noordijk et al. 2005), and the VEBEP regimen used in the trial by Picardi et al. (Picardi et al. 2007). Shahidi et al. retrospectively analyzed 61 patients with supradiaphragmatic HL treated with chemotherapy alone at Royal Marsden Hospital (Shahidi et al. 2006). The majority of patients received vinblastine, epirubicin, etoposide, and prednisolone (VEEP) or chlorambucil, vinblastine, procarbazine, and prednisone (ChlVPP). At a median follow-up of 6.5 years, there were a total 24 recurrences, resulting in a 5-year relapse rate of 40%. In a Phase II study conducted by the CALGB (Straus et al. 2007), patients with non-bulky early-stage HL were treated with six cycles of adriamycin, vinblastine, and gemcitabine (AVG) chemotherapy alone without radiation therapy. At a median follow-up of only 1.1 years, 11 of 99 patients relapsed, yielding a 2-year PFS rate of only 71%.

It therefore appears that less-effective or abbreviated chemotherapy, or alternatives to ABVD designed to limit chemotherapy-related toxicity, is not acceptable when radiation therapy is omitted. Toxicities associated with full course ABVD can be non-trivial, and these include myelosuppression, peripheral neuropathy, bleomycin lung toxicity, and cardiac toxicity. Of these ABVD-related toxicities, perhaps the most serious one is cardiac toxicity. In a study conducted by Aviles et al. on 399 HL patients treated with chemotherapy alone (Aviles et al. 2005), 163 patients received ABVD chemotherapy. Survivors were closely followed by cardiac examination and testing. At a median follow-up of 11.5 years, among the 163 patients treated with ABVD alone, six patients developed congestive heart failure, 10 had myocardial infarction, and a total of seven cardiac deaths were observed. Compared to the matched general population, the risk of cardiac deaths was significantly elevated at 46-fold, representing 39 excess cardiac deaths per 10,000 person-years of follow-up. A British study on 7,033 patients with HL survivors also demonstrated the independent effect of chemotherapy on risk of cardiac mortality (Swerdlow et al. 2007), although the relative risks were less dramatically elevated. The risk of cardiac mortality was separately analyzed for patients who received chemotherapy with mediastinal irradiation and chemotherapy without mediastinal irradiation. Among patients who received ABVD without mediastinal irradiation, a significantly elevated relative risk of cardiac mortality of 7.8 was observed ($p=0.01$). The relative risks of cardiac mortality after treatment with any adriamycin-based chemotherapy with and without mediastinal irradiation were 2.4 ($p=0.05$) and 3.2 ($p<0.001$), respectively.

2.3.2 Trials of Early PET Scans for Selecting Patients for Omission of Radiotherapy

Given the highly significant prognostic value of early PET response to chemotherapy, an intriguing question is if early PET response can be used as a tool to identify early-stage HL patients in whom radiation therapy can be omitted. The EORTC/GELA H10 trial is a randomized study designed to address this question. For patients with favorable disease, the standard arm consists of three cycles of ABVD followed by INRT while patients on the experimental arm receive two cycles of ABVD followed by PET scan. If the scan is negative, patients will receive two additional cycle of ABVD and then no further treatment. If the PET scan is positive, patients will receive two cycles of dose-escalated BEACOPP, followed by INRT. For patients with unfavorable disease, the standard arm consists of four cycles of ABVD followed by INRT while patients on the experimental arm receive two cycles of ABVD followed by PET scan. If the scan is negative, patients will receive four additional cycles of ABVD and then no further treatment. If the PET scan is positive, patients will receive two cycles of dose-escalated BEACOPP, followed by INRT. This trial is currently ongoing and results are not available.

In a British study in patients with CS IA and IIA without bulky disease, patients in complete or partial remission after three cycles of ABVD are examined with PET scan. If this scan is negative patients are randomized to IFRT or no further treatment. This trial has accrued the planned number of patients, but results will not be available for some time.

In a retrospective series by Barnes et al. (Barnes et al. 2008), 68 patients with non-bulky early-stage HL treated with anthracycline-based chemotherapy were reviewed. All patients underwent interim PET scan after two to three cycles of chemotherapy. A negative interim PET was observed in 51 patients and a positive interim PET in 17 patients. Sixty patients (88%) achieved a complete response to the chemotherapy. At a median follow-up of 32 months, six of the patients who achieved an initial complete response relapsed. Five of the six relapses were observed in patients treated with chemotherapy alone with negative interim PET, with the relapses occurring at the initial site(s) of disease. This is a small retrospective study with short follow-up, but the results raise the concern that chemotherapy alone may not be adequate even in the setting of initially non-bulky disease and a negative interim PET. It therefore appears that at the current time, there is no available data to support the omission of radiation therapy based on PET response or early-PET response in patients with early-stage HL.

2.3.3 Patterns of Failure After Chemotherapy for Early-Stage Hodgkin Lymphoma

Detailed patterns of failure analysis of the NCIC trial, which compared EFRT alone versus chemotherapy alone in low-risk patients, and compared combined modality therapy with two cycles of ABVD followed by IFRT with chemotherapy alone, were reported by MacDonald et al. (Macdonald et al. 2007). In patients randomized to receive chemotherapy alone, 88% of the relapses were in-field and would have been included in the EFRT. Although this study did not utilize IFRT, the authors found that 71% of the relapses in the chemotherapy-alone arm would have been included in an involved-field treatment.

In the randomized trial conducted by the CCG comparing chemotherapy alone based on risk group, and chemotherapy followed by IFRT, there were 34 relapses in the chemotherapy-alone arm (Nachman et al. 2002). In 29 of the 34 (85%) relapses, they were isolated relapses at initial sites of disease, which would have been covered by the IFRT.

Pattern of relapse data were also available in the randomized trial by Picardi et al. assessing whether radiation therapy can be eliminated based on PET response at the completion of the radiation therapy (Picardi et al. 2007). In the chemotherapy-alone arm, a total of 11 relapses were observed, all of which were at initial bulky site and/or contiguous nodal region. In contrast, only two relapses were observed in the combined modality therapy arm, one of which was in-field and the other one was out-of field.

In the study from Royal Marsden hospital on 61 patients with supradiaphragmatic HL treated with chemotherapy alone, of the 24 recurrences, 11 (45%) were in the same site, four (17%) were in new sites, and nine (38%) were in both old and new sites (Shahidi et al. 2006). The high relapse rate, including relapses at distant sites may be due to the inadequate chemotherapy, and the inclusion of patients with unfavorable factors such as large mediastinal adenopathy and B symptoms in the study.

2.4 Conclusion

Radiation therapy for early-stage HL has undergone substantial transformation over the last several decades. Its role evolved from being the sole treatment modality using large treatment fields to adjuvant local therapy directed to limited site(s) after systemic therapy. Given the well-documented patterns of relapse of the disease even after effective chemotherapy, and the failure thus far to reliably identify subgroups of early-stage patients in whom radiation therapy can be safely eliminated, radiation therapy remains an essential modality for the treatment of the disease. Continued advances in radiation therapy technology such as fusion with functional images, respiratory gating, and highly conformal techniques including IMRT and proton therapy will further improve targeting while sparing normal tissues (Ghalibafian et al. 2008; Girinsky et al. 2007; Girinsky and Ghalibafian 2007; Goodman et al. 2005; Yahalom 2005). In addition, if it is confirmed that reducing radiation field size and doses are safe and feasible as trial results become mature, further decrease in radiation-related toxicity will be anticipated. With the known toxicity of full-course chemotherapy which appears to be essential in the absence of radiation therapy, it appears that the treatment of choice for early-stage HL is abbreviated chemotherapy followed by limited radiation therapy, which will provide the best chance of cure up front while limiting acute and late effects.

References

Aviles A, Delgado S (1998) A prospective clinical trial comparing chemotherapy, radiotherapy and combined therapy in the treatment of early stage Hodgkin's disease with bulky disease. Clin Lab Haematol 20:95–99

Aviles A, Neri N, Nambo JM et al (2005) Late cardiac toxicity secondary to treatment in Hodgkin's disease. A study comparing doxorubicin, epirubicin and mitoxantrone in combined therapy. Leuk Lymphoma 46:1023–1028

Barnes JA, LaCasce AS, Toomey CE et al (2008) Early interim FDG-PET scan predicts outcome in non-bulky limited stage Hodgkin lymphoma, but may not guide use of consolidative radiotherapy. Blood (ASH Annual Meeting Abstracts) 112:518

Bloomfield CD, Pajak TF, Glicksman AS et al (1982) Chemotherapy and combined modality therapy for Hodgkin's disease: a progress report on Cancer and Leukemia Group B studies. Cancer Treat Rep 66:835–846

Bonadonna G, Zucali R, Monfardini S et al (1975) Combination chemotherapy of Hodgkin's disease with adriamycin, bleomycin, vinblastine, and imidazole carboxamide versus MOPP. Cancer 36:252–259

Bonadonna G, Bonfante V, Viviani S et al (2004) ABVD plus subtotal nodal versus involved-field radiotherapy in early-stage Hodgkin's disease: long-term results. J Clin Oncol 22:2835–2841

Brincker H, Bentzen SM (1994) A re-analysis of available dose-response and time-dose data in Hodgkin's disease. Radiother Oncol 30:227–230

Campbell BA, Voss N, Pickles T et al (2008) Involved-nodal radiation therapy as a component of combination therapy for limited-stage Hodgkin's lymphoma: a question of field size. J Clin Oncol 26:5170–5174

Canellos GP, Anderson JR, Propert KJ et al (1992) Chemotherapy of advanced Hodgkin's disease with MOPP, ABVD, or MOPP alternating with ABVD. N Engl J Med 327:1478–1484

Cheson BD, Horning SJ, Coiffier B et al (1999) Report of an international workshop to standardize response criteria for non-Hodgkin's lymphomas. NCI Sponsored International Working Group. J Clin Oncol 17:1244–1253

Cheson BD, Pfistner B, Juweid ME et al (2007) Revised response criteria for malignant lymphoma. J Clin Oncol 25:579–586

De Bruin ML, Sparidans J, Van't Veer MB et al (2009) Breast cancer risk in female survivors of Hodgkin's lymphoma: lower risk after smaller radiation volumes. J Clin Oncol 27:4239–4246

DeVita VT Jr, Serpick AA, Carbone PP (1970) Combination chemotherapy in the treatment of advanced Hodgkin's disease. Ann Intern Med 73:881–895

Duggan DB, Petroni GR, Johnson JL et al (2003) Randomized comparison of ABVD and MOPP/ABV hybrid for the treatment of advanced Hodgkin's disease: report of an intergroup trial. J Clin Oncol 21:607–614

Duhmke E, Franklin J, Pfreundschuh M et al (2001) Low-dose radiation is sufficient for the noninvolved extended-field treatment in favorable early-stage Hodgkin's disease: long-term results of a randomized trial of radiotherapy alone. J Clin Oncol 19:2905–2914

Eghbali H, Brice P, Creemers G-Y et al (2005) Comparison of three radiation dose levels after EBVP regimen in favorable supradiaphragmatic clinical stages (CS) I-II Hodgkin's lymphoma (HL): preliminary results of the EORTC-GELA H9-F trial. Blood (ASH Annual Meeting Abstracts) 106:240a

Eich H, Mueller R, Engert A et al (2005) Comparison of 30 Gy versus 20 Gy involved field radiotherapy after two versus four cycles ABVD in early stage Hodgkin's lymphoma: interim analysis of the German Hodgkin Study Group trial HD10. Int J Radiat Oncol Biol Phys 63:1–2

Eich HT, Muller RP, Engenhart-Cabillic R et al (2008) Involved-node radiotherapy in early-stage Hodgkin's lymphoma. Definition and guidelines of the German Hodgkin Study Group (GHSG). Strahlenther Onkol 184:406–410

Engert A, Schiller P, Josting A et al (2003) Involved-field radiotherapy is equally effective and less toxic compared with extended-field radiotherapy after four cycles of chemotherapy in patients with early-stage unfavorable Hodgkin's lymphoma: results of the HD8 trial of the German Hodgkin's Lymphoma Study Group. J Clin Oncol 21:3601–3608

Ferme C, Eghbali H, Meerwaldt JH et al (2007) Chemotherapy plus involved-field radiation in early-stage Hodgkin's disease. N Engl J Med 357:1916–1927

Franklin J, Paus M, Wolf J et al (2005) Chemotherapy, radiotherapy and combined modality for Hodgkin's disease, with emphasis on second cancer risk. The Cochrane Library Issue 4

Franklin J, Pluetschow A, Paus M et al (2006) Second malignancy risk associated with treatment of Hodgkin's lymphoma: meta-analysis of the randomised trials. Ann Oncol 17:1749–1760

Ghalibafian M, Beaudre A, Girinsky T (2008) Heart and coronary artery protection in patients with mediastinal Hodgkin lymphoma treated with intensity-modulated radiotherapy: dose constraints to virtual volumes or to organs at risk? Radiother Oncol 87:82–88

Girinsky T, Ghalibafian M (2007) Radiotherapy of hodgkin lymphoma: indications, new fields, and techniques. Semin Radiat Oncol 17:206–222

Girinsky T, van der Maazen R, Specht L et al (2006) Involved-node radiotherapy (INRT) in patients with early Hodgkin lymphoma: concepts and guidelines. Radiother Oncol 79:270–277

Girinsky T, Ghalibafian M, Bonniaud G et al (2007) Is FDG-PET scan in patients with early stage Hodgkin lymphoma of any value in the implementation of the involved-node radiotherapy concept and dose painting? Radiother Oncol 85:178–186

Girinsky T, Specht L, Ghalibafian M et al (2008) The conundrum of Hodgkin lymphoma nodes: to be or not to be included in the involved node radiation fields. The EORTC-GELA lymphoma group guidelines. Radiother Oncol 88:202–210

Goodman KA, Toner S, Hunt M et al (2005) Intensity-modulated radiotherapy for lymphoma involving the mediastinum. Int J Radiat Oncol Biol Phys 62:198–206

Hancock SL, Tucker MA, Hoppe RT (1993) Factors affecting late mortality from heart disease after treatment of Hodgkin's disease. JAMA 270:1949–1955

Heidenreich PA, Hancock SL, Lee BK et al (2003) Asymptomatic cardiac disease following mediastinal irradiation. J Am Coll Cardiol 42:743–749

Heidenreich PA, Hancock SL, Vagelos RH et al (2005) Diastolic dysfunction after mediastinal irradiation. Am Heart J 150:977–982

Heidenreich PA, Schnittger I, Strauss HW et al (2007) Screening for coronary artery disease after mediastinal irradiation for Hodgkin's disease. J Clin Oncol 25:43–49

Herbst C, Rehan FA, Brillant C et al (2010) Combined modality treatment improves tumour control and overall survival in patients with early stage Hodgkin lymphoma: a systematic review. Haematologica 95:494–500

Hodgson DC, Koh ES, Tran TH et al (2007) Individualized estimates of second cancer risks after contemporary radiation therapy for Hodgkin lymphoma. Cancer 110:2576–2586

Horwich A, Specht L, Ashley S (1997) Survival analysis of patients with clinical stages I or II Hodgkin's disease who have relapsed after initial treatment with radiotherapy alone. Eur J Cancer 33:848–853

Hull MC, Morris CG, Pepine CJ et al (2003) Valvular dysfunction and carotid, subclavian, and coronary artery disease in survivors of hodgkin lymphoma treated with radiation therapy. JAMA 290:2831–2837

ICRU (1993) Prescribing, recording and reporting photon beam therapy. Report 50.

Inskip PD, Robison LL, Stovall M et al (2009) Radiation dose and breast cancer risk in The Childhood Cancer Survivor Study. J Clin Oncol 27:3901–3907

Kaplan HS (1966) Evidence for a tumoricidal dose level in the radiotherapy of Hodgkin's disease. Cancer Res 26:1221–1224

Kaplan HS, Rosenberg SA (1966) The treatment of Hodgkin's disease. Med Clin N Am 50:1591–1610

Klimm BC, Engert A, Brillant C et al (2005) Comparison of BEACOPP and ABVD chemotherapy in intermediate stage Hodgkin's lymphoma: results of the fourth interim analysis of the HD 11 trial of the GHSG. J Clin Oncol 23 (Meeting Abstracts):561

Klimm B, Diehl V, Engert A (2007) Hodgkin's lymphoma in the elderly: a different disease in patients over 60. Oncology (Williston Park) 21:982–990

Kobe C, Dietlein M, Franklin J et al (2008) Positron emission tomography has a high negative predictive value for progression or early relapse for patients with residual disease after first-line chemotherapy in advanced-stage Hodgkin lymphoma. Blood 112:3989–3994

Kung FH, Schwartz CL, Ferree CR et al (2006) POG 8625: a randomized trial comparing chemotherapy with chemoradiotherapy for children and adolescents with Stages I, IIA, IIIA1 Hodgkin Disease: a report from the Children's Oncology Group. J Pediatr Hematol Oncol 28:362–368

Laskar S, Gupta T, Vimal S et al (2004) Consolidation radiation after complete remission in Hodgkin's disease following six cycles of doxorubicin, bleomycin, vinblastine, and dacarbazine chemotherapy: is there a need? J Clin Oncol 22:62–68

Lister TA, Crowther D, Sutcliffe SB et al (1989) Report of a committee convened to discuss the evaluation and staging of patients with Hodgkin's disease: Cotswolds meeting. J Clin Oncol 7:1630–1636

Macdonald DA, Ding K, Gospodarowicz MK et al (2007) Patterns of disease progression and outcomes in a randomized trial testing ABVD alone for patients with limited-stage Hodgkin lymphoma. Ann Oncol 18:1680–1684

Mendenhall NP, Rodrigue LL, Moore-Higgs GJ et al (1999) The optimal dose of radiation in Hodgkin's disease: an analysis of clinical and treatment factors affecting in-field disease control. Int J Radiat Oncol Biol Phys 44:551–561

Meyer RM, Gospodarowicz MK, Connors JM et al (2005) Randomized comparison of ABVD chemotherapy with a strategy that includes radiation therapy in patients with limited-stage Hodgkin's lymphoma: National Cancer Institute of Canada Clinical Trials Group and the Eastern Cooperative Oncology Group. J Clin Oncol 23:4634–4642

Nachman JB, Sposto R, Herzog P et al (2002) Randomized comparison of low-dose involved-field radiotherapy and no radiotherapy for children with Hodgkin's disease who achieve a complete response to chemotherapy. J Clin Oncol 20:3765–3771

Noordijk EM, Thomas J, Fermé C et al (2005) First results of the EORTC-GELA H9 randomized trials: the H9-F trial (comparing 3 radiation dose levels) and H9-U trial (comparing 3 chemotherapy schemes) in patients with favorable or unfavorable early stage Hodgkin's lymphoma (HL). J Clin Oncol 23 (Meeting Abstracts):561

O'Dwyer PJ, Wiernik PH, Stewart MB et al (1985) Treatment of early stage Hodgkin's disease: a randomized controlled trial of radiotherapy plus chemotherapy versus chemotherapy alone. In: Cavalli F, Bonadonna G, Rozencweig M (eds) Malignant lymphomas and Hodgkin's disease: Experimental and therapeutic advances. Proceedings of the Second International Conference on Malignant Lymphomas, Lugano, Switzerland, June 13–16, 1984, Martinus Nijhof, The Hague

Pavlovsky S, Maschio M, Santarelli MT et al (1988) Randomized trial of chemotherapy versus chemotherapy plus radiotherapy for stage I-II Hodgkin's disease. J Natl Cancer Inst 80:1466–1473

Peters MV (1950) A study of survivals in Hodgkin's disease treated radiologically. Am J Roentgenol 63:299–311

Picardi M, De Renzo A, Pane F et al (2007) Randomized comparison of consolidation radiation versus observation in bulky Hodgkin's lymphoma with post-chemotherapy negative positron emission tomography scans. Leuk Lymphoma 48:1721–1727

Schewe KL, Reavis J, Kun LE et al (1988) Total dose, fraction size, and tumor volume in the local control of Hodgkin's disease. Int J Radiat Oncol Biol Phys 15:25–28

Shahidi M, Kamangari N, Ashley S et al (2006) Site of relapse after chemotherapy alone for stage I and II Hodgkin's disease. Radiother Oncol 78:1–5

Somers R, Carde P, Henry-Amar M et al (1994) A randomized study in stage IIIB and IV Hodgkin's disease comparing eight courses of MOPP versus an alteration of MOPP with ABVD: a European Organization for Research and Treatment of Cancer Lymphoma Cooperative Group and Groupe Pierre-et-Marie-Curie controlled clinical trial. J Clin Oncol 12:279–287

Specht L (2003) Very long-term follow-up of the Danish National Hodgkin Study Group's randomized trial of radiotherapy (RT) alone vs. combined modality treatment (CMT) for early stage Hodgkin lymphoma, with special reference to second tumours and overall survival. Blood (ASH Annual Meeting Abstratcs) 102:637A

Specht L, Gray RG, Clarke MJ et al (1998) Influence of more extensive radiotherapy and adjuvant chemotherapy on long-term outcome of early-stage Hodgkin's disease: a meta-analysis of 23 randomized trials involving 3, 888 patients. International Hodgkin's Disease Collaborative Group. J Clin Oncol 16:830–843

Straus DJ, Portlock CS, Qin J et al (2004) Results of a prospective randomized clinical trial of doxorubicin, bleomycin, vinblastine, and dacarbazine (ABVD) followed by radiation therapy (RT) versus ABVD alone for stages I, II, and IIIA nonbulky Hodgkin disease. Blood 104:3483–3489

Straus D, LaCase A, Juweid M et al (2007) Doxorubicin, vinblastine and gemcitabine (AVG), a novel regimen excluding bleomycin for the treatment of early stage Hodgkin lymphoma (HL): results of CALGB 50203. Blood 110:70a–71a

Swerdlow AJ, Higgins CD, Smith P et al (2007) Myocardial infarction mortality risk after treatment for Hodgkin disease: a collaborative British cohort study. J Natl Cancer Inst 99:206–214

Thomas J, Fermé C, Noordijk EM et al (2007) Results of the EORTC-GELA H9 randomized trials: the H9-F trial (comparing 3 radiation dose levels) and H9-U trial (comparing 3 chemotherapy schemes) in patients with favorable or unfavorable early stage Hodgkin's lymphoma (HL). Haematologica 92(Suppl 5):27

Travis LB, Gospodarowicz M, Curtis RE et al (2002) Lung cancer following chemotherapy and radiotherapy for Hodgkin's disease. J Natl Cancer Inst 94:182–192

Travis LB, Hill DA, Dores GM et al (2003) Breast cancer following radiotherapy and chemotherapy among young women with Hodgkin disease. Jama-Journal of the American Medical Association 290:465–475

van Leeuwen FE, Klokman WJ, Stovall M et al (2003) Roles of radiation dose, chemotherapy, and hormonal factors in breast cancer following Hodgkin's disease. J Natl Cancer Inst 95:971–980

Vijayakumar S, Myrianthopoulos LC (1992) An updated dose-response analysis in Hodgkin's disease. Radiother Oncol 24:1–13

Yahalom J (2005) Transformation in the use of radiation therapy of Hodgkin lymphoma: new concepts and indications lead to modern field design and are assisted by PET imaging and intensity modulated radiation therapy (IMRT). Eur J Haematol 75(suppl 66):90–97

Yahalom J, Mauch P (2002) The involved field is back: issues in delineating the radiation field in Hodgkin's disease. Ann Oncol 13(Suppl 1):79–83

Yahalom J, Hoppe RT, Mauch PM (2007) Principles and techniques of radiation therapy for Hodgkin lymphoma. In: Hoppe RT, Mauch PM, Armitage JO et al (eds) Hodgkin lymphoma, 2nd edn. Lippincott Williams & Wilkins, Philadelphia

Background and Rationale for Radiotherapy in Advanced-Stage Hodgkin Lymphoma

3

Richard Hoppe and Berthe Aleman

Contents

R. Hoppe (✉)
Department of Radiation Oncology, Stanford University, 875 Blake Wilbur Dr, Rm CCG224, Stanford, CA 94305-5847, USA
e-mail: hoppe@reyes.stanford.edu

B. Aleman
Department of Radiotherapy, The Netherlands Cancer Institute, Plesmanlaan 121, Amsterdam 1066 CX, The Netherlands
e-mail: b.aleman@nki.nl

3.1 Historical Context, Treatment of Advanced Disease with Radiation Therapy Alone

Although the current standard treatments for stage III–IV HL emphasize the use of chemotherapy, prior to the introduction of mechlorethamine, vincristine, procarbazine, prednisone (MOPP) chemotherapy patients with advanced-stage HL were often treated with radiation therapy alone. With the introduction of effective chemotherapy, radiation therapy has been used in a consolidative fashion to initially involved sites, sites of bulky disease, or sites that failed to respond completely to chemotherapy.

In 1962, Henry Kaplan first introduced the concept of "total lymphoid irradiation" (TLI), which he employed in high dose (40–44 Gy) for patients with stage I–III disease (Kaplan and Rosenberg 1966). Patients with stage III were randomized to low-dose (15 Gy) palliative treatment to involved fields versus high-dose TLI. In 1968, he reported that four of five patients with stage IIIA and seven of 17 patients with stage IIIB disease were alive, without evidence of disease, as long as 5 years after TLI, and TLI was adopted as the standard treatment for these patients (Bagshaw et al. 1968). In the last analysis of this trial, the freedom from progression (FFP) was 41% and survival 35% at 20 years for the high-dose TLI group (Rosenberg and Kaplan 1985).

In1968, laparotomy with splenectomy was introduced as a routine staging procedure, and a randomized trial was initiated for patients with stage III disease comparing treatment with TLI to TLI followed by MOPP chemotherapy. FFP was superior after combined modality therapy in both stage IIIA and IIIB. In addition, the use of TLI alone in stage IIIB was clearly

L. Specht and J. Yahalom (eds.), *Radiotherapy for Hodgkin Lymphoma*,
DOI: 10.1007/978-3-540-78944-4_3, © Springer-Verlag Berlin Heidelberg 2011

inadequate, with a 15-year FFP of only 8%. However, in stage IIIA, the FFP was 70% after TLI alone (Rosenberg and Kaplan 1985). These results were mirrored in a large international data base that included 276 patients treated with irradiation alone who had laparotomy-documented stage IIIA disease, where the 5-year relapse-free survival was 64% (Henry-Amar et al. 1990a).

In the late 1970s, several groups of investigators looked more closely at the outcome of patients treated with irradiation alone in stage IIIA. Concepts of "anatomic substage" (Desser et al. 1977) or the extent of splenic involvement (Hoppe et al. 1980) were introduced in an effort to better identify patients with favorable stage IIIA, who could be managed with irradiation alone. This was done in an effort to avoid the toxicities of MOPP chemotherapy, especially sterility and secondary leukemia. However, the most reliable of these factors required staging laparotomy with splenectomy, which had fallen out of favor. In addition, Bonadonna and colleagues developed an alternative chemotherapy to MOPP, namely adriamycin, bleomycin, vinblastine, dacarbazine (ABVD), which was not associated with sterility or secondary myelodysplasia (Bonadonna et al. 1975).

The major question for management of these patients then became one of chemotherapy alone versus combined modality therapy. Argument for a combined modality approach was based on two important factors: (1) as noted, radiation therapy alone was curative in more than half of patients and (2) when patients with advanced disease relapsed, it was predominantly in sites of initial involvement (Young et al. 1978). Argument against the use of radiation therapy was based on the increased risk for complications. Arguments were strong on both sides of the issue. It was clear that the subject would be a fruitful one for investigation in randomized clinical trials.

3.2 Summary of the Literature on Advanced-Stage Hodgkin Lymphoma

Data on the optimal treatment strategy in advanced stages of HL are difficult to interpret. First, response to treatment has only recently been uniformly defined (Cheson et al. 2007). Although some investigators have defined PR as a ≥50% decrease, others have used a ≥75% decrease in the product of two perpendicular diameters in all measurable and evaluable lesions, in conjunction with negative bone marrow findings, no disease symptoms, and no new lesions. Furthermore, patients in partial remission after chemotherapy are often analyzed together with patients with primary progressive disease and those with early relapse after reaching complete remission with chemotherapy, with or without radiotherapy.

A meta-analysis of all randomized trials that were performed comparing chemotherapy alone versus chemotherapy plus radiotherapy was performed including 1,740 patients entered in trials between 1968 and 1988 (Loeffler et al. 1998). The trials were divided into two groups based on the design of the trial; (a) comparisons that were designed to evaluate the benefit of additional radiotherapy (RT) after the same chemotherapy (CT) (CT1 versus CT1 + RT; additional RT-design) and (b) comparisons that were designed to evaluate whether radiotherapy in a combined modality setting can be substituted by chemotherapy using either more cycles of the same chemotherapy or regimens that contain additional drugs (CT1 + CT2 versus CT1 + RT or CT1 versus CT2 + RT; parallel RT/CT design). Additional radiotherapy showed an 11% improvement in tumor control rate after 10 years ($P=0.0001$; 95% confidence interval 4–18%), but no difference in overall survival (OS) could be demonstrated ($P=0.57$). When combined modality treatment was compared to chemotherapy alone in the parallel RT/CT design, no difference in tumor control rate was demonstrated. Patients treated with a combination of chemotherapy and radiotherapy, however, had a significantly inferior long-term survival outcome than those treated with chemotherapy alone, provided an appropriate number of cycles of chemotherapy was given ($P=0.045$; 8% difference; 95% confidence interval 1–15%) (Loeffler et al. 1998). It is important to realize that the chemotherapy evaluated in this meta-analysis was MOPP or MOPP-like in the vast majority of the patients; only 230 patients received anthracycline-containing chemotherapy, nowadays considered standard.

Since this meta-analysis, however, new data were published. Chemotherapy schedules have been modified considerably. A selection of more recent trials evaluating patients with advanced HL is summarized in Table 3.1. Evidently, comparisons between trials must be made with caution because the characteristics

Table 3.1 Overview of publications including adult patients with advanced Hodgkin lymphoma

	Stage	Treatment	Time[a]	DFS/EFS/FFS/RFS		OS	
			years	%	P	%	P
Chemotherapy only							
CALGB (Canellos et al. 1992) $n=361$	IIIA2, IIIB and IVA or IVB	A:6–8 MOPP alone, no radiotherapy B:MOPP alternating with ABVD 12 cycles, no radiotherapy C:6–8 ABVD alone, no radiotherapy	5 5 5	50 65 61	B versus other 0.02	66 75 73	B versus other 0.28
CALGB/ECOG/SWOG/NCIC (Duggan et al. 2003) $n=856$	III_2A, IIIB or IV or relapse after definitive radiotherapy	A:8–10 ABVD, no radiotherapy B:8–10 MOPP-ABV hybrid, no radiotherapy	5 5	63 66	0.42	82 81	0.82
Chemotherapy with or without radiotherapy (by randomization)							
SWOG 7807 (Fabian et al. 1994) $n=278$	III or IV HL in CR after chemotherapy	A:6 MOP-BAP, no radiotherapy B:6 MOP-BAP+IFRT	5 5	66 74	>0.2	79 86	0.14
GELA H89 (Ferme et al. 2000; Ferme et al. 2006) $n=533$	IIIB/IV in CR or good PR after six cycles of chemotherapy	A:8 MOPP-ABV hybrid B:6 MOPP-ABV hybrid+(S)TNI C:8 ABVPP D:6 ABVPP+(S)TNI	10 10 10 10	76 79 70 76	0.09[b]	78 82 90 77	0.03[c]
EORTC 20884 (Aleman et al. 2003a) $n=739$	IIIA or IV in CR after chemotherapy	A:6–8 MOPP-ABV, no further treatment B:6–8 MOPP-ABV+IFRT	5 5	84 79	0.35	91 85	0.07
Chemotherapy and radiotherapy on indication							
Stanford V (Horning et al. 2000) $n=47$	III or IV or bulky mediastinal disease	Stanford V+radiotherapy in case of bulky mediastinal disease, nodal masses≥5 cm, macroscopic nodules in an intact spleen on CT scan	5	83	–	96	–
GHSG HD9 (Diehl et al. 2003; Diehl et al. 2004) $n=1,201$	unfavorable stage IIB or IIIA or stage IIIB or IV	A:COPP-ABVD+radiotherapy on originally bulky disease or residual tumor B:BEACOPP baseline+radiotherapy on originally bulky disease or residual tumor C:BEACOPP escalated+radiotherapy on originally bulky disease or residual tumor	7 7 7	67 75 84	A versus B versus C: <0.001	79 84 90	A versus B versus C: 0.004

(*continued*)

Table 3.1 (continued)

	Stage	Treatment	Time[a] years	DFS/EFS/FFS/RFS %	DFS/EFS/FFS/RFS P	OS %	OS P
British/Italian cooperation (Radford et al. 2002) $n=282$	unfavorable stage I or II HL or stage III or IV HL	ChlVPP-EVA hybrid + radiotherapy on originally bulky disease or residual abnormalities	5	78	0.0006	89	0.04
		VAPEC-B + radiotherapy on originally bulky disease or residual abnormalities	5	58		79	
Four Italian Cooperative Groups (Gobbi et al. 2005) $n=355$[d]	IIB,III or IV	A:ABVD + radiotherapy on previously bulky or partially remitting disease	5	78	B versus other <0.01	90	A versus C: 0.33
		B:Stanford V + radiotherapy on previously bulky or partially remitting disease	5	54		82	A versus B: 0.04
		C:MOPPEBVCAD + radiotherapy on previously bulky or partially remitting disease	5	81		89	B versus C: 0.33

[a] Time survival estimates

[b] Consolidation chemotherapy or radiotherapy $P = 0.07$

[c] Consolidation chemotherapy or radiotherapy $P = 0.29$

[d] Gruppo Italiano Studio Linfomi, Gruppo Multiregionale Studio Linfomi, Non-Hodgkin's Lymphoma Cooperative Study Group, and Gruppo Lombardo Studio Linfomi

[e] This regimen deviated from the original Stanford V schedule; radiation was only given to originally bulky sites and sites in partial remission after chemotherapy.

Abbreviations general

CALGB: Cancer and Leukemia Group B; CR(u): complete remission (unconfirmed); DFS: disease-free survival; ECOG: Eastern Cooperative Oncology Group; EFS: event-free survival; FFS: failure-free survival; GHSG: German Hodgkin Study Group; HL: Hodgkin lymphoma; (IF)radiotherapy: (involved-field) radiotherapy; N: number of patients; N.s.: not significant; OS: overall survival; PR: partial remission; RFS: relapse-free survival; (S)TNI: (sub) total nodal irradiation; SWOG: South West Oncology Group

Abbreviations chemotherapy

ABVD: doxorubicin, bleomycin, vinblastine, and dacarbazine; ABVPP: doxorubicin, bleomycin, vinblastine, procarbazine, prednisone; BEACOPP: bleomycin, etoposide, adriamycin, cyclophosphamide, vincristin, procarbazine, and prednisone; ChlVPP-EVA: chlorambucil, vinblastine, procarbazine, and prednisone/etoposide, vincristine, and doxorubicin; COPP-ABVD: cyclophosphamide, vincristine, procarbazine, and prednisone alternating with doxorubicin, bleomycin, vinblastine, and dacarbazine; MOPP: mechlorethamine, vincristine, procarbazine, prednisone; MOPP-ABV: mechlorethamine, vincristine, procarbazine, prednisone/doxorubicin, bleomycin, vinblastine; MOP-BAP: nitrogen mustard, vincristine, prednisone, bleomycin, doxorubicin, and procarbazine; MOPPEBVCAD: mechlorethamine, vincristine, procarbazine, prednisone, epidoxirubicin, bleomycin, vinblastine, lomustine, doxorubicin, and vindesine; Stanford V: doxorubicin, vinblastine, mechlorethamine, etoposide, vincristine, bleomycin, prednisone; VAPEC-B: doxorubicin, cyclophosphamide, etoposide, vincristine, bleomycin, and prednisolone of patients included in the trials may differ and for some trials the overall results are presented whereas for others results refer to patients with a certain response to chemotherapy only. Nevertheless, trials using chemotherapy only, irrespective of the response to chemotherapy, show slightly lower freedom from treatment failure rates as compared to those using a combination of chemotherapy and radiotherapy. The differences in OS rates between the studies using anthracycline-containing chemotherapy schedules are rather small. It is important, however, that although salvage therapy may be successful in terms of controlling HL, long-term complications may be increased after salvage therapy (Aleman et al. 2003b).

3.2.1 GELA

The Groupe d'Études des Lymphomes de l'Adulte (GELA) (Ferme et al. 2000) randomly assigned patients with stage IIIB/IV HL in complete remission or having achieved a good partial remission after six cycles of chemotherapy to two additional cycles of the same chemotherapy or to radiotherapy (H89). Usually subtotal nodal irradiation was given; inverted Y was only given in case of iliac or inguinal involvement. An elective dose of 30 Gy was given followed by a boost of 5 Gy to the initially involved areas and an additional 5 Gy to sites of residual mass after chemotherapy using conventional fractionation. Radiotherapy appeared not to be superior to consolidation chemotherapy after a doxorubicin-induced complete remission in patients with advanced HL (see Table 3.1).

3.2.2 EORTC

The European Organization for Research and Treatment of Cancer (EORTC) has also performed a randomized trial on the role of radiotherapy in the treatment of patients with advanced HL (E20884) between 1989 and 2000 (Aleman et al. 2003a). Patients with previously untreated stage III or IV HL who were in complete remission after hybrid chemotherapy with mechlorethamine, vincristine, procarbazine, prednisone, doxorubicin, bleomycin, and vinblastine (MOPP-ABV) were randomly assigned to receive either no further treatment or involved-field radiotherapy (IFRT). Radiotherapy consisted of 24 Gy to all initially involved nodal areas and 16–24 Gy to all initially involved extranodal sites. Patients in partial remission were treated with 30 Gy to nodal areas and 18–24 Gy to extranodal sites. IFRT started within 6–8 weeks after the first day of the last cycle of chemotherapy and was administered in one to three courses, depending on the extent of the original involvement. Patients in a complete remission after six to eight cycles of MOPP-ABV hybrid chemotherapy did not benefit from IFRT. Patients in partial remission after chemotherapy, however, probably benefited from radiotherapy since the event-free (EFS) and OS rates of these patients treated with IFRT were comparable to the EFS and OS rates in patients in complete remission after chemotherapy (Aleman et al. 2003a; Aleman et al. 2007). When comparing patients who reached a PR on CT and were irradiated with those who reached a complete remission, significantly more patients with bulky (mediastinal) disease at the start of treatment were found in the PR group. However, the only factor that correlated with final treatment outcome was response to radiotherapy. Important changes have occurred since the execution of this trial. MOPP-ABV hybrid chemotherapy is not considered to be the standard therapy by most and maybe more importantly possibilities to evaluate response to chemotherapy have improved tremendously (see Chap. 12).

3.2.3 GHSG

The German Hodgkin Study Group (GHSG) has performed several trials including patients with advanced HL. The randomized trial between 1993 and 1998 (HD9) compared cyclophosphamide, vincristine, procarbazine, and prednisone alternating with doxorubicin, bleomycin, vinblastine, and dacarbazine (COPP-ABVD), bleomycin, etoposide, adriamycin, cyclophosphamide, vincristin, procarbazine, and prednisone (BEACOPP) and escalated BEACOPP. After completion of chemotherapy, radiotherapy was give to sites of initial bulky disease (i.e., localizations at least 5 cm in diameter) to a dose of 30 Gy followed by a boost to any residual tumor to 40 Gy (Diehl et al. 2003). Escalated BEACOPP resulted in better tumor control and OS than COPP-ABVD also after prolonged follow-up (see Table 3.1).

In addition the GHSG performed the HD12 to test whether consolidative radiotherapy in the region of initial bulky disease and of residual disease is necessary after effective chemotherapy (Eich et al. 2007). Patients with previously untreated HL Stage IIB (large mediastinal mass and/or E-lesions) or Stage III to IV were randomized between 1999 and 2003 according to a factorial design between: eight escalated BEACOPP + radiotherapy (arm A), eight escalated BEACOPP non-radiotherapy (arm B), four escalated + four baseline BEACOPP + radiotherapy (arm C), four escalated + four baseline BEACOPP non-radiotherapy (arm D). A preliminary analysis showed that the freedom from treatment failure was not significantly different between the radiotherapy and the non-radiotherapy arms. The authors therefore concluded that radiotherapy can be reduced substantially after effective chemotherapy. However, because of the irradiation of 10% of patients in the non-radiotherapy arms, equivalent effectiveness of a non-radiotherapy strategy could not be proven (Eich et al. 2007).

3.2.4 Stanford

At Stanford during the 1970s and 1980s, approaches to combined modality therapy for advanced disease included novel sequencing of chemotherapy and radiotherapy (Hoppe et al. 1979) and the introduction of procarbazine, alkeran, vinblastine (PAVe), an alternative to the MOPP regimen, used in conjunction with radiation or alternating with ABVD (Horning et al. 1992). The stratification for these trials was somewhat complicated and the number of patients accrued was not sufficient to answer any of the clinical questions.

However, the Stanford team was committed to a combined modality approach. In addition, they wanted to abbreviate the duration of treatment and to minimize the toxicities of treatment by reducing the total dosages of drugs such as doxorubicin and bleomycin and using more limited radiation fields and lower doses of radiation (Bartlett et al. 1995). What evolved was the Stanford V program, which included brief, intensive chemotherapy followed by irradiation (36 Gy) to initially bulky (>5 cm) sites of disease. This 12-week chemotherapy program includes alternating weeks of myelosuppressive and non-myelosuppressive therapy. The total dose of doxorubicin is only ~40% and of bleomycin only ~20% of what would be included in eight cycles of ABVD. Radiotherapy is initiated 2–3 weeks following the end of chemotherapy to initial sites of bulky disease, including the spleen if focal nodules are seen in the spleen on CT. The prescribed dose is 36 Gy. More than 100 patients with stage III–IV have been treated in this fashion at Stanford. With a maximum follow-up of 14 years, the freedom from progression is 86% (S. Horning, personal communication 2009). In 1996, the Eastern Cooperative Oncology Group (ECOG) initiated a prospective randomized clinical trial comparing the Stanford V regimen (including radiation, as described above) with ABVD chemotherapy. On the ABVD arm, the only irradiation utilized was for large mediastinal masses.

The techniques of irradiation, as a component of the Stanford V regimen, are essential to its success. Variation in technique may explain, in part, why an Italian randomized trial of Stanford V versus ABVD versus mechlorethamine, vincristine, procarbazine, prednisone, epidoxorubicine, bleomycin, vinblastine, lomustine, doxorubicin, vindesine (MOPPEBVCAD) demonstrated an inferiority of the Stanford V regimen (Gobbi et al. 2005). As originally described, radiotherapy was to begin 1–3 weeks after the completion of chemotherapy (Bartlett et al. 1995). All sites of disease greater than 5 cm at the time of initial staging were to be included in the treatment fields. In addition, the bilateral low supraclavicular areas and pulmonary hilar regions were included as a component of the mediastinal treatment. The spleen was irradiated whenever there were focal nodules visible on the CT scan. In the Stanford series, more than 90% of patients qualified for consolidative irradiation.

In the Italian study, initial sites of disease greater than 6 cm (versus 5 cm) were considered for radiation and treatment was restricted to those patients who had only one or two sites to irradiate. Patients who achieved a complete response were not required to have any irradiation. Radiotherapy was delayed until 4–6 weeks (median 6 weeks) following the conclusion of chemotherapy (versus 1–3 weeks). Using these criteria, only two-thirds of patients received radiotherapy, a much smaller proportion than in the Stanford experience.

The current Stanford protocol calls for identification by pretreatment CT of all sites of disease >5 cm. The spleen is also evaluated carefully to detect focal splenic nodules. Shortly before the completion of chemotherapy, a CT simulation study is obtained and following the completion of chemotherapy a PET (positron emission tomography)-CT scan is performed. The pretreatment PET-CT is fused with the CT simulation study in order to localize the involved nodes. Superior and inferior margins of 2 cm are added to the involved nodes, based upon the initial PET-CT study. Three-dimensional planning is used to confirm that the 95% isodose volume includes all of the nodal regions of interest. The prescribed dose is 36 Gy and the daily dose is 1.5–1.8 Gy (almost always 1.5 Gy when the mediastinum is being irradiated). The treatment volume is extended to include the low supraclavicular regions and the bilateral hilar regions whenever the mediastinum is being irradiated. If treatment to the spleen is indicated, a 4-D planning scan is obtained and the spleen is treated with respiratory gating in order to minimize the volume of left lung and left kidney in the radiation field.

At the time of the post-chemotherapy PET-CT scan, if there is any residual PET avid disease, care is taken to include this in the radiation field, even if it was outside the volume initially intended for treatment (this is, in fact, quite rare).

3.3 Current Opinion

Over the years several groups have described prognostic scores and used these factors to tailor treatment. Hasenclever et al. have developed the International Prognostic Score for patients with advanced disease based on the following risk factors for: age >45 years, male sex, stage IV, hemoglobin <10.5 g/dl, albumin <4 g/dl, lymphocytes $<0.8\times10^9$/l or <6%, white blood count $>15\times10^9$/l (Hasenclever and Diehl 1998).

Choice of treatment is nowadays based not only on the knowledge on prognostic factors but also on late effects of treatment. There is a large spectrum of late effects varying from decreased fertility, hormonal disturbances, pulmonary problems and fatigue to serious morbidity and mortality from second cancers and cardiovascular diseases (Aleman et al. 2003b; Hancock and Hoppe 1996; Swerdlow et al. 2000; Swerdlow et al. 2007; van Leeuwen et al. 2000).

The occurrence of late effects is related to treatment intensity. The increased risk of second solid tumors is clearly related to radiation. A dose–effect relation has been shown for second breast cancer in women treated at young age for HL (Travis et al. 2003; van Leeuwen et al. 2003). Cardiotoxicity is evidently related to cumulative anthracycline dose (Kremer et al. 2001) and radiation dose to the heart (Moser et al. 2006).

Since a combination of chemotherapy and (extended-field) radiotherapy may, however, lead to an even greater risk of complications (Hancock and Hoppe 1996; Henry-Amar et al. 1990b; Klimm et al. 2007; Swerdlow et al. 2000; van Leeuwen et al. 2000) radiation volumes and radiation dose should be as limited as possible (Girinsky et al. 2006; Shahidi et al. 2006).

The risks of (late) toxicity of treatment must be balanced against the risk of treatment failure, since patients who have no response to initial therapy or who have an early relapse are not likely to be cured by salvage treatment (Ferme et al. 2002; Sureda et al. 2001)

3.3.1 *Treatment Recommendations Advanced-Stage Hodgkin Lymphoma*

Treatment should start with systemic therapy. In case of a complete remission after adequate chemotherapy like six to eight cycles of ABVD no further treatment is recommended. In case of a partial remission after ABVD-like chemotherapy, radiotherapy to residual abnormalities with a small margin is recommended. If, however, a treatment is used that has always included radiotherapy on indication, like Stanford V for instance, radiotherapy should still be used according to the specific protocol.

3.4 Future

The search for the optimal balance between treatments with high chances of control of the disease and treatments with low risks of long-term morbidity and mortality is expected to continue in the next decades. Better response evaluation will be of crucial importance.

Functional imaging techniques like Positron Emission Tomography using fluorine-18 (FDG-PET)-scans will probably become very important to adjust treatment depending on the evaluation of response on

PET. The best timing of the PET scan remains to be determined. Until now PET scans are usually used to evaluate response at the end of chemotherapy. The GHSG has integrated evaluation with PET scans in their new study in patients with advanced HL. In the recently started HD15 in advanced stages of HL eight cycles of BEACOPP escalated are compared to six courses of BEACOPP escalated and eight courses of BEACOPP-14. In this trial radiotherapy is given only to FDG-PET-positive residual tumors (Diehl et al. 2003). An interim analysis showed a significantly better progression-free survival at 12 months in PET-negative patients after chemotherapy. The authors concluded that radiotherapy following six or eight cycles of BEACOPP may be restricted to those patients who are PET-positive after chemotherapy (Kobe et al. 2008).

Improved diagnostic possibilities will have a major influence on radiotherapy. By limiting radiation volume and dose it is expected that cardiovascular toxicity (Hancock and Hoppe 1996) and the risk of second cancers will be reduced (Travis et al. 2003; van Leeuwen et al. 2003). What the influence of introducing more sophisticated radiation techniques would be on long-term effects is still difficult to predict. For instance, using intensity-modulated radiation therapy could in case of radiation of lymph nodes in the mediastinum lead to a lower dose to irradiated normal tissue but a larger volume of irradiated tissues may receive a low radiation dose. We expect a lower dose will decrease the risk of breast cancer, but so far no dose–volume relations have been described with regard to the risk of developing breast cancer (Travis et al. 2003; van Leeuwen et al. 2003).

In conclusion, for patients with advanced-stage HL, powerful chemotherapy is indicated, in case of a partial remission after chemotherapy, followed by radiotherapy to residual abnormalities using only a small margin.

References

Aleman BM, Raemaekers JM, Tirelli U et al (2003a) Involved-field radiotherapy for advanced Hodgkin's lymphoma. N Engl J Med 348:2396–2406

Aleman BM, Raemaekers JM, Tomisic R et al (2007) Involved-field radiotherapy for patients in partial remission after chemotherapy for advanced Hodgkin's lymphoma. Int J Radiat Oncol Biol Phys 67:19–30

Aleman BM, van den Belt-Dusebout AW, Klokman WJ et al (2003b) Long-term cause-specific mortality of patients treated for Hodgkin's disease. J Clin Oncol 21:3431–3439

Bagshaw MA, Kaplan HS, Rosenberg SA (1968) Extended-field radiation therapy in Hodgkin's disease. A progress report. Radiol Clin N Am 6:63–70

Bartlett NL, Rosenberg SA, Hoppe RT et al (1995) Brief chemotherapy, Stanford V, and adjuvant radiotherapy for bulky or advanced-stage Hodgkin's disease: a preliminary report. J Clin Oncol 13:1080–1088

Bonadonna G, Zucali R, Monfardini S et al (1975) Combination chemotherapy of Hodgkin's disease with adriamycin, bleomycin, vinblastine, and imidazole carboxamide versus MOPP. Cancer 36:252–259

Canellos GP, Anderson JR, Propert KJ et al (1992) Chemotherapy of advanced Hodgkin's disease with MOPP, ABVD, or MOPP alternating with ABVD. N Engl J Med 327:1478–1484

Cheson BD, Pfistner B, Juweid ME et al (2007) Revised response criteria for malignant lymphoma. J Clin Oncol 25:579–586

Desser RK, Golomb HM, Ultmann JE et al (1977) Prognostic classification of Hodgkin disease in pathologic stage III, based on anatomic considerations. Blood 49:883–893

Diehl V, Franklin J, Pfreundschuh M et al (2003) Standard and increased-dose BEACOPP chemotherapy compared with COPP-ABVD for advanced Hodgkin's disease. N Engl J Med 348:2386–2395

Diehl V, Thomas RK, Re D (2004) Part II: Hodgkin's lymphoma–diagnosis and treatment. Lancet Oncol 5:19–26

Duggan DB, Petroni GR, Johnson JL et al (2003) Randomized comparison of ABVD and MOPP/ABV hybrid for the treatment of advanced Hodgkin's disease: report of an intergroup trial. J Clin Oncol 21:607–614

Eich HT, Gossmann A, Engert A et al (2007) A Contribution to solve the problem of the need for consolidative radiotherapy after intensive chemotherapy in advanced stages of Hodgkin's lymphoma–analysis of a quality control program initiated by the radiotherapy reference center of the German Hodgkin Study Group (GHSG). Int J Radiat Oncol Biol Phys 69:1187–1192

Fabian CJ, Mansfield CM, Dahlberg S et al (1994) Low-dose involved field radiation after chemotherapy in advanced Hodgkin disease. A Southwest Oncology Group randomized study. Ann Intern Med 120:903–912

Ferme C, Mounier N, Casasnovas O et al (2006) Long-term results and competing risk analysis of the H89 trial in patients with advanced-stage Hodgkin lymphoma: a study by the Groupe d'Etude des Lymphomes de l'Adulte (GELA). Blood 107:4636–4642

Ferme C, Mounier N, Divine M et al (2002) Intensive salvage therapy with high-dose chemotherapy for patients with advanced Hodgkin's disease in relapse or failure after initial chemotherapy: results of the Groupe d'Etudes des Lymphomes de l'Adulte H89 Trial. J Clin Oncol 20:467–475

Ferme C, Sebban C, Hennequin C et al (2000) Comparison of chemotherapy to radiotherapy as consolidation of complete or good partial response after six cycles of chemotherapy for patients with advanced Hodgkin's disease: results of the groupe d'etudes des lymphomes de l'Adulte H89 trial. Blood 95:2246–2252

Girinsky T, van der Maazen R, Specht L et al (2006) Involved-node radiotherapy (INRT) in patients with early Hodgkin lymphoma: concepts and guidelines. Radiother Oncol 79:270–277

Gobbi PG, Levis A, Chisesi T et al (2005) ABVD versus modified Stanford V versus MOPPEBVCAD with optional and limited radiotherapy in intermediate- and advanced-stage Hodgkin's lymphoma: final results of a multicenter randomized trial by the Intergruppo Italiano Linfomi. J Clin Oncol 23:9198–9207

Hancock SL, Hoppe RT (1996) Long-term complications of treatment and causes of mortality after Hodgkin's disease. Semin Radiat Oncol 6:225–242

Hasenclever D, Diehl V (1998) A prognostic score for advanced Hodgkin's disease. International Prognostic Factors Project on Advanced Hodgkin's Disease. N Engl J Med 339:1506–1514

Henry-Amar M, Aeppli DM, Anderson J et al (1990a) Workshop statistical report. In: Somers R, Henry-Amar M, Meerwaldt JH et al (eds) Treatment strategy in Hodgkin's disease. INSERM/John Libbey Eurotext, London

Henry-Amar M, Hayat M, Meerwaldt JH et al (1990b) Causes of death after therapy for early stage Hodgkin's disease entered on EORTC protocols. EORTC Lymphoma Cooperative Group. Int J Radiat Oncol Biol Phys 19:1155–1157

Hoppe RT, Portlock CS, Glatstein E et al (1979) Alternating chemotherapy and irradiation in the treatment of advanced Hodgkin's disease. Cancer 43:472–481

Hoppe RT, Rosenberg SA, Kaplan HS et al (1980) Prognostic factors in pathological stage IIIA Hodgkin's disease. Cancer 46:1240–1246

Horning SJ, Ang PT, Hoppe RT et al (1992) The Stanford experience with combined procarbazine, Alkeran and vinblastine (PAVe) and radiotherapy for locally extensive and advanced stage Hodgkin's disease. Ann Oncol 3:747–754

Horning SJ, Williams J, Bartlett NL et al (2000) Assessment of the Stanford V regimen and consolidative radiotherapy for bulky and advanced Hodgkin's disease: Eastern Cooperative Oncology Group pilot study E1492. J Clin Oncol 18:972–980

Kaplan HS, Rosenberg SA (1966) Extended-field radical radiotherapy in advanced Hodgkin's disease: short-term results of 2 randomized clinical trials. Cancer Res 26:1268–1276

Klimm B, Eich H, Haverkamp H et al (2007) Poorer outcome of elderly patients treated with extended-field radiotherapy compared with involved-field radiotherapy after chemotherapy for Hodgkin's lymphoma: an analysis from the German Hodgkin Study Group. Ann Oncol 18:357–363

Kobe C, Dietlein M, Franklin J et al (2008) Positron emission tomography has a high negative predictive value for progression or early relapse for patients with residual disease after first-line chemotherapy in advanced-stage Hodgkin lymphoma. Blood 112:3989–3994

Kremer LC, van Dalen EC, Offringa M et al (2001) Anthracycline-induced clinical heart failure in a cohort of 607 children: long-term follow-up study. J Clin Oncol 19:191–196

Loeffler M, Brosteanu O, Hasenclever D et al (1998) Meta-analysis of chemotherapy versus combined modality treatment trials in Hodgkin's disease. International Database on Hodgkin's Disease Overview Study Group. J Clin Oncol 16:818–829

Moser EC, Noordijk EM, van Leeuwen FE et al (2006) Long-term risk of cardiovascular disease after treatment for aggressive non-Hodgkin lymphoma. Blood 107:2912–2919

Radford JA, Rohatiner AZ, Ryder WD et al (2002) ChlVPP/EVA hybrid versus the weekly VAPEC-B regimen for previously untreated Hodgkin's disease. J Clin Oncol 20:2988–2994

Rosenberg SA, Kaplan HS (1985) The evolution and summary results of the Stanford randomized clinical trials of the management of Hodgkin's disease: 1962-1984. Int J Radiat Oncol Biol Phys 11:5–22

Shahidi M, Kamangari N, Ashley S et al (2006) Site of relapse after chemotherapy alone for stage I and II Hodgkin's disease. Radiother Oncol 78:1–5

Sureda A, Arranz R, Iriondo A et al (2001) Autologous stem-cell transplantation for Hodgkin's disease: results and prognostic factors in 494 patients from the Grupo Espanol de Linfomas/Transplante Autologo de Medula Osea Spanish Cooperative Group. J Clin Oncol 19:1395–1404

Swerdlow AJ, Barber JA, Hudson GV et al (2000) Risk of second malignancy after Hodgkin's disease in a collaborative British cohort: the relation to age at treatment. J Clin Oncol 18:498–509

Swerdlow AJ, Higgins CD, Smith P et al (2007) Myocardial infarction mortality risk after treatment for Hodgkin disease: a collaborative British cohort study. J Natl Cancer Inst 99:206–214

Travis LB, Hill DA, Dores GM et al (2003) Breast cancer following radiotherapy and chemotherapy among young women with Hodgkin disease. JAMA 290:465–475

van Leeuwen FE, Klokman WJ, Stovall M et al (2003) Roles of radiation dose, chemotherapy, and hormonal factors in breast cancer following Hodgkin's disease. J Natl Cancer Inst 95:971–980

van Leeuwen FE, Klokman WJ, Veer MB et al (2000) Long-term risk of second malignancy in survivors of Hodgkin's disease treated during adolescence or young adulthood. J Clin Oncol 18:487–497

Young RC, Canellos GP, Chabner BA et al (1978) Patterns of relapse in advanced Hodgkin's disease treated with combination chemotherapy. Cancer 42:1001–1007

Salvage Therapy for Relapsed and Refractory Hodgkin Lymphoma

4

Joachim Yahalom, Andreas Rimner, and Richard W. Tsang

Contents

J. Yahalom (✉) and A. Rimner
Department of Radiation Oncology, Memorial Sloan-Kettering Cancer Center, 1275 York Ave, New York, NY 10021-6094, USA
e-mail: yahalomj@mskcc.org

R.W. Tsang
Department of Radiation Oncology, Princess Margaret Hospital, 610 University Ave, Toronto, ON M5G 2M9, Canada
e-mail: richard.tsang@rmp.uhn.on.ca

4.1 Introduction

The majority of patients with Hodgkin lymphoma (HL) should expect a cure with a standard initial treatment. Yet, in approximately 30–40% of patients who present at an advanced stage, HL remains refractory or relapses after obtaining a brief remission (Aleman et al. 2003; Canellos et al. 1992; Connors et al. 1997; Diehl et al. 1998; Duggan et al. 2003; Edwards-Bennett et al. 2010; Engert et al. 2009). In early-stage patients that are currently treated with combined-modality therapy, failure of treatment is expected in less than 10% of patients (Bonadonna et al. 2004; Engert et al. 2007; Meyer et al. 2005). However, a recent trend by some to treat early-stage patients with chemotherapy alone has increased the risk of failure of early-stage patients to approximately 20% (Yahalom 2009).

Primary refractory and relapsed HL is still curable in at least 50% of cases with programs that often combine re-induction of response with standard-dose chemotherapy salvage followed by high-dose chemoradiotherapy and autologous stem-cell transplantation (ASCT). However, if this "second chance" for cure is missed, the likelihood of obtaining a long-lasting additional remission is dismal (Bartlett et al. 2007; Moskowitz et al. 2009). Since many of the patients who require salvage after a failure of primary treatment have never been exposed to RT (although in most cases the relapses occurs in the primary site), the role of RT in salvage will be discussed in this chapter in more detail.

4.2 Salvage After Radiotherapy Alone

Nowadays, patients with classical HL are rarely treated with radiation alone. Yet, the treatment with

L. Specht and J. Yahalom (eds.), *Radiotherapy for Hodgkin Lymphoma*,
DOI: 10.1007/978-3-540-78944-4_4, © Springer-Verlag Berlin Heidelberg 2011

limited-field RT alone is still the standard of care in early-stage lymphocyte predominance HL and is also used for patients with early-stage classical HL who refuse or have contraindications to standard chemotherapy; extended-field RT alone remains for these patients a highly effective treatment option (Hoppe et al. 2008b).

Most of the experience with salvage after radiation alone was generated more than 2 decades ago, when extended-field RT alone was the standard primary treatment for all patients with early-stage and even stage III disease. This experience is still valuable today, but is relevant mostly in the special circumstances outlined above.

The relapse rate from primary RT alone for stage I–II disease is in the range of 20–35%. Most of the relapses will occur during the first 3 years (75–85%) (Yahalom 1996). Approximately 60% of relapses occur in unirradiated nodal areas and the remainder in extranodal sites such as lung and bone (Carde et al. 1988). Thus, the relapse represents a tumor that is neither radiotherapy resistant nor is chemotherapy resistant.

Most patients who fail to respond, or relapse, after RT alone can be salvaged successfully with standard-dose chemotherapy with or without additional RT. Favorable outcomes with long-term (5–10-year) overall survival (OS) rates between 57% and 89% have been reported with the use of combination chemotherapy (Cooper et al. 1984; Horwich et al. 1997; Ng et al. 2004; Olver et al. 1988; Roach, III et al. 1990; Ruffer et al. 2005; Santoro et al. 1986; Vinciguerra et al. 1986). Several large series with mature follow-up are shown in Table 4.1.

Younger age at diagnosis and longer initial remission interval were significant favorable factors for OS. In a favorable subset of patients with a long initial remission interval, an 85% complete response rate was observed with 20-year disease-free survival of 45% after mustargen, vincristine (Oncovin), procarbazine, and prednisone (MOPP) salvage chemotherapy. Patients without a complete response to salvage chemotherapy had a poor outcome (Longo et al. 1992). Horwich et al. reported 10-year OS after relapse of 63% (Horwich et al. 1997). On multivariate analysis, only age was a significant factor for OS; age, histologic subtype, and extranodal involvement at relapse were significant for cause-specific survival.

The German Hodgkin Study Group reported their experience with bleomycin, etoposide, doxorubicin (Adriamycin), cyclophosphamide, vincristine (Oncovin), procarbazine, and prednisone (BEACOPP) and COPP/ABVD as salvage treatment for 107 patients that were initially treated with primary extended-field RT for early-stage HL (Ruffer et al. 2005). With a median follow-up of 45 months, they observed a complete response in 87%, freedom from second failure (FF2F) of 81%, and OS of 89%. They identified an age >50 years, B symptoms, and extranodal involvement as significant adverse predictors for OS, and age, B symptoms, and salvage chemotherapy regimen for FF2F. Other examples of salvage chemotherapy regimen in relapsed HL include etoposide, vinblastine, and doxorubicin (EVA) with a complete response rate of 40% and a 3-year failure-free survival of 29% (Canellos et al. 1995).

RT-alone failures do not need to undergo high-dose therapy with ASCT; in fact, the long-term survival of such patients approaches that achieved with primary systemic therapy of de novo advanced disease. Both MOPP and ABVD combinations were effective as salvage regimens, but since ABVD's advantage over

Table 4.1 Salvage chemotherapy for relapse after radiation alone

Center	No. of patients	Chemotherapy	Overall survival
International Database (laparotomy staged) (Specht et al. 1994)	681	Various	70% (10 years)
International Database (non-laparotomy staged) (Horwich et al. 1997)	473	Various	63% (10 years)
Stanford (Roach, III et al. 1990)	99	MOPP	57% (10 years)
Peter McCallum (Olver et al. 1988)	70	MOPP	71% (10 years)
Instituto Nazionale Tumori (Santoro et al. 1986)	63	ABVD	80% (7 years)
Dana Farber (Ng et al. 2004)	100	ABVD	89% (10 years)

ABVD = adriamycin, bleomycin, vincristine, and dacarbazine; MOPP = mustargen, oncovin, procarbazine, and prednisone

MOPP in both efficacy and toxicity has been documented in the treatment of advanced-stage disease, ABVD has become the preferred regimen for salvage of RT failures. Adding involved-field RT to sites of relapse that were not included in the original radiation field (i.e., inguinal relapse after subtotal lymphoid irradiation) is recommended and, in the Stanford series, patients salvaged with a combination of chemotherapy and radiation have done significantly better than those salvaged with chemotherapy alone (Roach, III et al. 1990).

Having a combination of adverse factors such as B symptoms, extranodal, or stage IV disease carries a worse prognosis, and patients that relapse with these features should be considered for more intensive salvage. Following standard-dose chemotherapy for all RT failures, response should be evaluated with a positron emission tomography (PET)/computed tomography (CT) scan to verify a complete response and followed closely. Incomplete responders should be considered for salvage that includes HDT/ASCT.

4.3 Salvage of Patients Who Relapse or Remain Refractory After Chemotherapy Alone or Combined-Modality Therapy

Relapsed HL is defined as reappearance of HL after a variable disease-free interval following initial therapy with either chemotherapy alone, RT alone, or combined-modality therapy. Refractory disease or progressive disease is defined as the failure to achieve a significant response to initial therapy, or progression of disease as measured by clinical or radiographic methods within the first 90 days following the end of primary treatment.

All refractory/relapsed disease should be biopsy-proven since residual lumps or old or new imaging abnormalities may represent other malignancies, infectious, inflammatory, necrotic or fibrotic residual tissue, or other benign conditions. It is not rare to find, after treatment of HL, residual or new lesions with high PET uptake that represent non-Hodgkin lymphoma or sarcoidosis. Clinical restaging at the time of relapse is important for the selection of a treatment approach and for prognostic purposes.

There are several salvage options for relapsed and refractory HL following systemic treatment, including chemotherapy alone, RT alone, combined-modality treatment, and autologous or allogeneic bone-marrow transplantation. Yet, for most patients, the best second chance of cure is with a combination of initial standard-dose chemotherapy salvage regimen followed by high-dose therapy and ASCT with RT to selected sites integrated into the salvage program either before or after transplantation. Yet, some patients may be poor candidates for an HDT/ASCT program due to other morbidities or advanced age, and some may still be salvaged with radiation alone or standard-dose chemotherapy. These options are discussed below.

4.4 Salvage with Radiation Alone

A failure to respond to chemotherapy does not necessarily imply radiation resistance, and applying radiation judiciously in the salvage setting remains an important component of salvage therapy. In the late 1980s and early 1990s, before the routine and safer use of HDT and ASCT, selected patients who failed initial chemotherapy were treated with salvage RT alone (Brada et al. 1992; Campbell et al. 2005; Uematsu et al. 1993; Wirth et al. 1997). With the advent of ASCT, salvage RT alone has become less commonly used, because HL frequently presents in a more disseminated distribution at relapse and the risk for further relapse in systemic sites is relatively high. The salvage results with RT alone were clearly inferior to those of HDT/ASCT, possibly with the exception of highly selected patient groups.

Some patients, however, may still be eligible for this approach because they cannot undergo ASCT due to age or comorbidities; or they possess favorable clinical features that indicate a potential benefit with local therapy alone. Infrequently, some of the patients with localized nodal relapses after a long disease-free interval are potentially curable with salvage RT alone.

Relapses of HL following chemotherapy tend to recur in previously involved sites in up to 83%, particularly if the disease was bulky (Macdonald et al. 2007; Mundt et al. 1995; Shahidi et al. 2006). The radiation techniques used for salvage therapy varied from involved fields to extended fields such as mantle fields, to sometimes total lymphoid irradiation (TLI) given sequentially. Patients with predominately localized nodal relapses were selected to receive RT because the disease could be encompassed with typical RT fields. Excellent in-field control rates are achieved (70–90%), and approximately 25–40% of patients survived 5 years with control of disease (Brada et al. 1992; Campbell et al. 2005; Leigh et al. 1993; Pezner et al. 1994; Uematsu et al. 1993; Wirth et al. 1997). These studies, however, suffered from small numbers with only 14–100 patients per study and very variable patient characteristics; they are thus hard to compare. Table 4.2 summarizes the published experience from the largest series.

The largest published experience to date of salvage RT is of patients treated on German Hodgkin Study Group (GHSG) protocols from 1988 to 1999 (n = 4,754) (Josting et al. 2005a). Among the 624 patients with refractory or recurrent HL following initial therapy, 100 (16%) were selected to receive RT for salvage (in an era when HDT/ASCT was an available potential alternative). Eighty-five percent of the patients had progressed after cyclophosphamide, Oncovin, procarbazine, and prednisone (COPP)-ABVD or similar regimens, 8% after BEACOPP, and 7% had RT alone. RT salvage volumes consisted of involved-field RT in 37%, and extended-field techniques for the remainder (mantle, 43%; inverted Y, 8%; total nodal irradiation (TNI) or sub-TNI, 12%). The response rate to salvage RT (median dose, 40 Gy) was 81% (CR, 77%; partial response [PR], 4%); hence the majority being documented as CRs. The 5-year FF2F and OS rates were 28% and 51%, respectively, similar to that reported in the previous literature (Brada et al. 1992; Campbell et al. 2005; Uematsu et al. 1993; Wirth et al. 1997). Criticisms of this study include that the RT fields varied greatly; RT doses ranged from 15 to 50 Gy; the patient population represented a favorable subgroup, with most patients (87%) having limited-stage disease at relapse; biopsies of relapses were not mandatory; and the subsequent treatment modalities varied greatly, from palliative treatment to allogeneic transplantation.

Patients with disease-free interval more than 12 months from completion of initial chemotherapy are more likely to have a durable response (Brada et al. 1992; Josting et al. 2005a; Wirth et al. 1997). Other characteristics that predict for a favorable response to salvage RT include younger age, early stage at relapse, predominantly nodal distribution of disease, good performance status, and absence of constitutional (B) symptoms (Brada et al. 1992; Campbell et al. 2005; Josting et al. 2005a).

When salvage RT is being considered, care must be applied to take account of prior RT exposure, performance status of the patient, residual bone marrow function, the ability to encompass all sites of active disease, and the overall tolerance of the patient to the proposed treatment. Also, the merits of covering potential high-risk areas in contiguity with gross disease must be carefully weighed against treatment toxicity of wide-field radiation. To this end, ^{18}F-PET scans are very useful to define metabolically active disease that may not be abnormal on anatomic imaging alone. If extended fields are necessary (e.g., mantle, and paraaortic/spleen coverage, or inverted Y fields to cover pelvic nodal disease), particularly when both supra- and infradiaphragmatic coverage are required, sequential treatment is necessary with a treatment gap of 1–3 months for hematologic recovery. The total dose required to achieve a high degree of local control (≥90%) has been reported to be in the range of 30.0–37.5 Gy in an era of RT for chemotherapy-naive tumors (Vijayakumar and Myrianthopoulos 1992). Further analysis showed that, above 32.5 Gy, no dose–response relationship was apparent, although there was a suggestion that larger tumors required a higher dose (Brincker and Bentzen 1994). Logistic regression analysis showed that the dose required for 95% local control was 27 Gy for subclinical disease, 34 Gy for nodes <6 cm, and 35 Gy for nodes >6 cm. In the chemotherapy refractory or relapse setting, the control

Table 4.2 Salvage radiotherapy after relapse from chemotherapy

Center	No. of Patients	FFR of FFP (%)	% Survival
GHSG (Josting et al. 2005a)	100	28% (5 years)	51%
Peter MacCallum (Campbell et al. 2005)	81	33% (10 years)	46%
Royal Marsden (Brada et al. 1992)	25	23% (10 years)	40%

GHSG = German Hodgkin Lymphoma Study Group

rates with salvage RT approaches these levels with median dose of 36–40 Gy (Campbell et al. 2005; Josting et al. 2005a). Although the data on salvage RT cannot be directly compared with the results of ASCT, these studies nevertheless show that RT alone could salvage a significant proportion of patients who fail chemotherapy. Therefore, judicious use of RT is an option for selected patients who relapse after chemotherapy, particularly if there was a long disease-free interval. Due to the excellent CR and local control rates, RT remains one of the most potent agents for HL. The experience of salvage RT also forms the basis for more aggressive high-dose programs that incorporate RT in sequence with salvage CT and ASCT to maximize tumor control from both modalities of treatment.

4.5 Salvage of Systemic Chemotherapy Failures with Standard-Dose Chemotherapy Regimen

Prior to the advent of HDT/ASCT, salvage of systemic therapy failures of advanced-stage disease was attempted by either repeating the same regimen, switching to an alternative regimen (MOPP failures treated with ABVD and vice versa), or, for failures of combinations of two regimens (MOPP/ABVD), combinations of other agents.

Overall, approximately 10–30% of patients achieved lasting CRs to this approach. The most important factor that determined the success of a standard-dose salvage program was the duration of the original remission. Patients with a remission duration that was shorter than 1 year or were primary refractory had very poor outcomes. Other poor indicators were stage IV at primary diagnosis and B symptoms at relapse. In a study from British Columbia, the 5-year FF2F after salvage was only 17%, but was 82% if none of the adverse factors was present ($P < .001$) (Lohri et al. 1991). In a series from the National Cancer Institute of MOPP failures salvaged with MOPP, 24% of patients who had long original remissions survived beyond 10 years, but only 11% of those relapsing earlier than 1 year had long survival (Longo et al. 1992). In the CALGB randomized study that compared initial treatment with either MOPP, ABVD, or MOPP/ABVD, patients who failed to respond to ABVD and were salvaged with MOPP had a 5-year failure-free survival of 31% (Canellos et al. 1992).

In summary, depending on prognostic factors such as initial response duration, disease extent, and performance status, probably 10–30% of relapsed patients are still potentially curable with standard-dose chemotherapy.

4.6 High-Dose Therapy (HDT) and Autologous Stem-Cell Transplantation

Over the last 2 decades, HDT followed by ASCT has become the standard salvage program for patients with classical HL who failed chemotherapy alone or combined-modality therapy. Yet, for patients that failed radiation alone and for patients with lymphocytic predominant HL, less intensive salvage treatments are appropriate.

High-dose chemotherapy followed by an autologous bone marrow transplantation (ABMT) was first used in the early 1980s for refractory and relapsed HL. Many of the patients in the early series had already failed prior standard-dose salvage regimens and were probably more heavily pretreated than most patients that are salvaged today (Carella et al. 1985; Jagannath et al. 1986; Philip et al. 1986). Since then, the results and the safety of HDT/ASCT have continuously improved and the increase in its application stemmed simply from the clear advantage over the dismal results of standard-dose salvage (Horning et al. 1997; Rapoport et al. 2004; Reece et al. 1994; Wheeler et al. 1997; Yahalom et al. 1993).

4.6.1 The Randomized Trials

Two randomized trials have further established the role of ABMT/ASCT for relapsed and refractory HL (Linch et al. 1993; Schmitz et al. 2002; Schmitz et al. 2005). In the first small trial by the British National Lymphoma Investigation Group, Linch et al. demonstrated a 3-year event-free survival (EFS) and progression-free survival benefit with high-dose salvage chemotherapy (BEAM) followed by an ABMT compared to standard-dose chemotherapy (mini-BEAM) without an ABMT (EFS

53% versus 10%, respectively) (Linch et al. 1993). Only 20 patients were assigned to each arm and the trial closed early due to problems with accrual, as the patients preferred the more aggressive regimen.

Schmitz et al. randomized 161 patients to four cycles of conventional dose dexamethasone, carmustine, etoposide, cytarabine, and melphalan (Dexa-BEAM) compared with two cycles of Dexa-BEAM, high-dose Dexa-BEAM, and ABMT/ASCT (Schmitz et al. 2002; Schmitz et al. 2005). In 117 patients that were chemotherapy sensitive with a PR or CR to the first two cycles of Dexa-BEAM, 3-year FF2F in the high-dose chemotherapy arm was significantly improved compared with standard-dose chemotherapy (3-year FF2F, 55% versus 34%). In a subset analysis, the authors demonstrated that both early and late relapses benefited from high-dose therapy followed by ABMT/ASCT; particularly, the early relapses had a significantly improved FF2F. On long-term follow-up presented in abstract form only, the 7-year FF2F was improved in early and late first relapses, but not for those with multiple relapses (Schmitz et al. 2005). While the 7-year FF2F continued to be significantly different between the two arms, the OS was not significantly different.

Criticisms of this study include the lack of standardization for involved-field RT (IFRT), poor accrual, and early closure of the trial and high toxicity of the Dexa-BEAM regimen. Possible explanations for finding no difference in OS include the variable timing of high-dose therapy and transplantation in the course of the disease, and the use of various salvage regimens including transplantation for the patients in the non-transplantation arm after subsequent relapses. Similar findings were described in two case-control studies with superior outcomes for patients receiving HDT and ASCT when compared with conventional salvage therapy (André et al. 1999; Yuen et al. 1997).

4.6.2 Standard-Dose Salvage Prior to HDT/ASCT

In general, salvage therapy today is administered in two phases. Initially, a standard-dose chemotherapy regimen is given to induce a response in an attempt to achieve maximal reduction in the tumor bulk, optimally, a CR. This is usually followed by stem-cell mobilization and collection. IFRT when given pre-transplantation is normally given following collection and prior to the administration of the second phase that consists of the high-dose chemotherapy or chemoradiation regimen.

Many different standard-dose salvage chemotherapy regimens have been tested in preparation for ASCT, but none has emerged as a standard of care. These include dexamethasone, cisplatin, cytarabine (DHAP) (Josting et al. 2002), DEXA-BEAM (Josting et al. 1998), carmustine, etoposide, cytarabine, melphalan (Mini-BEAM) (Martin et al. 2001), ifosfamide, carboplatin, etoposide (ICE) (Moskowitz 2002; Moskowitz et al. 2001; Moskowitz et al. 2004), gemcitabine, dexamethasone, cisplatin (GDP) (Kuruvilla et al. 2006), and gemcitabine, vinorelbine, liposomal doxorubicin (GVD/GND) (Bartlett et al. 2007). No regimen has been proven superior to others in a randomized fashion, and the choice of the salvage chemotherapy regimen is mostly driven by institutional preference.

At Memorial Sloan-Kettering Cancer Center (MSKCC), we typically use ICE × 2 cycles followed by stem collection and pre-ASCT, and IFRT prior to HDT. In patients that do not respond with a PET-CR to ICE, we currently continue HDT with GND × 2 cycles to achieve maximal reduction of tumor burden prior to stem-cell rescue (Moskowitz et al. 2010). The response to standard-dose salvage chemotherapy has been found to be one of the most important prognostic factors (Yahalom et al. 1993). Originally, the response criteria were based primarily on CT scan responses. More recently, the role of PET scans in salvage of HL has been explored and found to be valuable (Castagna et al. 2009; Jabbour et al. 2007; Svoboda et al. 2006). In our experience pre-ASCT CR documented by normalization of functional imaging (most by FDG-PET, some by gallium) was associated with an EFS of 77%, compared with 33% if functional imaging remained positive ($P = 0.00004$) (Moskowitz et al. 2010). Therefore, a maximal effort to obtain a PET-CR pre-ASCT, including the addition of IFRT, is strongly recommended.

4.6.3 High-Dose Therapy Regimens and Stem-Cell Source

Standard-dose salvage chemotherapy is followed by high-dose therapy consisting of chemotherapy with or without RT. Similar to the variety of options with standard-dose salvage regimens, there is not a single preferred high-dose chemotherapy protocol. Commonly used combinations are the CBV regimen (cyclophosphamide and carmustine, VP-16) (Jagannath et al. 1986; Reece et al. 1994; Wheeler et al. 1997), Cy/VP-16 (cyclophosphamide and VP-16) (Moskowitz 2002; Yahalom et al. 1993), or high-dose BEAM (carmustine, etoposide, cytarabine, and melphalan) (Argiris et al. 2000; Chopra et al. 1993; Josting et al. 2005b).

After high-dose therapy, patients undergo stem-cell rescue with an autologous transplantation with an ABMT or ASCT. In the early days of autologous transplantation, bone-marrow-derived stem cells were used for stem-cell rescue after high-dose therapy (Carella et al. 1985; Jagannath et al. 1986; Philip et al. 1986). However, this involved multiple bone-marrow aspirations under general anesthesia and was associated with a slow recovery of blood counts following the transplantation. Patients in whom the pelvic bones had been involved by lymphoma or treated with RT posed a specific challenge for stem-cell collection from pelvic bones. Since the advent of hematopoietic growth factors in the early 1990s, peripheral stem cells have been used more commonly for transplantation after HDT, because they are easily collected after growth-factor stimulation, independent of prior treatment or involvement of the pelvic bones, allow a more rapid recovery of blood counts following the transplantation, and thus decrease the risk for short-term complications, transfusions, and duration of hospitalization (Majolino et al. 1997; Schmitz et al. 1996; Sureda et al. 2001). Overall, the therapeutic efficacy and long-term toxicity appear to be comparable to ASCT compared with ABMT.

4.6.4 Predictive Factors of HDT/ASCT Salvage Outcome

Several groups retrospectively identified prognostic factors that affected salvage outcome. In almost all series, time to relapse of less than a year was a strong adverse prognostic factor. Other adverse factors noted by most investigators were extranodal disease and B symptoms at relapse/refractory state.

The International Prognostic Factors Project for advanced Hodgkin's disease developed a score consisting of seven factors that predicted disease progression and OS in advanced HL (Hasenclever and Diehl 1998). It includes a serum albumin <4 g/dL, a hemoglobin <10.5 g/dL, male sex, an age of 45 years and higher, stage IV disease, a leukocyte count of ≥15,000/mm^3, and a lymphocyte count <600/mm^3, <8% of the white blood cell count, or both. This score has been successfully translated and simplified to predict the outcome of HL after ASCT by Bierman et al (Bierman et al. 2002). They describe that low albumin, low hemoglobin, greater age, and low lymphocyte counts were predictive for shorter EFS, while only low hemoglobin, higher age, and low lymphocyte counts predicted shorter OS. They did not confirm an association of stage IV, higher leukocyte count, or male sex with worse outcome.

The GHSG reported a new prognostic score based on 422 patients with relapsed HL (Josting et al. 2002). They identified duration of initial remission, stage of disease at relapse, and anemia as the three most important prognostic factors for additional relapses. Only 140 of 422 patients underwent an ASCT/ABMT as part of their salvage therapy, and 54 patients received salvage RT in some fashion. They reported a CR rate after salvage RT of 92% and a PR rate of 4% for an overall response rate of 96%, confirming the significant role of RT as a salvage treatment modality.

At MSKCC, a prognostic model for relapsed/refractory patients was developed following the analysis of a prospective intent-to-treat study, and it has later been utilized to tailor the intensity of treatment in the next institutional HDT/ASCT program (Moskowitz et al. 2001; Moskowitz et al. 2010). The prognostic model was based on three independent factors identified to be independently associated with an inferior outcome. These were refractory disease or relapse in less than 1 year, B symptoms at the time of relapse, and extranodal involvement at relapse. The favorable group consisted of patients with one or no adverse factors and at a median follow-up of 43 months; EFS in this group was 83%. The intermediate group included patients with two adverse factors and the EFS was 27%; the poor-prognosis group with three adverse factors had an EFS of only 10%.

The following MSKCC regimen was designed with augmentation of salvage program for the intermediate- and poor-prognosis groups. The intermediate group received augmented ICE as the initial salvage regimen and the poor-prognosis group received high-dose ICE with stem support. Interim evaluation was performed with functional imaging and the patients then proceeded to receive IFRT followed immediately by high-dose chemoradiotherapy and ASCT (Moskowitz et al. 2010). EFS in both groups markedly improved with the risk-tailored dose-escalation approach. Remarkably, the poor-prognosis group showed the most improvement, their EFS approached 40% (compared with 10% in the prior program). Functional imaging (FI) (done primarily with FDG-PET) pre-ASCT emerged as the most important prognostic predictor in this study; 4-year EFS in patients remaining FI positive was 33% compared with those who were FI negative, whose EFS was 77% ($P = 0.00004$). Adding more chemotherapy (such as GND) and possibly escalating the IFRT dose is currently evaluated at MSKCC in patients who remain PET-positive after ICE.

4.6.5 Incorporation of Radiotherapy into HDT/ASCT Programs

Although high-dose chemotherapy has significantly improved the salvage prospects of patients with refractory or relapsed HD, approximately 50% of patients who underwent transplant remain refractory or relapse shortly after BMT. In the absence of promising new agents for pre-ABMT high-dose chemotherapy and the inability to significantly escalate the doses of current combinations, it appears justified to encourage and optimize the integration of radiation, the most effective single agent in the treatment of HL, into HDT/ASCT salvage programs.

It is of interest to note that an increasing number of patients who failed primary treatment and are considered for salvage programs have never received radiation as part of their initial treatment. Many of these patients have most likely developed some degree of drug resistance or toxicity and are yet expected to require doses of drugs that may exceed the tolerance of critical organs. However, most of those patients do not exhibit a cross-resistance to radiation. This notion is supported by several reports indicating that approximately 30% of selected patients who relapsed after chemotherapy attain a lasting complete response to RT (see above).

An important argument in support of incorporating RT into high-dose salvage programs is the pattern of relapse after high-dose chemotherapy. It is similar to the pattern of relapse after chemotherapy-only programs for early-stage disease or for advanced-stage disease (Dhakal et al. 2009; Shahidi et al. 2006). Namely, patients relapse in sites of initial involvement, mostly nodal sites as was documented by several investigators (Reece et al. 1994). Therefore, these sites are predictable and amenable to effective treatment with RT as was documented by several groups (Mundt et al. 1995; Poen et al. 1996). Mundt et al. described that IFRT reduced the rate of local relapses in sites of prior HL involvement from 43% to 26% and improved 5-year local control rates in all sites, nodal sites, and sites that were persistent to high-dose chemotherapy (Mundt et al. 1995). A similar effect was observed by Poen et al. from Stanford, who reported only four local failures (out of 67) in irradiated sites (Poen et al. 1996). Other teams that used IFRT before BMT reported a significant decrease in the incidence of relapse in irradiated areas (Pezner et al. 1994; Reece et al. 1994).

The issues of optimal timing of RT in relation to BMT, the dose and schedule of RT, and the sites to be treated remain open and, unfortunately, are unlikely to be studied in a prospective manner in the near future (Yahalom 1995). At MSKCC, we have always preferred to schedule the delivery of radiation immediately before high-dose chemotherapy, assuming that it may have a beneficial "debulking" effect before "definitive" chemotherapy and may prevent unpredictable delays in giving RT later (post-transplantation) engendered by a potentially long engraftment period. Another hypothetical advantage to pre-BMT irradiation is that the re-infused stem cells are not exposed to a potentially leukemogenic treatment of radiation post-engraftment.

Another critical issue in the design of a comprehensive combined-modality approach to an HDT/ASCT salvage program is, "What sites should be irradiated? Bulky? Residual? All initially involved? Or all nodal sites?" (Argiris et al. 2000; Majhail et al. 2006; Rapoport et al. 2004; Reece et al. 1994). A concern regarding using RT prior to transplant emerged from the experience in the late 1980s at the Princess Margaret Hospital (Tsang et al. 1999). HL patients who received radiation to the chest (some received a full mantle field) as part of their initial or salvage therapy and proceeded within 50 days to BMT had a higher risk of pulmonary complications compared with patients who were irradiated post-transplant. The experience at MSKCC is different; the salvage programs for both HL and non-Hodgkin's lymphoma include accelerated IFRT pre-transplant, and the cumulative experience in over 600 patients in several salvage programs over 2 decades confirmed a high safety profile of the pre-transplant

IFRT (toxic mortality of less than 3%). Indeed, only very rarely severe complications could be attributed (even in part) to the IFRT component in our experience (Hoppe et al. 2008a; Hoppe et al. 2009; Moskowitz et al. 2001; Moskowitz et al. 2004; Moskowitz et al. 2010; Yahalom et al. 1993). It is suggested that the practice of initial reduction of the tumor bulk with standard-dose chemotherapy, particularly in the chest, allowed a limited conformal radiation volume pre-HDT/ASCT to spare most of the heart and lung, and thus avoid the toxicity of larger radiation fields.

Administering radiation beyond the involved relapse site remains a challenge in HDT programs. In a study by Mundt et al., less than 30% of known sites of irradiated patients were treated. It appears that relapse shifted from irradiated sites to unirradiated previously involved or uninvolved sites (Mundt et al. 1995; Mundt et al. 1999). Further, some patients who come to salvage therapy frequently have multiple sites of nodal or extranodal sites of involvement. Thus, standard-fractionation IFRT to all involved sites may require prolonged and potentially myelotoxic treatments. An alternative approach was to incorporate low-dose total body irradiation into the ASCT conditioning regimen. However, concerns of potential increased toxicity, especially in previously irradiated patients, have discouraged further evaluation of this combined-modality approach. There were also concerns regarding the tumoricidal value of the relatively low doses of radiation used for total body irradiation (10–14 Gy) (Yahalom 1996).

In the majority of patients, the most common sites of relapse are still nodal. This "mostly nodal" pattern of relapse suggests that the radiation technique of choice for incorporating RT into salvage programs for HD is TLI. This approach has been under study at MSKCC since 1985 (Yahalom et al. 1989; Yahalom et al. 1993). The approach at MSKCC has regarded RT in the salvage setting as a quasi-systemic therapy, but also provided an option to boost RT to clinically involved sites. This approach is feasible when given in an accelerated mode, thus assuring that the delivery of chemotherapy and stem-cell rescue is not delayed. The TLI field avoids the toxicity of total body irradiation while still providing effective RT to most lymph nodes, allows the delivery of doses above the limits of total body irradiation, and permits the exposure of selected involved extranodal sites. The experience at MSKCC using a TLI-based salvage program in previously unirradiated patients has been highly successful in both relapsed and refractory patients (Moskowitz et al. 2001; Moskowitz et al. 2010; Yahalom et al. 1993).

Previously irradiated patients may still receive effective dose radiation at relapse, albeit in doses lower than 36 Gy to sites that have previously been irradiated. In concurrence with this notion, the current approach at MSKCC maximizes the use of RT to include all salvage patients regardless of whether they have or have not been previously irradiated. Candidates for combined-modality high-dose therapy are first re-induced with ICE chemotherapy. Only responders to ICE proceed to high-dose therapy. ICE is also used with granulocyte-colony-stimulating factor to mobilize peripheral blood stem cells, which are retrieved and cryopreserved for later use. RT includes IFRT alone (to residual or previously bulky sites) in previously irradiated patients; the dose of IFRT ranges between 18 and 36 Gy. In previously unirradiated patients, IFRT (18 Gy) is immediately followed by TLI (18 Gy). All RT is administered twice a day within 2 weeks. This is followed by high-dose chemotherapy and peripheral blood stem-cell transplantation.

We recently updated information on all 186 previously unirradiated refractory (53%) and relapsed (47%) HL patients treated on MSKCC protocols that included IFRT followed by TLI as part of the conditioning regimen. At a median follow-up of 5 years (the program started in 1985), the 5- and 10-year OS was 68% and 56%, and the 5- and 10-year EFS was 62% and 56%, respectively. The safety profile of the TLI-based program has dramatically improved over time. Over the last 2 decades, only five of 133 patients (3%) died of early toxicity with only one event of death from infection (1.3%) during the last 10 years. These deaths (mostly of sepsis) were not necessarily related to RT.

In a prospective phase I/II randomized study of TLI and HDT/ASCT, Evens et al. from Northwestern University delivered accelerated hyperfractionated TLI in twice-daily fractions to a total dose of 1,500 cGy in 10 fractions combined with a boost to involved sites to a total combined dose of 3,000 cGy in 20 fractions (Evens et al. 2007). They showed a substantial 5-year EFS and OS benefit with the use of TLI (63% versus 6% and 61% versus 27%, respectively) compared with patients treated with HDT/ASCT and chemotherapy alone. TLI was found to be a predictor for improved EFS on multivariate analysis.

While most institutions still use high-dose chemotherapy-only salvage regimens, the experience from

MSKCC and Northwestern University supports the efficacy and the safety of integrating RT as either IFRT or in combination with TLI in salvage regimens, particularly in patients who have not had prior exposure to radiation.

Long-term follow-up of MSKCC patients salvaged mostly with programs that incorporated IFRT with or without TLI showed a relatively small increased risk of secondary solid tumors (Goodman et al. 2008). Myelodysplastic syndrome and leukemia risk was elevated compared with the general population and most likely reflected the multiple exposures that these patients had prior to entering the HDT/ASCT salvage programs. Other long-term morbidities were rare and the global quality of life parameters were comparable to those of the general population.

4.6.6 Salvage After ASCT Failure

Patients who fail salvage HDT with an ASCT have a dismal prognosis. Their salvage options after transplantation are severely limited by their tolerance for further therapy given multiple rounds of prior intense therapy as well as the treatment-resistant biology of their disease. The median survival for patients failing after ASCT ranges from 24 to 33 months (Crump 2008; Kewalramani et al. 2003). Recently, Moskowitz et al. reported OS rates of 23% in patients who failed after ASCT (Moskowitz et al. 2009). A small subset of patients with a good functional status, younger age, and a matching donor may be eligible for allogeneic BMT (Crump 2008). The transplantation-related mortality with allogeneic transplantations is substantial, up to 61% in early studies (Akpek et al. 2001; Milpied et al. 1996). Therefore, attempts are made to perform reduced-intensity allogeneic stem-cell transplantations. With such a regimen, OS rates of up to 59% have been described by Sureda et al. in a patient population that included 52% patients with prior ASCT (Sureda et al. 2008).

4.7 Role of RT in Local Control and Palliation

For HL patients who are not candidates for ASCT or have recurrent disease despite ASCT, radiation is a very effective modality for providing symptom relief and local control. The palliative role of RT for HL has not been extensively studied, and no phase III trials have been published to determine the optimal approach in terms of patient selection, dose-fractionation parameters, and radiation volume. It is likely that palliative RT has continually been underutilized in patients with disseminated HL because of a variety of systemic treatment options. When palliative RT is considered, it is important to establish the goal of therapy. Distinction should be made between local control of disease, i.e., radical RT given for permanent local control and possible long-term survival, or RT given purely for the relief of symptoms. In general, even non-curable HL patients may still have a longer life expectancy than those with non-Hodgkin lymphoma or solid tumors, and it is often worthwhile to deliver a moderately high-dose course of treatment (>30 Gy, conventional fractionation) to aim for local control. In a retrospective review of 56 patients who had progression or relapse of HL after ASCT treated with salvage RT ± chemotherapy, coverage of all disease sites with an intention for local control was possible in 70%, while 30% were treated to the symptomatic site(s) only (Tsang et al. 2009). Prior RT was given in 59% of the patients, as part of initial management or during the peri-transplant period where the indication to use IFRT was a bulky tumor 5 cm or more in diameter. Extended-field RT was not routinely given peri-transplant. With a salvage RT median dose of 35 Gy, the overall response rate was 84%, with a 2-year in-field local control rate of 69% (Tsang et al. 2009). At 5 years, the OS was 32%, and five patients (out of 56) achieved long-term (>5 years) disease-free survival with a salvage RT approach. Therefore, although salvage RT given in a post-ASCT setting is rarely curative, in selected cases durable long-term control of disease and survival can be achieved. However, the results are dependent on how extensively RT had been used previously, as the benefits of RT could be exploited in a more systematic integration with the high-dose ASCT program, i.e., with RT given in the peri-transplant period.

For end-stage patients with a short life expectancy and a poor performance status, symptom relief can be achieved with common palliative regimens such as 20 Gy in five fractions, or 25–30 Gy in 10–15 fractions. In deciding about the use of palliative RT, its dose and volumes of treatment, care must be exercised to take account of prior RT exposure, anticipated toxicity, hematologic tolerance, performance status of the patient, and the options of other systemic therapy.

4.8 Conclusion

ASCT has been established as the standard for aggressive salvage therapy in relapsed and refractory HL. ASCT has developed as a salvage modality with continuous improvement in outcome and toxicity profile. Many prognostic factors for risk stratification have been identified and allow the development of risk-stratified treatment approaches in the future. RT plays a crucial role in local control and relapse-free survival and should ideally be systematically included as an integral part of the salvage program.

References

Akpek G, Ambinder RF, Piantadosi S et al (2001) Long-term results of blood and marrow transplantation for Hodgkin's lymphoma. J Clin Oncol 19:4314–4321

Aleman BM, Raemaekers JM, Tirelli U et al (2003) Involved-field radiotherapy for advanced Hodgkin's lymphoma. N Engl J Med 348:2396–2406

André M, Henry-Amar M, Pico JL et al (1999) Comparison of high-dose therapy and autologous stem-cell transplantation with conventional therapy for Hodgkin's disease induction failure: a case-control study. Societe Francaise de Greffe de Moelle. J Clin Oncol 17:222–229

Argiris A, Seropian S, Cooper DL (2000) High-dose BEAM chemotherapy with autologous peripheral blood progenitor-cell transplantation for unselected patients with primary refractory or relapsed Hodgkin's disease. Ann Oncol 11:665–672

Bartlett NL, Niedzwiecki D, Johnson JL et al (2007) Gemcitabine, vinorelbine, and pegylated liposomal doxorubicin (GVD), a salvage regimen in relapsed Hodgkin's lymphoma: CALGB 59804. Ann Oncol 18:1071–1079

Bierman PJ, Lynch JC, Bociek RG et al (2002) The International Prognostic Factors Project score for advanced Hodgkin's disease is useful for predicting outcome of autologous hematopoietic stem cell transplantation. Ann Oncol 13:1370–1377

Bonadonna G, Bonfante V, Viviani S et al (2004) ABVD plus subtotal nodal versus involved-field radiotherapy in early-stage Hodgkin's disease: long-term results. J Clin Oncol 22:2835–2841

Brada M, Eeles R, Ashley S et al (1992) Salvage radiotherapy in recurrent Hodgkin's disease. Ann Oncol 3:131–135

Brincker H, Bentzen SM (1994) A re-analysis of available dose-response and time-dose data in Hodgkin's disease. Radiother Oncol 30:227–230

Campbell B, Wirth A, Milner A et al (2005) Long-term follow-up of salvage radiotherapy in Hodgkin's lymphoma after chemotherapy failure. Int J Radiat Oncol Biol Phys 63:1538–1545

Canellos GP, Anderson JR, Propert KJ et al (1992) Chemotherapy of advanced Hodgkin's disease with MOPP, ABVD, or MOPP alternating with ABVD. N Engl J Med 327:1478–1484

Canellos GP, Petroni GR, Barcos M et al (1995) Etoposide, vinblastine, and doxorubicin: an active regimen for the treatment of Hodgkin's disease in relapse following MOPP. Cancer and Leukemia Group B. J Clin Oncol 13:2005–2011

Carde P, Burgers JM, Henry-Amar M et al (1988) Clinical stages I and II Hodgkin's disease: a specifically tailored therapy according to prognostic factors. J Clin Oncol 6:239–252

Carella AM, Santini G, Santoro A et al (1985) Massive chemotherapy with non-frozen autologous bone marrow transplantation in 13 cases of refractory Hodgkin's disease. Eur J Cancer Clin Oncol 21:607–613

Castagna L, Bramanti S, Balzarotti M et al (2009) Predictive value of early 18F-fluorodeoxyglucose positron emission tomography (FDG-PET) during salvage chemotherapy in relapsing/refractory Hodgkin lymphoma (HL) treated with high-dose chemotherapy. Br J Haematol 145:369–372

Chopra R, McMillan AK, Linch DC et al (1993) The place of high-dose BEAM therapy and autologous bone marrow transplantation in poor-risk Hodgkin's disease. A single-center eight-year study of 155 patients. Blood 81:1137–1145

Connors JM, Klimo P, Adams G et al (1997) Treatment of advanced Hodgkin's disease with chemotherapy–comparison of MOPP/ABV hybrid regimen with alternating courses of MOPP and ABVD: a report from the National Cancer Institute of Canada clinical trials group. J Clin Oncol 15:1638–1645

Cooper MR, Pajak TF, Gottlieb AJ et al (1984) The effects of prior radiation therapy and age on the frequency and duration of complete remission among various four-drug treatments for advanced Hodgkin's disease. J Clin Oncol 2:748–755

Crump M (2008) Management of Hodgkin lymphoma in relapse after autologous stem cell transplant. In: Gewirtz AM, Muchmore EA, Burns LJ (eds) Hematology 2008. American Society of Hematology Education Program Book. American Society of Hematology, Washington

Dhakal S, Biswas T, Liesveld JL et al (2009) Patterns and timing of initial relapse in patients subsequently undergoing transplantation for Hodgkin's lymphoma. Int J Radiat Oncol Biol Phys 75:188–192

Diehl V, Franklin J, Hasenclever D et al (1998) BEACOPP, a new dose-escalated and accelerated regimen, is at least as effective as COPP/ABVD in patients with advanced-stage Hodgkin's lymphoma: interim report from a trial of the German Hodgkin's Lymphoma Study Group. J Clin Oncol 16:3810–3821

Duggan DB, Petroni GR, Johnson JL et al (2003) Randomized comparison of ABVD and MOPP/ABV hybrid for the treatment of advanced Hodgkin's disease: report of an intergroup trial. J Clin Oncol 21:607–614

Edwards-Bennett SM, Jacks LM, Moskowitz CH et al (2010) Stanford V program for locally extensive and advanced Hodgkin lymphoma: the Memorial Sloan-Kettering Cancer Center experience. Ann Oncol 21:574–581

Engert A, Franklin J, Eich HT et al (2007) Two cycles of doxorubicin, bleomycin, vinblastine, and dacarbazine plus extended-field radiotherapy is superior to radiotherapy alone in early favorable Hodgkin's lymphoma: final results of the GHSG HD7 trial. J Clin Oncol 25:3495–3502

Engert A, Diehl V, Franklin J et al (2009) Escalated-dose BEACOPP in the treatment of patients with advanced-stage Hodgkin's lymphoma: 10 years of follow-up of the GHSG HD9 study. J Clin Oncol 27:4548–4554

Evens AM, Altman JK, Mittal BB et al (2007) Phase I/II trial of total lymphoid irradiation and high-dose chemotherapy with autologous stem-cell transplantation for relapsed and refractory Hodgkin's lymphoma. Ann Oncol 18:679–688

Goodman KA, Riedel E, Serrano V et al (2008) Long-term effects of high-dose chemotherapy and radiation for relapsed and refractory Hodgkin's lymphoma. J Clin Oncol 26:5240–5247

Hasenclever D, Diehl V (1998) A prognostic score for advanced Hodgkin's disease. International Prognostic Factors Project on Advanced Hodgkin's Disease. N Engl J Med 339:1506–1514

Hoppe BS, Moskowitz CH, Filippa DA et al (2008a) Involved-field radiotherapy before high-dose therapy and autologous stem-cell rescue in diffuse large-cell lymphoma: long-term disease control and toxicity. J Clin Oncol 26:1858–1864

Hoppe RT, Advani RH, Ambinder RF et al (2008b) Hodgkin disease/lymphoma. J Natl Compr Canc Netw 6:594–622

Hoppe BS, Moskowitz CH, Zhang Z et al (2009) The role of FDG-PET imaging and involved field radiotherapy in relapsed or refractory diffuse large B-cell lymphoma. Bone Marrow Transplant 43:941–948

Horning SJ, Chao NJ, Negrin RS et al (1997) High-dose therapy and autologous hematopoietic progenitor cell transplantation for recurrent or refractory Hodgkin's disease: analysis of the Stanford University results and prognostic indices. Blood 89:801–813

Horwich A, Specht L, Ashley S (1997) Survival analysis of patients with clinical stages I or II Hodgkin's disease who have relapsed after initial treatment with radiotherapy alone. Eur J Cancer 33:848–853

Jabbour E, Hosing C, Ayers G et al (2007) Pretransplant positive positron emission tomography/gallium scans predict poor outcome in patients with recurrent/refractory Hodgkin lymphoma. Cancer 109:2481–2489

Jagannath S, Dicke KA, Armitage JO et al (1986) High-dose cyclophosphamide, carmustine, and etoposide and autologous bone marrow transplantation for relapsed Hodgkin's disease. Ann Intern Med 104:163–168

Josting A, Katay I, Rueffer U et al (1998) Favorable outcome of patients with relapsed or refractory Hodgkin's disease treated with high-dose chemotherapy and stem cell rescue at the time of maximal response to conventional salvage therapy (Dex-BEAM). Ann Oncol 9:289–295

Josting A, Rudolph C, Reiser M et al (2002) Time-intensified dexamethasone/cisplatin/cytarabine: an effective salvage therapy with low toxicity in patients with relapsed and refractory Hodgkin's disease. Ann Oncol 13:1628–1635

Josting A, Nogova L, Franklin J et al (2005a) Salvage radiotherapy in patients with relapsed and refractory Hodgkin's lymphoma: a retrospective analysis from the German Hodgkin Lymphoma Study Group. J Clin Oncol 23:1522–1529

Josting A, Rudolph C, Mapara M et al (2005b) Cologne high-dose sequential chemotherapy in relapsed and refractory Hodgkin lymphoma: results of a large multicenter study of the German Hodgkin Lymphoma Study Group (GHSG). Ann Oncol 16:116–123

Kewalramani T, Nimer SD, Zelenetz AD et al (2003) Progressive disease following autologous transplantation in patients with chemosensitive relapsed or primary refractory Hodgkin's disease or aggressive non-Hodgkin's lymphoma. Bone Marrow Transplant 32:673–679

Kuruvilla J, Nagy T, Pintilie M et al (2006) Similar response rates and superior early progression-free survival with gemcitabine, dexamethasone, and cisplatin salvage therapy compared with carmustine, etoposide, cytarabine, and melphalan salvage therapy prior to autologous stem cell transplantation for recurrent or refractory Hodgkin lymphoma. Cancer 106:353–360

Leigh BR, Fox KA, Mack CF et al (1993) Radiation therapy salvage of Hodgkin's disease following chemotherapy failure. Int J Radiat Oncol Biol Phys 27:855–862

Linch DC, Winfield D, Goldstone AH et al (1993) Dose intensification with autologous bone-marrow transplantation in relapsed and resistant Hodgkin's disease: results of a BNLI randomised trial. Lancet 341:1051–1054

Lohri A, Barnett M, Fairey RN et al (1991) Outcome of treatment of first relapse of Hodgkin's disease after primary chemotherapy: identification of risk factors from the British Columbia experience 1970 to 1988. Blood 77:2292–2298

Longo DL, Duffey PL, Young RC et al (1992) Conventional-dose salvage combination chemotherapy in patients relapsing with Hodgkin's disease after combination chemotherapy: the low probability for cure. J Clin Oncol 10:210–218

Macdonald DA, Ding K, Gospodarowicz MK et al (2007) Patterns of disease progression and outcomes in a randomized trial testing ABVD alone for patients with limited-stage Hodgkin lymphoma. Ann Oncol 18:1680–1684

Majhail NS, Weisdorf DJ, Defor TE et al (2006) Long-term results of autologous stem cell transplantation for primary refractory or relapsed Hodgkin's lymphoma. Biol Blood Marrow Transplant 12:1065–1072

Majolino I, Pearce R, Taghipour G et al (1997) Peripheral-blood stem-cell transplantation versus autologous bone marrow transplantation in Hodgkin's and non-Hodgkin's lymphomas: a new matched-pair analysis of the European Group for Blood and Marrow Transplantation Registry Data. Lymphoma Working Party of the European Group for Blood and Marrow Transplantation. J Clin Oncol 15:509–517

Martin A, Fernández-Jiménez MC, Caballero MD et al (2001) Long-term follow-up in patients treated with Mini-BEAM as salvage therapy for relapsed or refractory Hodgkin's disease. Br J Haematol 113:161–171

Meyer RM, Gospodarowicz MK, Connors JM et al (2005) Randomized comparison of ABVD chemotherapy with a strategy that includes radiation therapy in patients with limited-stage Hodgkin's lymphoma: National Cancer Institute of Canada Clinical Trials Group and the Eastern Cooperative Oncology Group. J Clin Oncol 23:4634–4642

Milpied N, Fielding AK, Pearce RM et al (1996) Allogeneic bone marrow transplant is not better than autologous transplant for patients with relapsed Hodgkin's disease. European Group for Blood and Bone Marrow Transplantation. J Clin Oncol 14:1291–1296

Moskowitz C (2002) Risk-adapted therapy for relapsed and refractory lymphoma using ICE chemotherapy. Cancer Chemother Pharmacol 49(Suppl 1):S9–S12

Moskowitz CH, Nimer SD, Zelenetz AD et al (2001) A 2-step comprehensive high-dose chemoradiotherapy second-line program for relapsed and refractory Hodgkin disease: analysis by intent to treat and development of a prognostic model. Blood 97:616–623

Moskowitz CH, Kewalramani T, Nimer SD et al (2004) Effectiveness of high dose chemoradiotherapy and autologous stem cell transplantation for patients with biopsy-proven primary refractory Hodgkin's disease. Br J Haematol 124:645–652

Moskowitz AJ, Perales MA, Kewalramani T et al (2009) Outcomes for patients who fail high dose chemoradiotherapy and autologous stem cell rescue for relapsed and primary refractory Hodgkin lymphoma. Br J Haematol 146:158–163

Moskowitz CH, Yahalom J, Zelenetz AD et al (2010) High-dose chemo-radiotherapy for relapsed or refractory Hodgkin lymphoma and the significance of pre-transplant functional imaging. Br J Haematol 148:890–897

Mundt AJ, Sibley G, Williams S et al (1995) Patterns of failure following high-dose chemotherapy and autologous bone marrow transplantation with involved field radiotherapy for relapsed/refractory Hodgkin's disease. Int J Radiat Oncol Biol Phys 33:261–270

Mundt AJ, Connell PP, Mansur DB (1999) What is the optimal treatment volume in Hodgkin's disease patients undergoing high-dose chemotherapy and adjuvant radiation therapy? Radiat Oncol Investig 7:353–359

Ng AK, Li S, Neuberg D et al (2004) Comparison of MOPP versus ABVD as salvage therapy in patients who relapse after radiation therapy alone for Hodgkin's disease. Ann Oncol 15:270–275

Olver IN, Wolf MM, Cruickshank D et al (1988) Nitrogen mustard, vincristine, procarbazine, and prednisolone for relapse after radiation in Hodgkin's disease. An analysis of long-term follow-up. Cancer 62:233–239

Pezner RD, Lipsett JA, Vora N et al (1994) Radical radiotherapy as salvage treatment for relapse of Hodgkin's disease initially treated by chemotherapy alone: prognostic significance of the disease-free interval. Int J Radiat Oncol Biol Phys 30:965–970

Philip T, Dumont J, Teillet F et al (1986) High dose chemotherapy and autologous bone marrow transplantation in refractory Hodgkin's disease. Br J Cancer 53:737–742

Poen JC, Hoppe RT, Horning SJ (1996) High-dose therapy and autologous bone marrow transplantation for relapsed/refractory Hodgkin's disease: the impact of involved field radiotherapy on patterns of failure and survival. Int J Radiat Oncol Biol Phys 36:3–12

Rapoport AP, Guo C, Badros A et al (2004) Autologous stem cell transplantation followed by consolidation chemotherapy for relapsed or refractory Hodgkin's lymphoma. Bone Marrow Transplant 34:883–890

Reece DE, Connors JM, Spinelli JJ et al (1994) Intensive therapy with cyclophosphamide, carmustine, etoposide +/- cisplatin, and autologous bone marrow transplantation for Hodgkin's disease in first relapse after combination chemotherapy. Blood 83:1193–1199

Roach M III, Brophy N, Cox R et al (1990) Prognostic factors for patients relapsing after radiotherapy for early-stage Hodgkin's disease. J Clin Oncol 8:623–629

Rüffer JU, Ballova V, Glossmann J et al (2005) BEACOPP and COPP/ABVD as salvage treatment after primary extended field radiation therapy of early stage Hodgkins disease – results of the German Hodgkin Study Group. Leuk Lymphoma 46:1561–1567

Santoro A, Viviani S, Villarreal CJ et al (1986) Salvage chemotherapy in Hodgkin's disease irradiation failures: superiority of doxorubicin-containing regimens over MOPP. Cancer Treat Rep 70:343–348

Schmitz N, Linch DC, Dreger P et al (1996) Randomised trial of filgrastim-mobilised peripheral blood progenitor cell transplantation versus autologous bone-marrow transplantation in lymphoma patients. Lancet 347:353–357

Schmitz N, Pfistner B, Sextro M et al (2002) Aggressive conventional chemotherapy compared with high-dose chemotherapy with autologous haemopoietic stem-cell transplantation for relapsed chemosensitive Hodgkin's disease: a randomised trial. Lancet 359:2065–2071

Schmitz N, Haverkamp H, Josting A et al (2005) Long term follow up in relapsed Hodgkin's disease (HD): updated results of the HD-R1 study comparing conventional chemotherapy (cCT) to high-dose chemotherapy (HDCT) with autologous haemopoetic stem cell transplantation (ASCT) of the German Hodgkin Study Group (GHSG) and the Working Party Lymphoma of the European Group for Blood and Marrow Transplantation (EBMT). J Clin Oncol 23 (Suppl. 16):6508

Shahidi M, Kamangari N, Ashley S et al (2006) Site of relapse after chemotherapy alone for stage I and II Hodgkin's disease. Radiother Oncol 78:1–5

Specht L, Horwich A, Ashley S (1994) Salvage of relapse of patients with Hodgkin's disease in clinical stages I or II who were staged with laparotomy and initially treated with radiotherapy alone. A report from the international database on Hodgkin's disease. Int J Radiat Oncol Biol Phys 30:805–811

Sureda A, Arranz R, Iriondo A et al (2001) Autologous stem-cell transplantation for Hodgkin's disease: results and prognostic factors in 494 patients from the Grupo Espanol de Linfomas/Transplante Autologo de Medula Osea Spanish Cooperative Group. J Clin Oncol 19:1395–1404

Sureda A, Robinson S, Canals C et al (2008) Reduced-intensity conditioning compared with conventional allogeneic stem-cell transplantation in relapsed or refractory Hodgkin's lymphoma: an analysis from the Lymphoma Working Party of the European Group for Blood and Marrow Transplantation. J Clin Oncol 26:455–462

Svoboda J, Andreadis C, Elstrom R et al (2006) Prognostic value of FDG-PET scan imaging in lymphoma patients undergoing autologous stem cell transplantation. Bone Marrow Transplant 38:211–216

Tsang RW, Gospodarowicz MK, Sutcliffe SB et al (1999) Thoracic radiation therapy before autologous bone marrow transplantation in relapsed or refractory Hodgkin's disease. PMH Lymphoma Group, and the Toronto Autologous BMT Group. Eur J Cancer 35:73–78

Tsang RW, Goda J., Massey C et al (2009) Hodgkin-lymphoma with relapsed or progressive disease after autologous stem cell transplantation: efficacy of salvage radiation therapy. Int J Radiat Oncol Biol Phys 75(Suppl): S64

Uematsu M, Tarbell NJ, Silver B et al (1993) Wide-field radiation therapy with or without chemotherapy for patients with Hodgkin disease in relapse after initial combination chemotherapy. Cancer 72:207–212

Vijayakumar S, Myrianthopoulos LC (1992) An updated dose-response analysis in Hodgkin's disease. Radiother Oncol 24:1–13

Vinciguerra V, Propert KJ, Coleman M et al (1986) Alternating cycles of combination chemotherapy for patients with recurrent Hodgkin's disease following radiotherapy. A prospectively randomized study by the Cancer and Leukemia Group B. J Clin Oncol 4:838–846

Wheeler C, Eickhoff C, Elias A et al (1997) High-dose cyclophosphamide, carmustine, and etoposide with autologous transplantation in Hodgkin's disease: a prognostic model for treatment outcomes. Biol Blood Marrow Transplant 3:98–106

Wirth A, Corry J, Laidlaw C et al (1997) Salvage radiotherapy for Hodgkin's disease following chemotherapy failure. Int J Radiat Oncol Biol Phys 39:599–607

Yahalom J (1995) Integrating radiotherapy into bone marrow transplantation programs for Hodgkin's disease. Int J Radiat Oncol Biol Phys 33:525–528

Yahalom J (1996) Management of relapsed and refractory Hodgkin's disease. Semin Radiat Oncol 6:210–224

Yahalom J (2009) Role of radiation therapy in Hodgkin's lymphoma. Cancer J 15:155–160

Yahalom J, Gulati S, Shank B et al (1989) Total lymphoid irradiation, high-dose chemotherapy and autologous bone marrow transplantation for chemotherapy-resistant Hodgkin's disease. Int J Radiat Oncol Biol Phys 17:915–922

Yahalom J, Gulati SC, Toia M et al (1993) Accelerated hyperfractionated total-lymphoid irradiation, high-dose chemotherapy, and autologous bone marrow transplantation for refractory and relapsing patients with Hodgkin's disease. J Clin Oncol 11:1062–1070

Yuen AR, Rosenberg SA, Hoppe RT et al (1997) Comparison between conventional salvage therapy and high-dose therapy with autografting for recurrent or refractory Hodgkin's disease. Blood 89:814–822

Principles of Chemotherapy in Hodgkin Lymphoma

5

Anu Batra and Carol S. Portlock

Contents

A. Batra (✉)
New York Medical College (Sound Shore), New Rochelle, New York, USA

C.S. Portlock
Memorial Sloan-Kettering Cancer Centre, 1275 York Ave, Mail Box 546, New York, NY 10021-6007, USA
e-mail: portlocc@mskcc.org

5.1 Introduction

Significant advances have been made in the chemotherapy regimens for Hodgkin Lymphoma (HL) over the last 40 years. New treatment concepts and drug combinations have continued to increase the cure rate and acute side effects have been reduced. HL was one of the first malignancies for which chemotherapy was investigated and was successful. It is interesting to know the timeline of events as they happened and evolved into the standard treatments we know today (Diehl 2007). Thomas Hodgkin first described HL in his 1832 paper, entitled "On Some Morbid Appearances of the Absorbent Glands and Spleen." Osler's textbook of medicine was the first publication to mention chemotherapy for lymphoma, in 1894; Fowler's solution, an arsenic-containing medicinal, was recognized to have some activity against HL. In World War II, an explosion in Bari, Italy, exposed servicemen to the toxic effects of mustard gases. Follow-up on their bone marrow revealed marrow and lymphatic suppression.

In 1947, Albert and Petersen first published the results of significant shrinkage in the size of tumor masses with nitrogen mustard in patients with HL and lymphosarcoma; and it was the development of the nitrogen mustard-containing mechlorethamine, vincristine, procarbazine, and prednisone (MOPP) combination by DeVita et al. that led to the reproducible curability of advanced HL in the 1960s (DeVita, Jr. et al. 1970).

At present, more than 80% of patients with newly diagnosed classical HL (cHL) are expected to be long-term survivors. Combination chemotherapy is now the preferred modality of treatment, often combined with involved-field irradiation. In nodular-lymphocyte-predominant HL, radiotherapy remains the mainstay of treatment, while chemotherapy is generally reserved

L. Specht and J. Yahalom (eds.), *Radiotherapy for Hodgkin Lymphoma*,
DOI: 10.1007/978-3-540-78944-4_5, © Springer-Verlag Berlin Heidelberg 2011

for systemic relapse (Schlembach et al. 2002). Rituximab is a new monoclonal antibody that is being explored in all subtypes of HL and this will be briefly reviewed below. We will now discuss the various standard combination chemotherapy regimens and their side-effect profiles.

5.2 Common Chemotherapy Regimens in Classical Hodgkin Lymphoma

5.2.1 *MOPP Chemotherapy*

In advanced HL, De Vita et al. first reported the results of MOPP in 1967. Long-term follow-up of these 188 patients, published in 1980, revealed a complete remission rate of 84% and an estimated overall survival of 50% at 10 years (Longo et al. 1986).

MOPP is an acronym for four drugs, mechlorethamine, vincristine, procarbazine, and prednisone. Each drug is given in full dose as per the following schedule.

Mechlorethamine	6 mg/m^2	Day 1 and 8
Vincristine	1.4 mg/m^2	Day 1 and 8 (now capped at 2 mg)
Procarbazine	100 mg/m^2	Days 1–14
Prednisone	40 mg/m^2	Days 1–14

The cycle is repeated every 28 days and prednisone is administered on cycles 1 and 4 only. Patients are treated with two additional monthly cycles after clinical complete remission is achieved. All patients received at least 6 monthly cycles unless they had lymphoma progression.

5.2.1.1 Side-Effect Profile

MOPP therapy was associated with both acute and long-term toxicity. The major acute side effects included, but were not limited to, nausea, vomiting, bone-marrow suppression, alopecia, fatigue, or allergic reactions (more frequently associated with procarbazine).

Even though nausea and vomiting are often listed as the most common side effects of all chemotherapy regimens, they are no longer dose limiting in the modern era, as they were with MOPP in 1967 (Hesketh 2008). Neurotoxicity is associated with vincristine, including peripheral neuropathy, autonomic neuropathy, and muscular weakness in the hands and feet if the drug is not discontinued. For this reason, vincristine is capped at 2 mg per dose and is monitored closely; doses are reduced for symptoms and discontinued for any muscle weakness or significant numbness/paresthesias. Constipation is also a common problem and daily bowel movements are essential. Obstipation can be profound, if dosing is not adjusted as needed, and vincristine should be discontinued in the setting of adynamic ileus. Foods with high amounts of tyramine should be avoided as they can exacerbate the monoamine oxidase inhibitory effect of procarbazine. Moreover, drug interactions are numerous and should be carefully evaluated prior to treatment. The most common toxicity of this interaction is an Antabuse (disulfiram)-type reaction with alcohol, and this must be carefully avoided. Prednisone side effects include susceptibility to infection, gastrointestinal distress, diabetes, and sleeplessness/personality changes.

5.2.1.2 Long-Term Side Effects of MOPP

Infertility in females: In a cohort study by De Bruin et al., the risk of premature menopause with chemotherapy was 12.3-fold higher than with radiotherapy as observed in a 9.4-year follow-up cohort. Strongest associations were observed with alkylating agents like procarbazine and cyclophosphamide, which appeared to be dose related (De Bruin et al. 2008). MOPP is associated with at least a 50% rate of primary ovarian failure and is age-related and cumulative-dose-related. In the modern era, protection of ovarian function can be attempted with gonadotropin-releasing hormone agonists, although the effectiveness has not yet been proven (Falorio et al. 2008; van der Kaaij et al. 2010).

The majority of male survivors of HL receiving MOPP develop azoospermia or severe oligospermia (van der Kaaij et al. 2007). Recovery is less frequent and slower with the use of alkylating-agent chemotherapy. Fertility can be secured after nonalkylating chemotherapy for HL, such as adriamycin (doxorubicin), bleomycin, vinblastine, and dacarbazine (ABVD; see below) (van der Kaaij et al. 2007). Hence all men should be counseled on sperm banking prior to chemotherapy.

Another significant long-term side effect of MOPP therapy was the development of myelodysplastic syndrome or acute leukemia with a maximum risk between 3–5 years following treatment (Pedersen-Bjergaard et al. 1987).

Due to the significant acute side effects associated with MOPP, a number of attempts were made to modify it, including MVPP (vinblastine substituted for vincristine in MOPP) or B-CVPP (bleomycin and cyclophosphamide substitution for nitrogen mustard in MOPP). However, these regimens failed to increase the overall disease-free survival over MOPP. As discussed below, MOPP has been abandoned for other regimens with fewer acute and late side effects.

5.2.2 ABVD

ABVD was first developed by Bonadonna et al. in the 1970s (Bonadonna et al. 1975). Every drug in this combination was non-cross resistant with the drugs constituting MOPP. Initially it was used in MOPP failures; however, it is now the standard chemotherapy for patients with cHL.

This regimen consists of adriamycin (doxorubicin), bleomycin, vinblastine, and dacarbazine given every 2 weeks as per the following schedule.

Doxorubicin	25 mg/m^2	Days 1 and 15
Bleomycin	10 units/m^2	Days 1 and 15
Vinblastine	6 mg/m^2	Days 1 and 15
Dacarbazine	375 mg/m^2	Days 1 and 15

The cycle is repeated every 28 days; thus, one cycle contains two treatments.

Prior to chemotherapy, a compete blood count along with kidney and liver function should be obtained. A baseline electrocardiogram (EKG) and echocardiogram or multiple gated acquisition (MUGA) scan should be obtained before treatment, as doxorubicin is known to be potentially cardiotoxic. Similarly, chest X-ray or computed tomography (CT) chest and pulmonary function tests (including diffusing capacity of the lung for carbon monoxide [DLCO]) must be used to assess the lungs prior to the use of bleomycin.

ABVD alone can cure many patients with cHL Unlike MOPP, it has acceptable acute toxicity in the modern era, and few late side effects (infertility and second malignancies are uncommon) if used carefully.

Results from a prospective, randomized trial by The Cancer and Leukemia Group B (CALGB) comparing MOPP with ABVD or MOPP alternating with ABVD suggested that ABVD therapy for 6–8 months was as effective as 12 months of MOPP alternating with ABVD, and both were superior to MOPP alone in the treatment of advanced Hodgkin's disease. ABVD was less myelotoxic than MOPP or ABVD alternating with MOPP (Canellos et al. 1992).

5.2.2.1 Side-Effect Profile

Potential acute side effects include fatigue, nausea, vomiting, mild alopecia, and myelosuppresion. Tingling and numbness in fingers and toes are common after several treatments and disappear after vinblastine is stopped at the end of all chemotherapy (it is very rare that this drug needs to be discontinued for neuropathic complaints). Constipation and ileus are modest side effects caused by vinblastine, unlike vincristine. Stool softeners are usually needed to maintain regular bowel movements. Itching and red rash at the injection site may occur secondary to doxorubicin, bleomycin, and vinblastine. Doxorubicin and vinblastine are vesicants and extreme care is needed with intravenous administration. Patients should be informed to protect the skin from overexposure to the sun and use a sunscreen with a sun protection factor (SPF) of 15 or greater. Tanning and thickening of skin along with darkening of nails may occur due to bleomycin. These skin changes are slowly reversible after therapy. Potential cardiac toxicity is possible with doxorubicin, but the cumulative dose of 300 mg/m^2 with six cycles is well below concern in the majority. Bleomycin may cause pulmonary toxicity manifested by chest tightness, dry/non-productive cough, chest discomfort, shortness of breath, and change in pulmonary function tests. One must be alert to these symptoms and findings, as the resultant pulmonary toxicity and fibrosis may not be reversible. If these symptoms are detected early, the drug is discontinued and the patient can be successfully treated with steroids with a slow taper. It is generally wise to repeat the pulmonary function tests following four cycles of ABVD, or sooner if patients become symptomatic. There is a small but growing literature that suggests that growth factor support using granulocyte colony-stimulating factor (G-CSF) may contribute to this toxicity, but this is not fully established. Pulmonary toxicity may also be more problematic in those patients receiving ABVD following mediastinal radiotherapy (which is rarely done currently). ABVD may also be associated with a rare anaphylactoid reaction with the initial dose. Test doses are no longer employed, as these are not predictive. Fatal complications may occur with the acute reaction as well as with the cumulative toxicity. Unfortunately, stopping bleomycin may not alter a fatality and this toxicity is the greatest potential hazard of the regimen.

ABVD is associated with a lower long-term risk of infertility in men and amenorrhea/ovarian failure in women. In one study, the incidence of azoospermia occurred in 36% of patients with ABVD versus 97% in MOPP. Recovery of spermatogenesis is higher in patients with ABVD compared with MOPP (van der Kaaij et al. 2007).

Second malignancies associated with ABVD alone are rare (Valagussa et al. 1986).

5.2.3 BEACOPP

BEACOPP is a more recent chemotherapy regimen for poor risk cHL. In BEACOPP, the total chemotherapy dose is increased with the addition of etoposide and administration of chemotherapy every 21 days instead of 28 days.

Etoposide alone has been reported to have a 20–60% response rate in refractory HL.

The German Hodgkin's Lymphoma study group (GHSG) developed the BEACOPP regimen based upon mathematical modeling. Patients typically receive treatment in cycles of 21 days with no chemotherapy drugs given on days 16–21. Treatment consists of six to eight cycles. In Germany and Austria it has become standard therapy. BEACOPP appears to result in a higher cure rate in advanced HL (Diehl et al. 1997). BEACOPP is more expensive as it requires G-CSF support. This regimen has not been adopted in the USA, as there is no prospective trial directly comparing its use with ABVD alone, the US standard regimen, and as discussed below it is associated with secondary myelodysplasia (MDS)/AML.

BEACOPP is given per the following schedule.

Cyclophosphamide	650 mg/m²	IV	Day 1
Adriamycin	25 mg/m²	IV	Day 1
Etoposide	100 mg/m²	IV	Days 1–3
Vincristine	1.4 mg/m² (max 2 mg)	IV	Day 8
Bleomycin	10 mg/m²	IV	Day 8
Procarbazine	100 mg/m²	orally	Day 1–14
Prednisone	40 mg/m²	orally	Day 1–14

BEACOPP escalated is given according to the following schedule.

Cyclophosphamide	1,250 mg/m²/day	IV	Day 1
Adriamycin	35 mg/m²	IV	Day 1
Etoposide	200 mg/m²	IV	Days 1–3
Vincristine	1.4 mg/m² (max 2 mg)	IV	Day 8
Bleomycin	10 mg/m²	IV	Day 8
Procarbazine	100 mg/m²	Orally	Day 1–7
Prednisone	40 mg/m²	Orally	Day 1–14

In escalated BEACOPP, the doses of cyclophosphamide, etoposide, and doxorubicin are increased and require the use of G-CSF or pegfilgrastim on day 8.

In a study (HD 9) trial by GHSG conducted from 1993 to 1998, 1,201 patients with newly diagnosed cHL in unfavorable stages IIB, III, or IV were randomly assigned to receive eight cycles of COPP-ABVD, or BEACOPP, or escalated BEACOPP each followed by radiotherapy for disease more than 5 cm in diameter at the time of diagnosis or for residual disease after eight cycles of chemotherapy (Diehl et al. 2003).

Of the 1,195 patients finally evaluated, increased-dose BEACOPP was associated with a lower incidence of induction failure (2% versus 8% and 10%). Rate of freedom from treatment failure at 5 years was 69% in the COPP-ABVD group, 76% in the BEACOPP group, and 87% in the escalated BEACOPP group, and the 5-year overall survival rates were 83%, 88%, and 91%, respectively (with a statistically significant difference only between escalated BEACOPP and COPP-ABVD). Seventy-one percent of patients in the two BEACOPP groups received radiotherapy compared with 64% of patients in the COPP-ABVD group. Escalated BEACOPP is more expensive than COPP-ABVD.

Like ABVD, before BEACOPP chemotherapy is started, a complete blood count as well as kidney and liver function should be done. An EKG and echocardiogram or MUGA, chest X-ray, and pulmonary function tests should be obtained prior to initiating chemotherapy. Growth factors (G-CSF or Neupogen [filgrastim]) are routinely required with BEACOPP

5.2.3.1 Acute Side Effects

A decrease in blood counts is very common. Grade 4 leukopenia and anemia are more common with BEACOPP, especially escalated BEACOPP. Thrombocytopenia is also seen, but it is less severe. Other side effects are those of the individual drugs as described above for MOPP and ABVD. Cyclophosphamide is used rather than nitrogen mustard. Its side effects are similar, with less nausea and vomiting. Cyclophosphamide may occasionally cause hemorrhagic cystitis.

Like MOPP, long-term side effects of BEACOPP include infertility and second neoplasms including MDS and acute myeloid leukemia (AML). The overall rates of second malignancy were 6.8%, 8.9%, and 6.7% of patients treated with escalated BEACOPP, baseline BEACOPP, and COPD-ABVD, respectively, in the study mentioned above.

Dysspermia is another significant side effect of BEACOPP, though there is no significant difference between BEACOPP and escalated BEACOPP. Sperm banking should be offered to all males prior to chemotherapy and all childbearing females who have not completed families should be placed on oral contraceptive pills and/or gonadotropin-releasing hormone agonist in an effort to preserve fertility during chemotherapy.

Recently BEACOPP has been further modified to BEACOPP-14, in which treatment is given over 14 days with G-CSF (Sieber et al. 2003). Escalated BEACOPP is associated with an increased risk of secondary malignancies; therefore, the risk-benefit ratio is poor. A risk-adapted approach to treatment intensity has been formulated, and this is expected to reduce this late effect.

5.2.4 Stanford V

Like BEACOPP, Stanford V is a combined modality regimen used in the treatment of advanced cHL. Stanford V chemotherapy involves delivering a 3-month weekly drug schedule, followed by involved-field radiation therapy in patients with bulky stage II, as well as advanced stage III and IV disease.

It consists of seven drugs, alternating myelosuppressive medications with non-myelosuppressive ones, according to the following schedule.

Doxorubicin	25 mg/m^2	IV	Days 1 and 15
Mechlorethamine	6 mg/m^2	IV	Day 1
Vinblastine	6 mg/m^2	IV	Days 1 and 15
Bleomycin	5 units/m^2	IV	Day 8 and 22
Vincristine	1.4 mg/m^2	IV	Day 8 and 22 (cap 2 mg)
Etoposide	60 mg/m^2	IV	Day 15
Etoposide	120 mg/m^2	IV	Day 16
Prednisone	40 mg/m^2	Orally	Every other day, start taper at week 10

Stanford V cycles are repeated every 28 days for three cycles.

The potential side-effect profile of the drugs in Stanford V have been described above. Etoposide may cause nausea, vomiting, facial flushing, loss of appetite, and myelosuppression. Rarely, etoposide may cause acute leukemia. Unlike BEACOPP, Stanford V does not contain procarbazine, and this means that infertility and second neoplasms are potentially less prevalent with this regimen. Nevertheless, as a combined modality regimen, Stanford V may have late second neoplasms related to the involved-field radiotherapy, as does BEACOPP. The doses of bleomycin and doxorubicin are lower than that in ABVD or escalated BEACOPP (5 units/m^2 rather than 10 per dose; 150 mg/m^2 per course rather than 300 mg/m^2 for ABVD and 210 mg/m^2 for escalated BEACOPP) and, as expected, pulmonary and cardiac toxicities are therefore less of a concern.

Stanford V has been found to be a highly efficacious regimen in advanced cHL and to have a good side-effect profile. A prospective comparison of Stanford V and ABVD is completed and mature results are awaited. Late effects of Stanford V appear to be better than BEACOPP, with somewhat greater infertility risk than ABVD, but no major secondary malignancy risk to date (Horning et al. 2002).

5.2.5 Rituximab

Rituximab is a monoclonal antibody against the CD20 antigen on B cells, and is FDA approved for the treatment of B-cell non-HL. Rituximab is now used in the relapse treatment of nodular-lymphocyte-predominant HL (nLPHL) (Nogova et al. 2006) and is being investigated in combination with ABVD for cHL. It is given in a dose of 375 mg/m^2 IV once a week for 4–8 weeks, depending upon the clinical circumstance; maintenance therapy may also be administered (four doses once every 6 months or one dose every 3 months; duration is generally 2 years).

The side-effect profile for Rituximab includes acute infusion reactions (usually occurring during the infusion) such as mild muscle aches, joint aches, chills, low-grade fever, mild skin rash, and mild headache. Severe reactions such as angioedema, hypotension, cardiac arrhythmias, and wheezing/shortness of breath warrant discontinuation of treatment. Intravenous steroids may be utilized in pretreatment or as needed to reduce side effects, and the infusion can sometimes be reinstituted successfully. All patients are pretreated with Tylenol and Benadryl.

Since rituximab is known to cause hypotension, patients may be advised not to take antihypertensive medications 12 h prior to treatment.

Liver-function tests should be monitored in patients who receive Rituximab and hepatitis serologies should be obtained in all patients prior to therapy.

Patients with serologic evidence of prior or current Hepatitis B may experience reactivation of the virus and this may become a life-threatening complication.

The risk of reactivation is present for up to 1 year after treatment. Therefore, this drug is not recommended for those with measurable virus prior to treatment. All others should be considered for antiviral suppression. Routine blood counts and renal function tests should also be done on a regular basis as needed.

Rare side effects of Rituximab include progressive multifocal leukoencephalopathy, allergic mucocutaneous reactions, and bowel perforation.

5.2.6 Bendamustine

Bendamustine is a bifunctional mechlorethamine derivative containing a benzimidazole ring that forms DNA cross links leading to cell apoptosis and also prevents replication of cells. It was first approved by the FDA in March 2008 for the treatment of chronic lymphocytic leukemia. In October 2008, the FDA extended the approval to indolent B-cell non-HL refractory to rituximab.

There is limited data on the efficacy of bendamustine in HL. A small phase II study in heavily pretreated, relapsed, and refractory Hodgkin lymphoma, following autologous or non-myeloablative allogeneic stem-cell transplant failures or patients not candidates for transplant, revealed 12 of 16 patients with objective response, six with complete responses, six with partial responses, and one with stable disease (Moskowitz et al. 2009).

The side-effect profile of bendamustine includes nausea, vomiting, fatigue, fever, and, rarely, infusion reactions and anaphylaxis. Premedication with antipyretics and corticosteroids may be needed in patients with mild previous infusion reactions. Hematological toxicities include neutropenia, anemia, and thrombocytopenia. Patients with myelosuppresion are more prone to infections, particularly pneumonia. Skin reactions vary from a rash to bullous exanthema, which may require discontinuation of the drug. Bendamustine is not recommended for patients with moderate to severe hepatic impairment or renal impairment (glomerular filtration rat less than 40).

5.2.7 SGN-35

SGN-35 is an antibody-drug conjugate of monomethyl auristatin E and anti CD30 monoclonal antibody that interferes with the growth of CD30-positive tumors, particularly HL and anaplastic large-cell lymphoma. The antibody-drug conjugate is internalized into the target cells and leads to the release of monomethyl auristatin E, a potent antimitotic drug, into the cytoplasm, which eventually induces G2/M-phase growth arrest and cell death.

In a phase I trial by Younis et al., 45 patients with refractory or recurrent CD30-positive hematologic malignancies, including HL ($n = 42$), systemic anaplastic large-cell lymphoma ($n = 2$), and angioimmunoblastic

T-cell lymphoma ($n = 1$) were treated with SGN-35 ranging from 0.1 to 3.6 mg/kg every 3 weeks. There were 23% complete regressions and 45% complete and partial regressions among evaluable patients. The most common side effects reported to date for SGN-35 include peripheral neuropathy, fatigue, nausea, diarrhea, dizziness, pyrexia, and neutropenia (Fanale et al. 2009; Younes et al. 2008).

5.3 Late Side Effects of Chemotherapy

Patients who are free of cHL for 5 years post-therapy are considered cured. The late side effects of chemotherapy include development of malignancies and cardiac and/or pulmonary toxicity. There are three main types of late malignancies associated with classic HL therapy: MDS and acute leukemia, non-HL, and second solid tumors. The risk of the kind of late complication depends on the type of prior treatment.

5.3.1 Myelodysplasia and Acute Myeloid Leukemia

The relative risk of AML in patients treated for HL is 0–80-fold higher than in the general population. Alkylating agents are associated with the development of these secondary leukemias. ABVD has almost no risk for leukemia while maintaining its therapeutic effectiveness; thus, it has been adopted over MOPP-type regimens. Increasing the number of MOPP cycles was associated with a higher risk of AML. Substituting/omitting mechlorethamine in MOPP lowered the risk of AML substantially. Standard BEACOPP is associated with a lower risk of AML compared with escalated BEACOPP (2.5%). BEACOPP contains the alkylating agents cyclophosphamide and procarbazine, as well as etoposide. These three agents are all associated with MDS/AML risk. Likewise, Stanford V has a lower risk of MDS/AML when utilizing only three doses of nitrogen mustard during the 3-month regimen. It also contains etoposide; so, it is not free of this potential late hazard.

Development of MDS/AML after HL is associated with an extremely poor prognosis, and is considered to be almost always fatal. The GHSG reported no benefit of stem-cell transplantation in such patients.

5.3.2 Non-Hodgkin Lymphoma

The relative risk of NHL compared with the general population ranges between 6% and 36%. The risk is higher in patients treated with combined modality versus radiation alone, suggesting an important role for chemotherapy induction. Intermediate or aggressive B-cell lymphomas are the most common subtypes found in patients with a second NHL. Some authors suggest that transformation to NHL might be a part of the natural history of cHL as it is in nLPHL (Bennett et al. 1991; Rueffer et al. 2001).

5.3.3 Solid Tumors

The late development of solid tumors in patients with HL treated with chemotherapy include lung cancer, breast cancer, and gastrointestinal cancer. Smokers with HL receiving radiotherapy and/or chemotherapy are at a higher risk of developing lung cancer compared with nonsmokers (Travis et al. 2002). Thus, patients should be advised to avoid smoking. The cost-effectiveness and survival advantage of screening such patients with chest X-ray or CT scan remain to be investigated. Also, the relationship of newer chemotherapy regimens (including ABVD) with the development of solid tumors needs to be further investigated. In general, ABVD alone is not associated with an increased risk of solid tumors.

Exposure to radiation in young women (age less than 35 years) increases the risk of breast cancer. Thus, women who have been treated with radiation should undergo annual breast physical exams and breast imaging starting 8–10 years after radiation or at the age of 40. Due to the increased density of breast tissue in young females, breast MRI is thought to be more sensitive and hence considered as a better screening tool for such patients.

5.4 Follow-Up

Follow-up of patients with HL includes physical examination along with routine lab studies including complete blood count, liver and renal function, and imaging (usually CXR alternating with CT of the torso) every

3–4 months for the first 2 years and biannually until 5 years. Annual thyroid function tests should be performed in patients who have received prior radiation to the neck and mediastinum.

Annual visits should include careful health maintenance follow-up including mammogram, Pap smear, colonoscopy, prostate monitoring, and skin screening. All patients should get annual flu shots. Patients who undergo splenectomy or receive involved-field radiotherapy to the spleen should get pneumococcal vaccine every 5 years.

References

Bennett MH, MacLennan KA, Vaughan HG et al (1991) Non-Hodgkin's lymphoma arising in patients treated for Hodgkin's disease in the BNLI: a 20-year experience. British National Lymphoma Investigation. Ann Oncol 2(Suppl 2):83–92

Bonadonna G, Zucali R, Monfardini S et al (1975) Combination chemotherapy of Hodgkin's disease with adriamycin, bleomycin, vinblastine, and imidazole carboxamide versus MOPP. Cancer 36:252–259

Canellos GP, Anderson JR, Propert KJ et al (1992) Chemotherapy of advanced Hodgkin's disease with MOPP, ABVD, or MOPP alternating with ABVD. N Engl J Med 327:1478–1484

De Bruin ML, Huisbrink J, Hauptmann M et al (2008) Treatment-related risk factors for premature menopause following Hodgkin lymphoma. Blood 111:101–108

DeVita VT Jr, Serpick AA, Carbone PP (1970) Combination chemotherapy in the treatment of advanced Hodgkin's disease. Ann Intern Med 73:881–895

Diehl V (2007) Hodgkin's disease – from pathology specimen to cure. N Engl J Med 357:1968–1971

Diehl V, Sieber M, Ruffer U et al (1997) BEACOPP: an intensified chemotherapy regimen in advanced Hodgkin's disease. The German Hodgkin's Lymphoma Study Group. Ann Oncol 8:143–148

Diehl V, Franklin J, Pfreundschuh M et al (2003) Standard and increased-dose BEACOPP chemotherapy compared with COPP-ABVD for advanced Hodgkin's disease. N Engl J Med 348:2386–2395

Falorio S, Angrilli F, Fioritoni G (2008) Gonadotropin-releasing hormone analog treatment for the prevention of treatment-related ovarian failure and infertility in women of reproductive age with Hodgkin lymphoma. Leuk Lymphoma 49:1087–1093

Fanale M, Bartlett NL, Forero-Torres A et al (2009) The antibody-drug conjugate Brentuximab Vedotin (SGN-35) induced multiple objective responses in patient with relapsed or refractory CD30-positive lymphomas in a phase 1 weekly dosing study. Blood 114

Hesketh PJ (2008) Chemotherapy-induced nausea and vomiting. N Engl J Med 358:2482–2494

Horning SJ, Hoppe RT, Breslin S et al (2002) Stanford V and radiotherapy for locally extensive and advanced Hodgkin's disease: mature results of a prospective clinical trial. J Clin Oncol 20:630–637

Longo DL, Young RC, Wesley M et al (1986) Twenty years of MOPP therapy for Hodgkin's disease. J Clin Oncol 4:1295–1306

Moskowitz AJ, Hamlin PA, Gerecitano J et al (2009) Bendamustine is highly active in heavily pre-treated relapsed and refractory Hodgkin lymphoma and serves as a bridge to allogeneic stem cell transplant. Blood 114

Nogova L, Rudiger T, Engert A (2006) Biology, clinical course and management of nodular lymphocyte-predominant Hodgkin lymphoma. In: Berliner N, Linker C, Schiffer CA (eds) Hematology 2006. American Society of Hematology Education Program Book. American Society of Hematology, Washington

Pedersen-Bjergaard J, Specht L, Larsen SO et al (1987) Risk of therapy-related leukaemia and preleukaemia after Hodgkin's disease. Relation to age, cumulative dose of alkylating agents, and time from chemotherapy. Lancet 2:83–88

Rueffer U, Josting A, Franklin J et al (2001) Non-Hodgkin's lymphoma after primary Hodgkin's disease in the German Hodgkin's Lymphoma Study Group: incidence, treatment, and prognosis. J Clin Oncol 19:2026–2032

Schlembach PJ, Wilder RB, Jones D et al (2002) Radiotherapy alone for lymphocyte-predominant Hodgkin's disease. Cancer J 8:377–383

Sieber M, Bredenfeld H, Josting A et al (2003) 14-day variant of the bleomycin, etoposide, doxorubicin, cyclophosphamide, vincristine, procarbazine, and prednisone regimen in advanced-stage Hodgkin's lymphoma: results of a pilot study of the German Hodgkin's Lymphoma Study Group. J Clin Oncol 21:1734–1739

Travis LB, Gospodarowicz M, Curtis RE et al (2002) Lung cancer following chemotherapy and radiotherapy for Hodgkin's disease. J Natl Cancer Inst 94:182–192

Valagussa P, Santoro A, Fossati-Bellani F et al (1986) Second acute leukemia and other malignancies following treatment for Hodgkin's disease. J Clin Oncol 4:830–837

van der Kaaij MA, Heutte N, Le SN et al (2007) Gonadal function in males after chemotherapy for early-stage Hodgkin's lymphoma treated in four subsequent trials by the European Organisation for Research and Treatment of Cancer: EORTC Lymphoma Group and the Groupe d'Etude des Lymphomes de l'Adulte. J Clin Oncol 25:2825–2832

van der Kaaij MAE, van Echten-Arends J, Simons AHM et al (2010) Fertility preservation after chemotherapy for Hodgkin lymphoma. Hematol Oncol

Younes A, Forero-Torres A, Bartlett NL et al (2008) Multiple complete responses in a phase 1 dose-escalation study of the antibody-drug conjugate SGN-35 in patients with relapsed or refractory CD30-positive lymphomas. Blood 112:370

Management of Lymphocyte Predominant Hodgkin Lymphoma

6

Ronald C. Chen and Peter M. Mauch

Contents

R.C. Chen
3239 SW Arrowhead Road, Topeka, KS 66614-4023, USA
e-mail: rcchen@partners.org

P.M. Mauch (✉)
Department of Radiation Oncology, Brigham & Women's Hospital, 75 Francis St, ASB1 L2, Boston, MA 02115, USA
e-mail: pmauch@lroc.harvard.edu

Abbreviations

ABVD	doxorubicin, bleomycin, vinblastine, dacarbazine
CHL	classical Hodgkin lymphoma
CR	complete response
CT	computed tomography
EFRT	extended-field radiation therapy
ETFL	European Task Force on Lymphoma
FFTF	freedom from treatment failure
GHSG	German Hodgkin Study Group
HL	Hodgkin lymphoma
IFRT	involved-field radiation therapy
L&H	lymphocytic proliferation with histiocytes
LPHL	lymphocyte-predominant Hodgkin lymphoma
MOPP	mechlorethamine, vincristine, procarbazine, prednisone
NCCN	National Comprehensive Cancer Network
NHL	non-Hodgkin lymphoma
NOVP	mitoxantrone, vincristine, vinblastine, prednisone
PET	positron emission tomography
REAL	Revised European-American Lymphoma
RT	radiation therapy
WHO	World Health Organization

6.1 Introduction

Lymphocyte-predominant Hodgkin lymphoma (LPHL) is a rare subtype of Hodgkin lymphoma (HL), accounting for 3–8% of all patients diagnosed with HL in the USA and Europe (Diehl et al. 1999), or approximately 500 new cases annually in the USA. LPHL has pathological characteristics and a natural history distinctly different from classical Hodgkin lymphoma (CHL). Because of its

L. Specht and J. Yahalom (eds.), *Radiotherapy for Hodgkin Lymphoma*,
DOI: 10.1007/978-3-540-78944-4_6, © Springer-Verlag Berlin Heidelberg 2011

indolent course and typically early presentation, LPHL is managed uniquely compared with CHL, and treatment considerations over time have focused on reducing primary treatment and its associated long-term sequelae.

This chapter describes the histological characteristics, clinical presentation, prognosis, and management of LPHL. Because of the rarity of this disease, information has largely come from single-institution or pooled, multi-institutional retrospective analyses.

6.2 Histopathology

The classification of HL has become increasingly sophisticated over time. In 1944, Jackson and Parker used morphological criteria to classify HL into three subtypes (Parker 1944), one of which, paragranuloma, was known to have a more indolent course than the others. Prior to the development of curative treatment for HL, the 5-year survival of patients with paragranuloma was 53–95%, compared with 0–37% for the other two subtypes (Hanson 1964; Parker 1944; Smetana and Cohen 1956; Wright 1960). In 1966, the nomenclature proposed by Lukes and Butler described two subtypes of HL characterized by a predominant lymphocytic proliferation with histiocytes (L&H), and relative rare Reed–Sternberg cells: L&H diffuse and L&H nodular (Lukes and Butler 1966). The diffuse subtype commonly has a prominent histiocytic component, while in the nodular subtype, lymphocytes typically predominate, and nodular patterns are seen in areas of cellular proliferation (Lukes and Butler 1966). At the Rye Symposium that same year, the two L&H subtypes were simplified into LPHL.

With the development of immunohistochemistry, LPHL was further validated as a distinct entity that differs from other HL subtypes not only in natural history and morphology, but immunophenotypically as well. In 1994, the Revised European-American Lymphoma (REAL) classification characterized LPHL as a single entity with a nodular background composed of proliferating non-neoplastic small B lymphocytes, with or without areas of diffuse architecture, that consist mainly of T cells. With the use of anti-B-cell or anti-FDC antibodies, which enhance the identification of nodules, purely diffuse patterns were rarely seen (Harris et al. 1994). The neoplastic cells of LPHL are the atypical L&H cells, which are thought to originate from mature B cells (Re et al. 2005), while Reed–Sternberg cells are rarely seen. Atypical L&H cells have vesicular, polylobated nuclei and small nucleoli, and are sometimes called "popcorn" cells because of the morphological appearance of the nucleus (Harris et al. 1994). On immunohistochemistry, the neoplastic cells of LPHL are positive for B-cell-associated antigens (CD19, 20, 22, 79a), B-cell-specific transcription factors (Pax-5, Oct-2, and Bob-1), and leukocyte common antigen (CD45), and negative for CD15 and CD30. In contrast, other subtypes of HL – mixed cellularity, nodular sclerosing, lymphocyte-rich, and lymphocyte depleted – which are collectively called CHL, typically express CD15 and CD30 but not CD20 or CD45 (Table 6.1) (Harris et al. 1994). In 2001, the World Health Organization (WHO) classification system was published, and is currently the "gold standard" for categorizing hematologic malignancies. According to the WHO classification, at least a partial or minimal nodular pattern is required for diagnosis of LPHL (Jaffe et al. 2001). After careful review, if no nodular pattern is seen on a pathologic specimen, then other possible diagnoses should be considered, including diffuse large B-cell lymphoma or T-cell-rich B-cell lymphoma, which may have a histologic appearance similar to LPHL.

The increasing sophistication of diagnostic tools used in the classification of HL has allowed an improved reproducibility of results that was not possible previously. The European Task Force on

Table 6.1 Diagnostic characteristics of lymphocyte-predominant Hodgkin lymphoma versus classical Hodgkin lymphoma (Modified from Table 6 of REAL classification (Harris et al. 1994))

	LPHL	CHL
CD15	Negative	Usually positive
CD30	Usually negative	Usually positive
CD20	Usually positive	Usually negative
CD45	Positive	Usually negative
Tumor cells	L&H cells	Reed–Sternberg cells
Reed–Sternberg cells	Rare	Always
EMA	Often positive	Usually negative
EBV in large cells	Usually negative	Positive 20–70%

LPHL, lymphocyte-predominant Hodgkin lymphoma; CHL, classical Hodgkin lymphoma; L&H, lymphocytic and histiocytic; EMA, epithelial membrane antigen; EBV, Epstein–Barr virus

Lymphomas (ETFL) collected the pathologic specimens of 426 cases of presumed LPHL from 17 European and American institutions for review of the diagnosis by expert pathologists (Diehl et al. 1999). Using strict morphologic and immunophenotypic criteria as defined by the REAL classification, 51% of cases were confirmed to be LPHL, while 27% were reclassified as lymphocyte-rich CHL, 5% CHL, 3% non-Hodgkin lymphoma (NHL), 3% reactive lesions, and 11% could not be classified due to inadequate sample. Two other series using CD15 and CD30 immunohistochemistry showed reclassification rates of 16–41% (Bodis et al. 1997; Feugier et al. 2004). These findings emphasize the importance of using immunohistochemistry in the diagnosis and classification of HL, as well as reevaluation of prior diagnoses of LPHL in patients with recurrent disease or in examination of treatment outcomes from earlier series.

6.3 Clinical Presentation

LPHL commonly presents as chronic, asymptomatic lymphadenopathy in individual who may have had prior lymph node biopsies that revealed reactive follicular hyperplasia or progressive transformation of germinal centers (Miettinen et al. 1983; Orlandi et al. 1997). LPHL tends to present in the peripheral lymph node sites above or below the diaphragm (Bodis et al. 1997; Mauch et al. 1993). In an analysis of 719 patients with HL who uniformly underwent staging laparotomy with splenectomy, Mauch et al. found that LPHL commonly presented at peripheral sites and less commonly in the mediastinum (8%), lung hila (right 3%, left 5%), or upper abdomen (5%) (Mauch et al. 1993).

Most patients with LPHL present with stage I or II disease, approximately 80% in multiple series (Table 6.2) (Chera et al. 2007; Crennan et al. 1995; Diehl et al. 1999; Ha et al. 1999; Nogova et al. 2008; Orlandi et al. 1997; Pappa et al. 1995). B symptoms (fever, drenching night sweats, weight loss) occur in less than 10% of patients. In contrast, only about 60% of CHL presents as early-stage disease, and approximately 40% report B symptoms at presentation (Nogova et al. 2008). In addition, patients with LPHL less commonly than CHL present with involvement of three nodal areas (28% versus 55% in patients from the German Hodgkin Study Group [GHSG]), abnormal erythrocyte sedimentation rate (4% versus 45%), elevated lactate dehydrogenase (16% versus 32%), and mediastinal bulky tumor (31% versus 55%) (Nogova et al. 2008). Extranodal involvement is uncommon in LPHL: spleen is most common (8%), followed by liver (3%), bone marrow (1%), lung

Table 6.2 Clinical presentation of lymphocyte-predominant Hodgkin lymphoma versus classical Hodgkin lymphoma

	N	Median age	Male (%)	Stage (%)				
				I	II	III	IV	B Symptoms (%)
(Nogova et al. 2008)	394	37	75	63% early favorable, 16% early unfavorable		21		9
(Diehl et al. 1999)	219	35	74	53	28	14	6	10
(Chen et al. 2010)	125	27	82	57	34	8	2	5
(Orlandi et al. 1997)	68	35	68	51	24	13	12	15
(Crennan et al. 1995)	64	29	81	55	27	17	2	9
(Hansmann et al. 1984)[a]	145	~40	73	50	21	22	7	10
(Ha et al. 1999)[a]	70	25	79	60	36	3	1	7
(Chera et al. 2007)[a]	34	24	85	53	47	6	0	3
(Pappa et al. 1995)[a]	50	36	86	52	26	16	6	NA
Classical Hodgkin lymphoma (Nogova et al. 2008)	7,904	33	56	22% early favorable, 39% early unfavorable		39		40

[a]CD15/CD30 immunohistochemical review of pathological specimens to confirm LPHL diagnosis was not performed

(1%), skeleton (1%), and other organs (2%) (Diehl et al. 1999). There is a bimodal age distribution, one in children and one in adults, the latter with a median age of 30–40 years. LPHL affects more male than female subjects, with a male-to-female ratio of approximately 3:1 to 4:1.

6.4 Diagnosis and Staging Work-Up

LPHL diagnosis is made by lymph node biopsy and requires careful histopathologic and immunohistochemical analysis by an experienced hematopathologist. Once diagnosis is confirmed, staging evaluation is similar to that for CHL, and uses the Ann Arbor staging classification (Carbone et al. 1971). A detailed history should be taken to document presence or absence of B symptoms, and physical examination should include evaluation of all lymph node stations. Blood work is necessary to provide prognostic information via calculation of the International Prognostic Score (IPS) and to evaluate for involvement of bone, liver, or kidneys. Recommended studies include complete blood count with differential, calcium, blood urea nitrogen, creatinine, serum alkaline phosphatase, aspartate aminotransferase, alanine aminotransferase, lactate dehydrogenase, albumin, and erythrocyte sedimentation rate.

Because bone-marrow involvement is rare in LPHL, occurring in only 1–3% of patients (Diehl et al. 1999; Khoury et al. 2004; Pappa et al. 1995), a bone-marrow biopsy is recommended only for patients with stage IIB to IV disease. Staging laparotomy with splenectomy is no longer a standard part of the staging evaluation, as available data suggest that upstaging from this morbid procedure occurs infrequently. In a single-institutional series of 57 patients with clinical stage I or II LPHL who underwent staging laparotomy, seven were upstaged (13%): one of 27 patients with clinical stage IA (4%), five of 28 with clinical stage IIA (18%), and one of two patients with clinical stage IIB (Bodis et al. 1997). In another study by Ha et al., 23 patients with clinical stage I or II LPHL and negative lymphograms underwent staging laparotomy (Ha et al. 1999). No patient was upstaged. In a third study where 57 patients underwent staging splenectomy ($N=54$) or biopsy ($N=3$), only three patients who did not have splenomegaly were found to have splenic involvement histologically (Hansmann et al. 1984).

Contrast-enhanced computed tomography (CT) to evaluate the neck, chest, abdomen, and pelvis is a standard component of the staging work-up, while the role for positron emission tomography (PET) is unclear. As compared to CHL, the 18-fluorodeoxyglucose avidity of LPHL is lower (Hutchings et al. 2006), and may be similar to background 18-fluorodeoxyglucose avidity of benign, reactive lymphadenopathy or progressive transformation of germinal centers. Whether PET imaging provides additional useful information over CT scans for LPHL is being explored by some institutions (Ansquer et al. 2008).

6.5 Treatment and Outcomes for Stage I/II Disease

Historically, treatment for LPHL mirrored that for CHL, using combined chemotherapy and large-field radiation therapy (RT). Over time, however, it was recognized that LPHL is highly responsive to treatment, with over 90% of patients achieving CR from RT and/or chemotherapy (Table 6.3). LPHL also has a more indolent course and better prognosis compared with CHL, and is infrequently fatal, and more patients died from iatrogenic complications of therapy than from LPHL. Therefore, treatment regimens for LPHL have

Table 6.3 Complete response rates from LPHL treatment

	N	Treatments received	Stages of patients	CR (%)
(Diehl et al. 1999)	219	RT and/or CT	I–IV	96
(Nogova et al. 2008)	394	RT and/or CT	I–IV	87.5
(Feugier et al. 2004)	42	RT and CT	IA or IIA	98
(Ha et al. 1999)	70	RT and/or CT	I–IV	100
(Orlandi et al. 1997)	68	RT and/or CT	I–IV	93

CR, complete response; CT, chemotherapy; RT, radiation therapy become gradually less aggressive. Because of the rarity of LPHL, randomized trials to guide treatment decisions are lacking, and retrospective studies have been the main source of information regarding the outcomes of patients treated less aggressively, with RT alone, or more limited treatment fields such as involved-field RT (IFRT). The National Comprehensive Cancer Network has formulated a distinct treatment algorithm for patients with LPHL based on currently available data and consensus clinical experience (Table 6.4) (National Comprehensive Cancer 2009).

The clinical course and treatment outcomes differ for early (Stage I or II) and advanced (Stage III or IV) LPHL. In an analysis by the ETFL project, outcomes of 219 patients with LPHL from 17 European and American institutions treated with RT and/or chemotherapy were examined. The 8-year freedom from treatment failure (FFTF) rate for those with stage I LPHL was 85%, compared with 71% (stage II), 62% (stage III), and 24% (stage IV) (Diehl et al. 1999). Similarly, overall survival differed for early versus advanced disease: 99% (stage I), 94% (stage II), 94% (stage III), and 41% (stage IV). In addition, recurrences continue to develop even after 10 years, showing the importance of long-term follow-up for studies to fully capture the outcomes of this indolent disease. The GHSG also demonstrated different disease control and survival outcomes in early and advanced LPHL patients (Nogova et al. 2008).

The ETFL and GHSG studies have sufficiently large numbers of patients to examine predictors of treatment outcome using multivariable models (Diehl et al. 1999; Nogova et al. 2008). Both utilized immunohistochemical staining and expert pathological review to confirm LPHL diagnoses in all cases. In both studies, older age and advanced stage were associated with worsened survival; in the GHSG study, low hemoglobin level (<10.5 g/dL) was also a significant predictor. Advanced stage, low hemoglobin, and lymphopenia were significantly associated with a higher risk of treatment failure (Nogova et al. 2008).

Table 6.4 National Comprehensive Cancer Network (NCCN) guidelines (version 2 2009) for treatment of lymphocyte-predominant HL

Clinical stage	Recommended primary treatment
I–IIA	Involved-field RT or regional RT
I–IIB (rare)	Chemotherapy followed by involved-field RT
III–IVA	Chemotherapy with or without RT Or observation (controversial) Or local RT (palliation only)
III–IVB	Chemotherapy with or without RT

RT, radiotherapy

6.5.1 Outcomes from Combined-Modality Treatment

Patients with early-stage LPHL treated with chemotherapy and extended-field RT achieve high rates of CR and disease-specific survival. In a report of 42 patients with stage IA or IIA LPHL treated with 1–3 cycles of chemotherapy followed by extended-field RT (all patients were irradiated to the spleen and lumboaortic area), 98% achieved a CR (Feugier et al. 2004). The 15-year freedom from progression rate was 79.6%, and overall survival rate was 85.7%. Only one patient, who did not respond to initial therapy, died from HL (15-year HL mortality rate 2.4%). These excellent results do not appear to be different from series reporting data with RT alone.

In addition, this aggressive combined-modality treatment led to significant long-term adverse effects. Two patients developed secondary hematological malignancies (one non-Hodgkin lymphoma (NHL) and one leukemia), and three developed solid tumors (adenocarcinoma of unknown primary, prostate cancer, and breast cancer). These malignancies are potentially treatment related, as solid tumors are likely within the extended fields of RT. The 15-year rate of developing secondary hematologic malignancies was 6.3%, and solid tumors 19.1%. No cardiac mortality was observed.

6.5.2 Role of Chemotherapy in the Treatment of Stage I/II Disease

Wirth et al. performed a multicenter review of 202 stage I or II LPHL patients treated in Australia with RT alone (Wirth et al. 2005). Although pathology was not centrally reviewed, this study has a median follow-up of 15 years. The 10- and 15-year freedom from disease progression rates were 88% and 82%, while overall

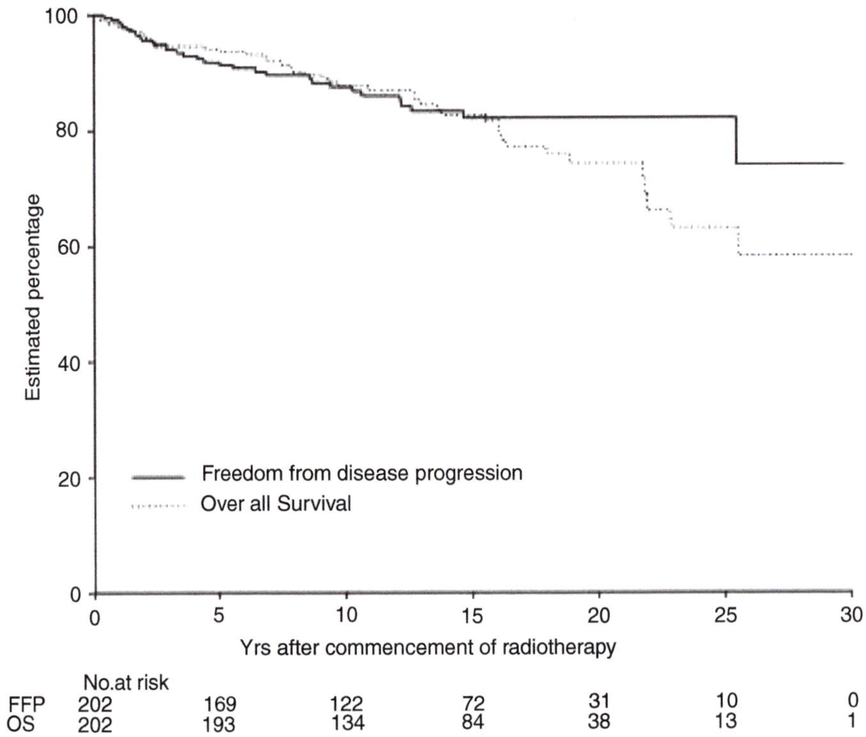

Fig. 6.1 Freedom from progression and overall survival rates for stage I and II patients treated with RT alone (From Wirth et al. 2005)

survival rates were 88% and 83% (Fig. 6.1). This large study shows that, for early LPHL, excellent outcomes can be achieved with RT alone. This trial with a large number of patients is a good baseline for future studies.

Nogova et al. examined the GHSG experience, comparing the outcomes of patients with stage IA LPHL treated with extended-field RT (EFRT), IFRT, or combined-modality treatment (RT and two to four cycles of chemotherapy) (Nogova et al. 2005). The CR rate from treatment was similar in all three groups, and ranged from 98–100%. This study is limited by short follow up, especially for the IFRT group (17 months), but the 2-year FFTF outcomes appeared promising for limited treatments: 100% for EFRT, 92% IFRT, and 97% combined modality (Fig. 6.2a). Overall survival at 24 months was 100% in all groups (Fig. 6.2b).

Similarly, in a retrospective review of 48 patients who had very favorable or favorable LPHL as defined by the European Organization for Research and Treatment of Cancer (EORTC)-Group d'Etude des Lymphomes de l'Adulte (GELA) (Tubiana et al. 1989), patients who received RT alone had outcomes similar to those who underwent induction chemotherapy followed by RT (Wilder et al. 2002). Recurrence-free survival rates at 10 years were 77% (RT alone) and 68% (chemotherapy and RT, $P = .89$); overall survival rates were 90% and 100%, respectively ($P = .43$).

On the other hand, a recent study from British Columbia, available only in abstract form, found that doxorubicin, bleomycin, vinblastine, dacarbazine (ABVD) chemotherapy with or without RT led to superior outcomes compared with RT alone for stage IA or IIA LPHL (Savage et al. 2007). Patients treated with RT alone ($N = 54$, median follow-up 16.5 years) had 5- and 10-year progression-free survival of 82% and 71%, while those who received ABVD ($N = 38$, median follow-up 4 years) had 5-year progression-free survival of 100%. The investigators concluded that ABVD is an essential part of treatment for limited-stage LPHL, though the poor outcomes of patients treated with RT alone from this study differ from what has been reported by other series (Wirth et al. 2005), and the longer median follow-up in the radiation-alone group potentially biases the conclusions.

Table 6.5 summarizes the rates of relapse in selected series of patients with stage I or II LPHL treated with RT alone, chemotherapy alone, or combined-modality therapy. Given favorable outcomes in patients treated with radiation alone, which are similar to those who received combined-modality treatment, the contribution

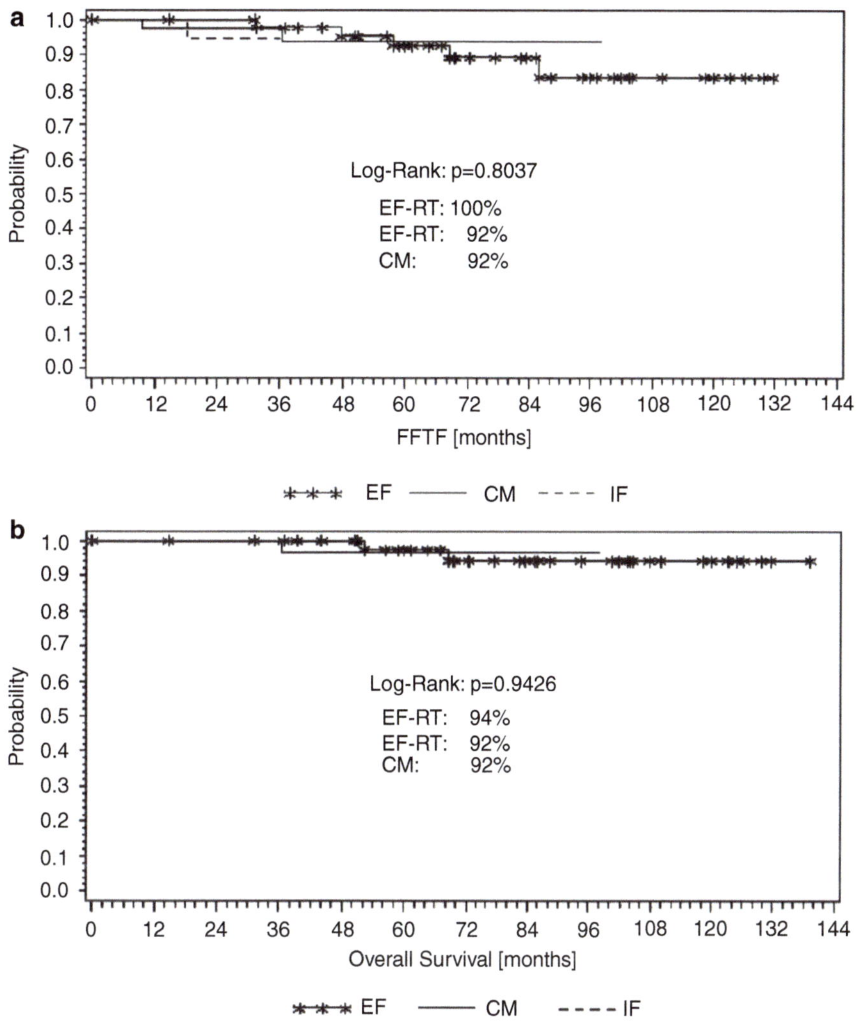

Fig. 6.2 (**a**) Freedom from treatment failure (FFTF) for stage IA patients treated with extended-field radiation therapy (EFRT), involved-field radiation therapy (IFRT), or combined modality (CM). (**b**) Overall survival for stage IA patients treated with EFRT, IFRT, or CM (From Nogova et al. 2005)

Table 6.5 Rate of relapse in Stage I–II LPHL treated with radiation therapy alone, chemotherapy alone, or combined-modality treatment

	Median follow-up (years)	IHC reviewed	Radiation therapy		Chemotherapy		Combined modality	
			No.	%	No.	%	No.	%
(Chen et al. 2010)	12	Yes	17/93	18	6/7	86	NA	NA
(van Grotel et al. 2006)	4.2	No	NA	NA	3/7	43	NA	NA
(Nogova et al. 2005)	3.6	Yes	5/90	6	NA	NA	1/41	2
(Feugier et al. 2004)	NA	Yes	NA	NA	NA	NA	6/42	10
(Wirth et al. 2005)	15	No	30/202	15	NA	NA	NA	NA
(Wilder et al. 2002)	9.3	Some	9/37	24	NA	NA	4/11	36
Total			61/422	14	9/14	62	11/94	12

IHC, CD15/CD30 immunohistochemistry reviewed to confirm LHPL diagnosis; LPHL, lymphocyte-predominant Hodgkin lymphoma from systemic therapy in the initial management of patients with early-stage LPHL is unclear. Very few patients receiving chemotherapy alone have been reported in the literature, though high relapse rates were reported in two small series, suggesting that chemotherapy may be less effective for this subtype compared with CHL (Bodis et al. 1997; van Grotel et al. 2006).

6.5.3 RT Technique

Radiation treatment is highly effective for LPHL. Few patients develop recurrent LPHL within the previously irradiated anatomical areas (Table 6.6). Wirth et al., in a series of 202 patients with stage I or II LPHL treated with radiation alone, estimate the 15-year cumulative incidence of in-field disease progression to be 2% (Wirth et al. 2005). A similar finding was reported by Wilder et al. (Wilder et al. 2002).

For stage I or II LPHL, limited-field RT appears to result in disease-control outcomes similar to EFRT (Bodis et al. 1997; Chera et al. 2007; Nogova et al. 2005; Schlembach et al. 2002; Wirth et al. 2005). In the Australian study by Wirth, a subset analysis was performed on 146 patients with supradiaphragmatic disease without mediastinal involvement (Wirth et al. 2005). No significant difference in outcome was seen between patients who had limited-field RT (without inclusion of the mediastinum) versus those treated with larger fields (mediastinum included), after controlling for disease location and number of involved sites (P =.18). Schlembach et al., in a series of 36 patients treated with RT alone for stage IA or IIA LPHL, found no significant difference in relapse-free or overall survival in patients who received limited/regional field RT versus subtotal or total nodal irradiation (Schlembach et al. 2002). Other studies have shown similar findings (Table 6.7).

Table 6.6 In-field recurrent disease as a proportion of all recurrences after radiation therapy for LPHL

	IHC reviewed	In-field recurrence	
		No.	%
(Nogova et al. 2005)	Yes	1/6	17
(Wirth et al. 2005)	No	4/24	17
(Chera et al. 2007)	No	2/6	33
(Schlembach et al. 2002)	Some	2/7	29
Total		9/43	21

IHC, CD15/CD30 immunohistochemistry reviewed to confirm LHPL diagnosis; LPHL, lymphocyte-predominant Hodgkin lymphoma

Table 6.7 Rate of relapse in Stage I–II LPHL treated with limited- or extended-field radiation therapy

	Median follow-up (years)	IHC reviewed	Limited-field		Extended-field	
			No.	%	No.	%
(Bodis et al. 1997)	10.8	Yes	2/19	11	6/41	15
(Regula, Jr. et al. 1988)	9.4	No	7/19	37	3/20	15
(Feugier et al. 2004)	NA	Yes	NA	NA	6/42	10
(Nogova et al. 2005)	3.6	Yes	1/45	2	4/45	9
(Chera et al. 2007)[a]	12.3	No	0/5	0	6/29	21
(Schlembach et al. 2002)	8.8	Some	5/28	18	2/8	25
Total			15/115	13	27/185	15

[a] Includes two patients with Stage III disease

IHC, CD15/CD30 immunohistochemistry reviewed to confirm LHPL diagnosis; LPHL, lymphocyte-predominant Hodgkin lymphoma

The optimal dose of radiation is unclear. Most studies of LPHL have reported dosages of 30–36 Gy to the involved regions (Bodis et al. 1997; Chera et al. 2007; Nogova et al. 2008; Wirth et al. 2005), which is also the recommended dose in the National Comprehensive Cancer Network (NCCN) guidelines (National Comprehensive Cancer 2009). Doses of 30 Gy are generally sufficient in patients whose nodal disease has been completely excised, while Bodis et al. report boosting sites of bulky disease to 42 Gy. Few studies have examined how radiation dose affects treatment outcome. In the largest series of patients treated with radiation alone for stage I or II LPHL, Wirth et al. examined the rates of in-field recurrences in patients who received 30–35 Gy versus those who received 36–40 Gy (Wirth et al. 2005). No significant difference was found.

6.5.4 Treatment-Related Complications

LPHL is rarely fatal, and most patients after treatment die from other causes (Table 6.8). Many causes of death may be treatment related, including some second cancers (leukemia in patients treated with chemotherapy, solid tumors in patients who received RT) and fatal coronary heart disease. However, not all second cancers developed after initial LPHL are treatment related. NHL may develop in approximately 3% of LPHL patients (Pellegrino et al. 2003), even in patients who received no chemotherapy or RT (Miettinen et al. 1983), and are thought to represent part of the natural history of LPHL. In addition, many solid tumors develop outside the radiation field (Hansmann et al. 1984; Schlembach et al. 2002; Wilder et al. 2002; Wirth et al. 2005), though few studies detail the location of second cancer in relation to irradiated areas. Wirth et al. estimate the 15-year cumulative incidence of in-field second cancers to be 3% (Wirth et al. 2005). Similar results were reported by Ha et al. (Ha et al. 1999). These data, as well as reports showing excellent disease-control outcomes from RT alone and from limited-field versus EFRT, support the use of less-aggressive treatment for early-stage LPHL. More details on acute- and long-term complications of therapy are described in Chap. 14.

6.5.5 Observation or Minimal Treatment After Surgical Resection

Two early retrospective series showed that, following surgical resection of nodal disease, observation or minimal treatment may be a reasonable option (Hansmann et al. 1984; Miettinen et al. 1983). Miettinen et al. examined the outcomes of 31 patients with LPHL who were originally misdiagnosed as having a non-malignant disease, thus left untreated initially. Five-year and 10-year actuarial survival were 93% and 80%, respectively (Miettinen et al. 1983). In another study, 34 patients with stage I or II LPHL underwent nodal biopsy or resection without further primary treatment (Hansmann et al. 1984). Of the 24

Table 6.8 Causes of death in patients treated for LPHL

	N	Stages	Median follow-up (years)	Causes of death			
				HL	Second cancer	Cardiac	Other
(Bodis et al. 1997)	71	I–IV	10.8	1	5	2	1
(Diehl et al. 1999)	219	I–IV	6.8	8	10	4	9
(Nogova et al. 2005)	131	IA	3.6	0	1	1	1
(Feugier et al. 2004)	42	IA/IIA	NA	1	2	0	0
(Chera et al. 2007)	34	I–IV	12.3	0	0	1	8
(Ha et al. 1999)	70	I–IV	12.3	4	0	0	9
(Orlandi et al. 1997)	68	I–IV	6.3	6	4	2	3
Total				20	22	10	31

LPHL, lymphocyte-predominant Hodgkin lymphoma; HL, Hodgkin lymphoma patients with stage I LPHL, 15 developed recurrent disease (63%); the majority were local or in neighboring nodal regions. Only one patient died from LPHL. On the other hand, of the 10 stage II patients in this study, five (50%) developed recurrent disease and died from LPHL.

These early results, plus a desire to spare children from the long-term adverse effects from chemotherapy and/or RT (including growth retardation, infertility, hypothyroidism, cardiopulmonary complications, and second malignancies) (Murphy et al. 2003), led some to selectively treat younger patients with surgery alone with little or no adjuvant therapy. The largest series of children treated with surgical resection alone without adjuvant therapy came from the European Network Group of Pediatric Hodgkin Lymphoma (Mauz-Korholz et al. 2007). Of 54 patients with stage IA LPHL, 18 developed recurrent disease (11 had local recurrence, and seven had a higher disease stage upon recurrence). One of two patients with stage IIA disease recurred. Progression-free survival differed significantly between patients who achieved a CR after surgery versus those who did not (67% versus 0%, p =.01). Overall survival in this cohort is 100% after a median follow-up of 43 months. In a second study from Children's Memorial Hospital, of 12 LPHL patients aged two to 17 who underwent surgery alone (if stage I and complete resection achieved) or surgery followed by 9 weeks of vincristine/doxorubicin/cyclophosphamide/prednisone (if stage II and/or incomplete resection) only one patient recurred (Murphy et al. 2003). The recurrence occurred in the only patient in this cohort with stage II disease. All patients are alive and without evidence of disease at the time of report, and no one developed a second malignancy, but median follow-up of this study was less than 6 years.

These data suggest that, for children with stage IA LPHL, two-thirds who undergo a complete resection of disease may remain disease-free for up to 4 years without adjuvant therapy. A potential disadvantage of this approach is that patients may ultimately develop recurrences that have a less favorable presentation and thus diminished potential for cure. In the two recent studies above, salvage therapies were successful and overall survival is 100%. Longer follow-up, as well as prospective studies, is needed to confirm these results. Currently, observation without treatment following surgical excision is considered experimental, and should be reserved for highly selected patients, such as those with poor performance status or those not able to tolerate RT. For patients with stage II or higher LPHL, observation is not appropriate given the high risk of recurrent disease and mortality from LPHL.

6.6 Treatment and Outcomes for Stage III/IV Disease

The best data on treatment outcomes for patients with advanced-stage LPHL are from the ETFL study (Diehl et al. 1999). In a pool of 219 patients with LPHL from 17 institutions, 20% presented with stage III or IV disease. The majority of these patients received chemotherapy with or without RT. For stage III patients, 8-year HL-specific survival and failure-free survival were 94% and 62%, respectively. For stage IV patients, the rates were 41% and 24%.

There are limited data comparing the outcomes of RT alone, chemotherapy alone, and combined-modality treatment in advanced-disease LPHL. Because of the systemic nature of advanced disease, chemotherapy is commonly used. In addition, the relative effectiveness of various chemotherapeutic regimens is unclear. Typically used regimens include MOPP (mechlorethamine, vincristine, procarbazine, prednisone) (Bodis et al. 1997; Chera et al. 2007; Diehl et al. 1999; Orlandi et al. 1997; Wilder et al. 2002), ABVD (doxorubicin, bleomycin, vinblastine, dacarbazine) (Bodis et al. 1997; Chera et al. 2007; Diehl et al. 1999; Nogova et al. 2008; Orlandi et al. 1997), MOPP/ABVD hybrid (Bodis et al. 1997; Chera et al. 2007; Diehl et al. 1999; Orlandi et al. 1997), epirubicin, bleomycin, vinblastine, methotrexate (Feugier et al. 2004), and NOVP (mitoxantrone, vincristine, vinblastine, prednisone) (Wilder et al. 2002). In addition, RT can be given for the purposes of palliation, when bulky sites of disease are causing pain or compromising critical organs. Conventional courses of RT to a dose of 30–36 Gy may provide rapid and durable response and alleviation of symptoms. In addition, Haas et al. have reported the successful treatment of six patients with recurrent LPHL using the short-course regimen (200 cGy × 2), designed for low-grade NHL (Haas et al. 2005). More data are needed to confirm the palliative efficacy of low-dose RT in LPHL patients.

6.7 Role of Monoclonal Antibody Therapy for LPHL

Therapy with an anti-CD20 antibody (such as rituximab) is logical for LPHL, because the malignant L&H cells express CD20, and this treatment may cause less toxicity than chemotherapy or radiation treatments. Two studies have examined the efficacy and toxicity of rituximab treatment for LPHL (Ekstrand et al. 2003; Rehwald et al. 2003). In a Phase II study by Ekstrand et al., 12 patients with de novo LPHL and 10 patients with relapsed disease were treated with rituximab monotherapy (Ekstrand et al. 2003). The pathology from all patients was reviewed, with immunohistochemistry performed to confirm the LPHL diagnosis. Ten patients (45%) achieved a CR, and 12 (55%) a partial response. The sample size of this study limited the ability to investigate whether disease burden (lymph node size, number of nodal regions involved) correlated with treatment response, but patients with de novo and recurrent disease appeared to respond similarly. With a median follow-up of 13 months, nine patients have relapsed, including two who initially achieved CR and seven who had partial response to rituximab. Five of the relapsed patients underwent a repeat biopsy; while three had recurrent LPHL, one demonstrated transformation to diffuse large B-cell lymphoma and another to T-cell-rich B-cell lymphoma, emphasizing the importance of obtaining tissue in patients with recurrent disease.

In another study performed by the GHSG, 15 patients with recurrent LPHL were treated with rituximab monotherapy (Schulz et al. 2008). All pathology was centrally reviewed, and at least 30% of tumor cells need to stain positive for CD20 for a patient to be eligible for this study. Eight patients (53%) achieved a CR, and six (40%) partial response; one patient with stage IV disease progressed on rituximab and died from LPHL. At a median follow-up of 63 months, the median time-to-progression after rituximab was 33 months.

Rituximab therapy is well tolerated. Toxicity usually occurred with the first infusion, and included chills (71% of patients), fever (50%), rhinitis (21%), nausea (21%), pruritis (21%), leucopenia (14%), and dizziness (14%) (Rehwald et al. 2003). Most (94%) of the described toxicity was grade 1–2, and no severe hematologic effects were seen (Ekstrand et al. 2003; Rehwald et al. 2003).

From these early reports, it appears that rituximab is a highly effective and tolerable treatment for LPHL, with initial response rates greater than 90%. However, durable response is not achieved with monotherapy, and the role of rituximab may be in its combination with other treatment modalities such as IFRT to increase response duration.

6.8 Follow-Up After Treatment Completion

Recurrent LPHL may occur more than 10 years after treatment (Chera et al. 2007; Diehl et al. 1999; Hansmann et al. 1984; Orlandi et al. 1997; Regula, Jr. et al. 1988; Schlembach et al. 2002; Wirth et al. 2005), and treatment-related complications such as second malignancies or cardiac disease also often occur more than 10 years after treatment. Therefore, long-term follow-up is needed. NCCN guidelines recommend routine physical examination, blood work (including complete blood count, erythrocyte sedimentation rate if initially elevated, chemistry profile), and CT scans of initially involved sites (National Comprehensive Cancer 2009).

For monitoring of late effects from therapy, patients who had neck or upper mediastinal disease should have thyroid-function tests annually to rule out hypothyroidism. Women who received chest or axillary irradiation (age 35 or younger at treatment) need to have annual mammography or breast magnetic resonance imaging beginning 8–10 years after RT to screen for secondary breast cancer. In addition, because of the long-term risk of cardiac disease, patients who received mediastinal irradiation should have a baseline stress echocardiography 10 years after treatment.

6.9 Treatment and Outcomes for Recurrent Disease

Successful salvage treatment can often be rendered in patients with recurrent LPHL. Salvage therapy usually consists of chemotherapy, but may also include RT if initial therapy did not include RT or if recurrent disease is located outside the prior

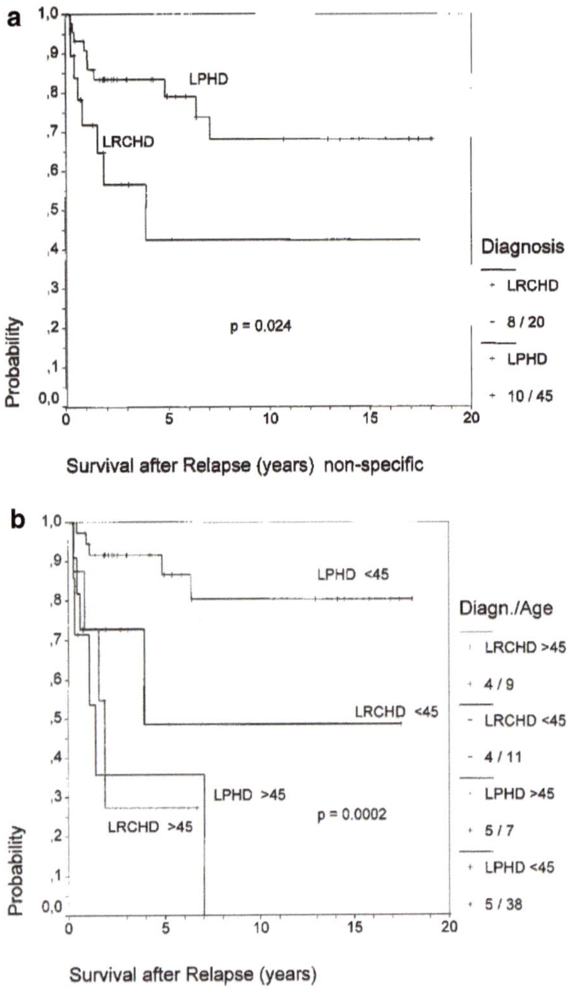

Fig. 6.3 (**a**) Overall survival after relapsed lymphocyte-predominant Hodgkin lymphoma (LPHL). (**b**) Overall survival after relapsed LPHL by age group (From Diehl et al. 1999)

radiation fields. In one of the largest reported series, 21% of LPHL patients developed recurrent disease after initial therapy (*N*=45), about one-fourth of whom (12 of 45 patients, 27%) had multiple relapses (Diehl et al. 1999). Five- and 10-year overall survivals after recurrence are approximately 80% and 70%, respectively (Fig. 6.3a). Patients younger than 45 years old may have better survival than older patients (Fig. 6.3b).

As shown in Table 6.8, LPHL patients more commonly die of iatrogenic or other causes than from progressive HL.

6.10 Conclusion

LPHL is a rare disease that is distinct from other types of HL histologically and clinically. LPHL is typically diagnosed in the male patient, and approximately 80% present in early stages. Historically, LPHL was treated similar to CHL. However, over time, it was recognized that LPHL is highly responsive to treatment (>90% achieve CR) and rarely fatal. More LPHL patients die from other causes, including iatrogenic causes such as secondary cancers and fatal coronary heart disease, than from HL. Therefore, gradual attempts have been made to decrease the aggressiveness of LPHL treatment.

Currently available evidence suggests that, for patients with early-stage disease, limited-field RT and EFRT are similarly effective, with the caution regarding differences in median follow-up times between these modalities, and the need for longer follow-up data. The use of more limited fields will reduce the risk of second malignancies. The role of chemotherapy for early-stage disease is unclear. For advanced-stage LPHL, patients are commonly treated with chemotherapy with or without RT. One recent study (Chen et al. 2010) of 113 stage I–II patients from a single institution, treated primarily with radiation therapy alone, reported 10-year progression-free survival (PFS) rates of 85% for stage I and 61% for stage II disease. Ten year overall survival rates were 94% and 97%, respectively. The extent of radiation delivered was not associated with PFS.

Newer treatment regimens under investigation include the use of rituximab to target the CD20-positive malignant cells, and a watch-and-wait strategy for highly selected pediatric patients who had complete resection of nodal disease.

Because of the potential for late recurrences, as well as risk for second cancers and/or treatment-related cardiac disease, long-term follow-up is necessary. Salvage treatment for recurrent disease is often successful, with 10-year survival after recurrence reaching 70% in one large series.

References

Ansquer C, Hervouet T, Devillers A et al (2008) 18-F FDG-PET in the staging of lymphocyte-predominant Hodgkin's disease. Haematologica 93:128–131

Bodis S, Kraus MD, Pinkus G et al (1997) Clinical presentation and outcome in lymphocyte-predominant Hodgkin's disease. J Clin Oncol 15:3060–3066

Carbone PP, Kaplan HS, Musshoff K et al (1971) Report of the Committee on Hodgkin's Disease Staging Classification. Cancer Res 31:1860–1861

Chen RC, Chin MS, Ng AK et al (2010) Early-stage, lymphocyte-predominant Hodgkin's lymphoma: patient outcomes from a large, single-institution series with long follow-up. J Clin Oncol 28:136–141

Chera BS, Olivier K, Morris CG et al (2007) Clinical presentation and outcomes of lymphocyte-predominant Hodgkin disease at the University of Florida. Am J Clin Oncol 30:601–606

Crennan E, D'Costa I, Liew KH et al (1995) Lymphocyte predominant Hodgkin's disease: a clinicopathologic comparative study of histologic and immunophenotypic subtypes. Int J Radiat Oncol Biol Phys 31:333–337

Diehl V, Sextro M, Franklin J et al (1999) Clinical presentation, course, and prognostic factors in lymphocyte- predominant Hodgkin's disease and lymphocyte-rich classical Hodgkin's disease: report from the European Task Force on Lymphoma Project on Lymphocyte-Predominant Hodgkin's Disease. J Clin Oncol 17:776–783

Ekstrand BC, Lucas JB, Horwitz SM et al (2003) Rituximab in lymphocyte-predominant Hodgkin disease: results of a phase 2 trial. Blood 101:4285–4289

Feugier P, Labouyrie E, Djeridane M et al (2004) Comparison of initial characteristics and long-term outcome of patients with lymphocyte-predominant Hodgkin lymphoma and classical Hodgkin lymphoma at clinical stages IA and IIA prospectively treated by brief anthracycline-based chemotherapies plus extended high-dose irradiation. Blood 104:2675–2681

Ha CS, Kavadi V, Dimopoulos MA et al (1999) Hodgkin's disease with lymphocyte predominance: long-term results based on current histopathologic criteria. Int J Radiat Oncol Biol Phys 43:329–334

Haas RL, Poortmans P, de JD et al (2005) Effective palliation by low dose local radiotherapy for recurrent and/or chemotherapy refractory non-follicular lymphoma patients. Eur J Cancer 41:1724–1730

Hansmann ML, Zwingers T, Boske A et al (1984) Clinical features of nodular paragranuloma (Hodgkin's disease, lymphocyte predominance type, nodular). J Cancer Res Clin Oncol 108:321–330

Hanson TA (1964) Histological classification and survival in Hodgkin's disease; a study of 251 cases with special reference to nodular sclerosing Hodgkin's disease. Cancer 17:1595–1603

Harris NL, Jaffe ES, Stein H et al (1994) A revised European-American classification of lymphoid neoplasms: a proposal from the International Lymphoma Study Group. Blood 84:1361–1392

Hutchings M, Loft A, Hansen M et al (2006) Different histopathological subtypes of Hodgkin lymphoma show significantly different levels of FDG uptake. Hematol Oncol 24:146–150

Jaffe ES, Harris NL, Stein H, Vardiman JW (2001) World Health Organization classification of tumours. Pathology and genetics of tumours of haematopoietic and lymphoid tissues, IARC Press, Lyon 2001.

Khoury JD, Jones D, Yared MA et al (2004) Bone marrow involvement in patients with nodular lymphocyte predominant Hodgkin lymphoma. Am J Surg Pathol 28: 489–495

Lukes RJ, Butler JJ (1966) The pathology and nomenclature of Hodgkin's disease. Cancer Res 26:1063–1083

Mauch PM, Kalish LA, Kadin M et al (1993) Patterns of presentation of Hodgkin disease. Implications for etiology and pathogenesis. Cancer 71:2062–2071

Mauz-Korholz C, Gorde-Grosjean S, Hasenclever D et al (2007) Resection alone in 58 children with limited stage, lymphocyte-predominant Hodgkin lymphoma-experience from the European network group on pediatric Hodgkin lymphoma. Cancer 110:179–185

Miettinen M, Franssila KO, Saxen E (1983) Hodgkin's disease, lymphocytic predominance nodular. Increased risk for subsequent non-Hodgkin's lymphomas. Cancer 51:2293–2300

Murphy SB, Morgan ER, Katzenstein HM et al (2003) Results of little or no treatment for lymphocyte-predominant Hodgkin disease in children and adolescents. J Pediatr Hematol Oncol 25:684–687

National Comprehensive Cancer Network (2009) Clinical practice guidelines in oncology. www.nccn.org

Nogova L, Reineke T, Eich HT et al (2005) Extended field radiotherapy, combined modality treatment or involved field radiotherapy for patients with stage IA lymphocyte-predominant Hodgkin's lymphoma: a retrospective analysis from the German Hodgkin Study Group (GHSG). Ann Oncol 16:1683–1687

Nogova L, Reineke T, Brillant C et al (2008) Lymphocyte-predominant and classical Hodgkin's lymphoma: a comprehensive analysis from the German Hodgkin Study Group. J Clin Oncol 26:434–439

Orlandi E, Lazzarino M, Brusamolino E et al (1997) Nodular lymphocyte predominance Hodgkin's disease: long-term observation reveals a continuous pattern of recurrence. Leuk Lymphoma 26:359–368

Pappa VI, Norton AJ, Gupta RK et al (1995) Nodular type of lymphocyte predominant Hodgkin's disease. A clinical study of 50 cases. Ann Oncol 6:559–565

Parker GH (1944) Hodgkin's disease II. Pathology N Engl J Med 231:34–44

Pellegrino B, Terrier-Lacombe MJ, Oberlin O et al (2003) Lymphocyte-predominant Hodgkin's lymphoma in children: therapeutic abstention after initial lymph node resection–a Study of the French Society of Pediatric Oncology. J Clin Oncol 21:2948–2952

Re D, Kuppers R, Diehl V (2005) Molecular pathogenesis of Hodgkin's lymphoma. J Clin Oncol 23:6379–6386

Regula DP Jr, Hoppe RT, Weiss LM (1988) Nodular and diffuse types of lymphocyte predominance Hodgkin's disease. N Engl J Med 318:214–219

Rehwald U, Schulz H, Reiser M et al (2003) Treatment of relapsed CD20+ Hodgkin lymphoma with the monoclonal antibody rituximab is effective and well tolerated: results of a phase 2 trial of the German Hodgkin Lymphoma Study Group. Blood 101:420–424

Savage KJ, Hoskins P, Klasa R et al (2007) ABVD chemotherapy is essential for optimal treatment of limited stage nodular lymphcyte predominant Hodgkin lymphoma. Haematologica 92(Suppl 5):27–28

Schlembach PJ, Wilder RB, Jones D et al (2002) Radiotherapy alone for lymphocyte-predominant Hodgkin's disease. Cancer J 8:377–383

Schulz H, Rehwald U, Morschhauser F et al (2008) Rituximab in relapsed lymphocyte-predominant Hodgkin lymphoma: long-term results of a phase 2 trial by the German Hodgkin Lymphoma Study Group (GHSG). Blood 111:109–111

Smetana HF, Cohen BM (1956) Mortality in relation to histologic type in Hodgkin's disease. Blood 11:211–224

Tubiana M, Henry-Amar M, Carde P et al (1989) Toward comprehensive management tailored to prognostic factors of patients with clinical stages I and II in Hodgkin's disease. The EORTC Lymphoma Group controlled clinical trials: 1964–1987. Blood 73:47–56

van Grotel M, Lam KH, de MR et al (2006) High relapse rate in children with non-advanced nodular lymphocyte predominant Hodgkin's lymphoma (NLPHL or nodular paragranuloma) treated with chemotherapy only. Leuk Lymphoma 47:1504–1510

Wilder RB, Schlembach PJ, Jones D et al (2002) European Organization for Research and Treatment of Cancer and Groupe d'Etude des Lymphomes de l'Adulte very favorable and favorable, lymphocyte-predominant Hodgkin disease. Cancer 94:1731–1738

Wirth A, Yuen K, Barton M et al (2005) Long-term outcome after radiotherapy alone for lymphocyte-predominant Hodgkin lymphoma: a retrospective multicenter study of the Australasian Radiation Oncology Lymphoma Group. Cancer 104:1221–1229

Wright CJ (1960) The "benign" form of Hodgkin's disease (Hodgkin's paragranuloma). J Pathol Bacteriol 80:157–171

Pediatric Hodgkin Lymphoma, the Rationale for Radiation Therapy

7

David C. Hodgson, Melissa M. Hudson, and Louis S. Constine

Contents

D.C. Hodgson (✉)
Radiation Medicine Program, Princess Margaret Hospital, University Health Network, and Dept. of Radiation Oncology, University of Toronto, 610 University Ave, Toronto, ON M5G 2M9, Canada
e-mail: david.hodgson@rmp.uhn.on.ca

M.M. Hudson
Department of Clinical Oncology, St Jude Children's Research Hospital, and the University of Tennessee College of Medicine, 332 N Lauderdale St, Mailstop 735, Memphis, TN 38105-2729, USA
e-mail: melissa.hudson@stjude.org

L.S. Constine
Departments of Radiation Oncology and Pediatrics, James P. Wilmot Cancer Center, University of Rochester Medical Center, P.O. Box 647, Rochester, NY 14642, USA
e-mail: louis_constine@urmc.rochester.edu

7.1 Treatment of Pediatric Hodgkin Lymphoma

The current era of risk-adapted response-based therapy for pediatric Hodgkin lymphoma (HL) presents several critical issues regarding the role of radiation therapy (RT):

- Can RT be eliminated while maintaining (for low-risk patients) or even augmenting (for high-risk patients) the curability of pediatric HL? Embedded in this question are the relative toxicities of curative chemotherapy (CT) versus less CT plus RT.
- Can the rapidity and the completeness of the response to CT define the use of RT, and will functional imaging enhance the precision of this approach?
- When RT is administered, then what is the appropriate target volume? Can RT be restricted to initially involved lymph nodes rather than chains (or regions) of nodes? In what settings should RT be directed to areas of initial bulk disease or residual post-CT disease? Should involved organs, such as the liver, lung, and heart, ever be irradiated?
- If we use RT, what is the appropriate dose? Should this be dependent on the initial or post-CT extent of disease, bulk of disease, organ at risk, age of the patient?

Inherent in these questions is the recognition that RT is effective in locally controlling pediatric HL but provokes a dose-dependent spectrum of toxicities. Most profound are musculoskeletal growth inhibition, coronary artery disease and cardiomyopathy, pulmonary fibrosis, infertility, and subsequent malignancies. However, eliminating RT necessitates more toxic chemotherapy (either agents or amounts). Discerning the ideal balance will maximize cure while minimizing toxicity. We address these questions in this chapter.

L. Specht and J. Yahalom (eds.), *Radiotherapy for Hodgkin Lymphoma*,
DOI: 10.1007/978-3-540-78944-4_7, © Springer-Verlag Berlin Heidelberg 2011

7.1.1 Radiation Therapy

Prior to the advent of effective chemotherapy regimens, extended-field RT to doses of 35–44 Gy produced 5-year overall survival rates among HL patients (both adults and children) exceeding 80% (Bayle-Weisgerber et al. 1984; Donaldson et al. 1976; Gehan et al. 1990; Mauch et al. 1979), thereby curing what had previously been a highly lethal malignancy. However, children receiving this treatment developed significant musculoskeletal growth impairment such as clavicular shortening and hypoplasia of the soft tissues in the neck and chest (Donaldson and Kaplan 1982; Mauch et al. 1983). The risk of second cancers (SC) was also increased in the long-term survivors of HL treated with full-dose RT (Aleman et al. 2003b; Alm El-Din et al. 2009; Bhatia et al. 2003; Constine et al. 2008; Hodgson et al. 2003; Metayer et al. 2000; Travis et al. 2005). For example, the Late Effects Study Group estimated the 30-year cumulative incidence of SC to be 26.3% among survivors diagnosed before age 16 (Bhatia et al. 2003). The relative risk (RR) of most forms of solid cancer are elevated in most studies of survivors, with breast cancer accounting for the greatest excess number of SC cases among females.

Full-dose mediastinal RT is also associated with an increased risk of atherosclerotic heart disease, valvular dysfunction, and pericardial disease, generally occurring >8–10 years following treatment (Adams et al. 2004; Hancock et al. 1993; Hull et al. 2003).

Moreover, full-dose mediastinal RT is associated with deterioration in pulmonary function tests, particularly diffusion capacity, although this is generally asymptomatic (Catane et al. 1979; Marina et al. 1995; Villani et al. 2000). In addition, dose-dependent thyroid toxicity including hypothyroidism, hyperthyroidism, benign and malignant thyroid nodules have been reported among long-term survivors of HL. Children receiving neck RT also appear to be at greater risk of hypothyroidism than adults receiving comparable treatment (Constine et al. 1984; Sklar et al. 2000).

7.1.2 Chemotherapy

The development of effective anthracycline-based chemotherapy regimens has led to a dramatic improvement in the survival of HL patients. However, a major challenge of treating pediatric HL is that chemotherapy may also produce significant delayed morbidity not seen among adult patients. For example, it is recognized that doxorubicin causes dose-dependent myocardial damage (Lipshultz et al. 1991; Pihkala et al. 1996; Polliack 1995), which in adults may lead to heart failure, typically seen during or shortly after treatment with doses exceeding 550 mg/m^2. In children, however, much lower doses of doxorubicin may impair myocardial growth, and have been associated with late declines in ventricular function (Kremer et al. 2001; Kremer et al. 2002; Lipshultz et al. 1991; Lipshultz et al. 1995). Further, preservation of fertility is a major issue in the management of pediatric HL, necessitating limitation of exposure to alkylating agents, particularly cyclophosphamide and procarbazine (Bramswig et al. 1990; Ortin et al. 1990; van den Berg et al. 2004). Alkylating agents have also been associated with an increased risk of leukemia (Metayer et al. 2000; Schonfeld et al. 2006) and, among adult survivors, lung cancer (Swerdlow et al. 2000; Travis et al. 2002). Children and adolescents treated with ABVD (doxorubicin, bleomycin, vinblastine, dacarbazine) are also at risk for bleomycin lung toxicity, which often emerges during treatment (Fryer et al. 1990; Hunger et al. 1994; Marina et al. 1995).

7.1.3 Combined-Modality Treatment

In order to maintain or improve high cure rates, while limiting the toxicities of chemotherapy and RT, a series of pediatric-specific protocols have been developed in which RT doses are limited to 15–25 Gy, delivered following chemotherapy, with excellent event-free survival (EFS) and overall survival (OS) for most patients (Donaldson 1981; Hudson et al. 1993; Hunger et al. 1994; Oberlin et al. 1992; Weiner et al. 1991). Contemporary standard treatment for pediatric HL typically employs a risk-adapted approach, in which combination chemotherapy is used alone or followed by low-dose involved field radiotherapy (IFRT). Treatment is intensified among those with high-risk (i.e., poor prognosis) disease, while reducing chemotherapy and radiation exposure among those with more favorable features. Different risk strata have been developed by different clinical trial groups, typically accounting for disease bulk, B-symptoms, and anatomic extent.

Table 7.1 Risk groups employed in selected trials of pediatric Hodgkin lymphoma

Study group/trial	Low risk	Intermediate risk	High risk
Children's Oncology Group	IA/IIA no bulk or extranodal extension	IA bulk or "E" extension IB IIA bulk or "E" extension IIB IIIA IVA	IIIB, IVB
German Multicenter Studies (Schellong et al. 1999; Ruhl et al. 2001)	IA/B IIA	IIB IIIEA IIIB	IIEB IIIEA/B IIIB IVA/B
St. Jude/Stanford/Dana Farber[b] (Donaldson et al. 2002; Hudson et al. 2004)	IA/IIA no bulk	IA bulk IB IIA bulk IIB III IV	
Children's Cancer Group 5942 (Nachman et al. 2002)	IA/B patients no adverse features[a] IIA patients no adverse features[a]	IA/B patients with adverse features[a] IIA patients with adverse features[a] IIB IIIA/B	IV

[a] Adverse factors include hilar lymphadenopathy, >4 sites of nodal disease, or bulky disease.

[b] Patients categorized as favorable or unfavorable risk

Although male gender, anemia, elevated total leukocyte count, and lymphopenia have been identified as adverse risk factors, these have not generally been incorporated into risk strata for purposes of treatment selection in pediatric protocols (Bader et al. 1993; Bonadonna et al. 1985; Gobbi et al. 1985; Hasenclever and Diehl 1998; Maity et al. 1992; Smith et al. 2003; Specht 1996). In contrast to many trials in adults, most treatment strata for children segregate patients into low, intermediate, and high-risk categories (Table 7.1). The overall goal of risk-adapted protocols has been to employ the judicious use of both CT and RT to achieve cure while limiting exposure to anthracyclines, alkylating agents, and irradiation of normal tissues.

7.2 Rationale for Radiotherapy

7.2.1 Favorable Risk Disease

Most children with stage IA/IIA non-bulky HL can be cured with abbreviated chemotherapy followed by 15–25 Gy IFRT (Table 7.2). Donaldson et al. reported the outcome of 110 children with stage I/IIA HL treated with four cycles of VAMP (vinblastine, doxorubicin, methotrexate, prednisone) chemotherapy followed by 15 Gy (for complete responders) or 25 Gy (for good partial responders) IFRT. Five-year OS and EFS were 99%, and 93%, respectively (Donaldson et al. 2002). The Children's Cancer Group (CCG) 5942 trial randomized complete responders to 21 Gy IFRT or no further treatment following four to six cycles of COPP/ABV (cyclofosfamide, vincristine, procarbazine, prednisone, doxorubicin, bleomycin, vinblastine) chemotherapy. The 3-year EFS and OS among favorable risk patients receiving combined-modality therapy were 97% and 100%, respectively (Nachman et al. 2002). The German Multicenter GPOH-HD 95 study treated patients with stage IA/B and IIA HL with two cycles of OPPA (vincristine, procarbazine, prednisolone, doxorubicin; for girls) or OEPA (vincristin, etoposide, prednisolone, doxorubicin; for boys). RT was omitted among those achieving a CR to chemotherapy (27% of treated patients); the remaining patients received 20–35 Gy IFRT. With a median follow-up of 38 months, the EFS was 94%

Table 7.2 Selected trials of combined-modality therapy in favorable risk pediatric Hodgkin lymphoma

Study group/trial	Sample size	Treatment	Event-free or disease-free survival	Overall survival	Follow-up (years)
Stanford (Hunger et al. 1994)	44 (CS/PSI-III)	3 MOPP/3 ABVD+15–25.5 Gy IFRT	100	100	10
French Society of Pediatric Oncology (Oberlin et al. 1992)	65 67	4 ABVD+20–40 Gy IFRT 2 MOPP/2 ABVD+20–40 Gy IFRT	90 87		4 4
St. Judes Children's Research Hospital (Hudson et al. 1993)	28 (CSII)	5 COP(P)/4 ABVD+20 Gy IFRT	96	96	5
French Society of Pediatric Oncology MDH-90 (Landman-Parker et al. 2000)	202	4 VBVP+20 Gy IFRT (good responders) 4VBVP+1–2 OPPA+20–40 Gy IFRT (poor responders)	91 78	97.5 (all)	5 5
Stanford/St. Jude/Dana Farber (Donaldson et al. 2002)	110	4 VAMP+15–25.5 Gy IFRT	93	99	5
U.S. Children's Cancer Group (Nachman et al. 2002)	294	4 COPP/ABV+21 Gy IFRT	100 (IFRT)	100 (IFRT)	3
German Multi-center HD-90 (Schellong et al. 1999)	267	2 OPPA/OEPA + 20–35 Gy IFRT	94	99.6	5
German Multi-center HD-95 (Ruhl et al. 2001; Dorffel et al. 2003; Ruhl et al. 2004)	281	2 OPPA/OEPA+20–35 Gy IFRT	94	NA	5
U.S. Pediatric Oncology Group (Tebbi et al. 2006)	46	4 DBVE+25.5 Gy IFRT	91	98	6
U.S. Pediatric Oncology Group (Kung et al. 2006)	247	4 MOPP/ABVD+25.5 Gy IFRT 6 MOPP/ABVD	91 83	97 94	3

CS, clinical stage; *IFRT*, involved field radiotherapy; *PS*, pathologic stage; *ABVD*, doxorubicin, bleomycin, vinblastine, and dacarbazine; *COP(P)*, *CCNU*, vincristine, procarbazine, prednisone; *MOPP*, nitrogen mustard, oncovin, procarbazine, and prednisone; *OEPA*, oncovin, etoposide, prednisone, doxorubicin; *OPPA*, oncovin, procarbazine, prednisolone, and doxorubicin; *VBVP*, vinblastine, bleomycin, etoposide, and prednisone; *VAMP*, vinblastine, doxorubicin, methotrexate, and prednisone; *DBVE*, doxorubicin, bleomycin, vinciristine, etoposide

among favorable risk patients (Ruhl et al. 2001). These studies, and others (Landman-Parker et al. 2000), indicate that the use of 15–25 Gy IFRT as part of treatment following a CR to two to four cycles chemotherapy cures the large majority of patients with favorable risk HL.

7.2.2 Intermediate and Unfavorable Risk Disease

Patients with unfavorable risk factors benefit from intensification of chemotherapy. In the GPOH-HD 95 trial, intermediate- and high-risk patients were treated with two cycles of OPPA or OEPA, followed by an additional two or four cycles of COPP (cyclophosphamide, vincristine, procarbazine, prednisone). IFRT was used for patients not achieving a complete response. With a median follow-up of 38 months, the EFS for intermediate- and high-risk patients were 91%, and 84%, respectively (Ruhl et al. 2001; Ruhl et al. 2004). Patients with intermediate-risk disease on CCG 5942 protocol were treated with six cycles of COPP/ABV. High-risk disease was treated with two courses of intensive multidrug chemotherapy with cytarabine/etoposide, COPP/ABV, and cyclophosphamide, vincristine, doxorubicin and methylprednisolone/prednisone followed by granulocyte colony-stimulating factor support. Three-year EFS rates in intermediate and high-risk patients receiving IFRT were 88% and 91%, respectively (Nachman et al. 2002). Other investigators have reported excellent EFS and OS using low-dose IFRT following chemotherapy for intermediate-risk disease (Table 7.3) (Hunger et al. 1994; Schellong et al. 1999), demonstrating that intensified chemotherapy followed by low-dose IFRT can overcome the adverse prognostic features associated with intermediate and high-risk disease.

The use of RT in the treatment of advanced-stage pediatric HL currently differs from the usual practice for adult HL. While RT typically has a limited role for adults with advanced-stage HL, in both the GOPH HD-95 and CCG 5942, the benefit of IFRT was most pronounced among high-risk patients (Nachman et al. 2002; Ruhl et al. 2001). Consequently, IFRT remains a component of treatment of intermediate- and high-risk disease in most multiinstitutional pediatric protocols. This is in contrast to the standard treatment for adult HL, for which trials have not found a benefit to IFRT among patients with advanced-stage disease achieving a CR after chemotherapy (Aleman et al. 2003a). However, bulk disease is often not controlled for, and patients achieving a PR are often administered consolidative radiotherapy and have similar outcomes to patients who had achieved a CR without chemotherapy. As noted below, careful analysis of patterns of failure among high-risk patients, and possibly distinction between different "high risk" features (e.g., bulk versus advanced stage), may help to identify those patients who truly benefit from RT.

7.2.3 Omission of Radiotherapy

In order to avoid the late toxicity associated with RT, some pediatric trials have evaluated treatment with chemotherapy alone (Hutchinson et al. 1998; Nachman et al. 2002; Sackmann-Muriel et al. 1981; Weiner et al. 1997). The POG 8265 treated 247 patients with favorable risk HL with four courses of alternating MOPP/ABVD (mechlorethamine, vincristine, procarbazine, prednisone, doxorubicin, bleomycin, vinblastine, dacarbazine) and randomized patients achieving CR and PR to either two more courses of the same chemotherapy or 25.5 Gy IFRT (159 (66%) of patients were randomized). Although the 8-year EFS among patients receiving IFRT was superior (91.1% versus 82.6%), this difference was not statistically significant due to the small sample size ($p=0.151$). There was no significant difference in OS (96.8% after combined-modality therapy, 93.6% after chemotherapy alone) (Kung et al. 2006). Similarly, the POG 8725 study randomized patients with intermediate or high- risk disease (clinical stage IIB, III, and IV) to eight cycles of MOPP/AVBD with or without total- or subtotal nodal RT. Event-free survival and OS in the two treatment arms were not significantly different (Weiner et al. 1997). However, conclusions derived from this study must be made cautiously because long-term toxicities were not assessed.

These studies show that intensive chemotherapy regimens can offset the benefit of RT; however, the exposure to anthracyclines and alkylating agents in these protocols exceeds the desirable limits for many pediatric patients. In the POG 8725 study for example, two patients died of sepsis, 38% experienced severe myleosuppression, and five developed hematologic second malignancies. In addition to the significant acute toxicity, it is not clear that the late effects of six to eight cycles of MOPP/ABVD are preferable to those seen with less intense chemotherapy plus IFRT.

The CCG 5942 study treated patients with risk-adapted chemotherapy (primarily COPP/ABV) and randomized complete responders to 21 Gy IFRT or no further therapy. In all risk strata, IFRT was associated with better EFS, with overall EFS of 91% for those receiving IFRT and 86% for those who did not. Overall survival, however, was not significantly different between the treatment arms (Nachman et al. 2002).

Table 7.3 Selected trials of combined-modality therapy in intermediate- or high-risk pediatric Hodgkin lymphoma

Study group/trial	Sample size	Treatment	Event-free or disease-free survival (%)	Overall survival (%)	Follow-up (years)
St. Jude Children's Research Hospital (Hudson et al. 1993)	30 (CS III) 27 (CSIV)	5 COP(P)/4 ABVD+20 Gy IFRT	97 85	100 86	5
Stanford (Hunger et al. 1994)	13 (CS/PS IV)	3 MOPP/3 ABVD+15–25.5 Gy IFRT	69	85	10
German Multi-center HD-90 (Schellong et al. 1999)	124 (IR) 179 (HR)	2 OEPA/OPPA+2 COPP+20–35 Gy IFRT 2 OEPA/OPPA+4 COPP+20–35 Gy IFRT	93 86	97 94	5
Pediatric Oncology Group (Weiner et al. 1997)	179	4 MOPP/4 ABVD +/– 21 Gy TNI/subTNI	79	92	5
Stanford/St. Jude/ Dana Farber (Friedmann et al. 2002)	56	6 VEPA+15–25 Gy IFRT	67.8	81.9	5
U.S. Children's Cancer Group (Nachman et al. 2002)	394 141	6 COPP/ABV +/– 21 Gy IFRT (IR) COPP/ABV+CHOP+Ara-C/VP-16+/– 21 Gy IFRT (HR)	88 (IFRT) 91 (IFRT)	95 100	3 3
German Multi-center HD-95 (Ruhl et al. 2001; Dorffel et al. 2003; Ruhl et al. 2004)	224 (IR) 280 (HR)	2 OPPA/OEPA+2 COPP+20–35 Gy IFRT 2 OPPA/OEPA+4 COPP+20–35 Gy IFRT	91 84	97% (all)	3
Stanford/St. Jude/ Dana Farber (Hudson et al. 2004)	159	3 VAMP/3 COP+15–25.5 Gy IFRT	75.5	92.7	5

HR, high risk; *IFRT*, involved-field radiation therapy; *IR*, intermediate risk; *TNI*, total nodal irradiation; *ABVD*, doxorubicin, bleomycin, vinblastine, and dacarbazine; *CVPP*, cyclophosphamide, vinblastine, procarbazine, prednisone; *COP(P)*, cyclophosphamide, oncovin, prednisone, and procarbazine; *COPP/ABV*, cyclophosphamide, oncovin, procarbazine, prednisone/doxorubicin, bleomycin, vinblastine; *MOPP*, nitrogen mustard, oncovin, procarbazine, and prednisone; *OEPA*, oncovin, etoposide, prednisone, Doxorubicin; *OPPA*, oncovin, procarbazine, prednisolone, and doxorubicin: *VAMP*, vinblastine, doxorubicin, methotrexate, and prednisone; *VEPA*, vinblastine, etoposide, prednisone, doxorubicin

In the GPOH-HD 95 trial described previously, IFRT was associated with significantly better EFS among intermediate- and high-risk patients (92% versus 77%), but not among low-risk patients (Ruhl et al. 2004).

In summary, following risk-adapted chemotherapy, IFRT appears to improve EFS without any early improvement in OS, in part due to the ability to salvage relapses after chemotherapy alone. Also, patients may live for long periods with multiply relapsed disease; so lengthy follow-up is required to document the impact of relapse on overall survival and the quality of that survival. If very intensive chemotherapy is used,

IFRT can be omitted without any reduction in disease control, although it is not clear that toxicity is reduced with this approach.

To further improve the treatment of HL, ongoing clinical research is generally taking two approaches that relate to RT: first, more sophisticated approaches to selecting patients that would benefit from RT are being evaluated. Second, there is increasing utilization of technical advances in imaging, target volume definition, and RT delivery that allow delivery of RT with less exposure of normal tissues.

7.2.4 Response-Adapted Therapy

A large proportion of pediatric HL patients can achieve long-term disease control without RT. A major clinical challenge is how to identify these patients reliably. One means of further refining treatment intensity is to modify treatment according to the response to the initial few cycles of chemotherapy, so-called *response-adapted* therapy. This approach is based on the premise that rapid early response (RER) to chemotherapy reflects the overall chemosensitivity of a patient's disease and is a predictor of good long-term disease control (Kung et al. 2006; Weiner et al. 1997). Rather than define a full course of treatment at the outset, the latter part of treatment is reduced in intensity or duration among those with RER to reduce toxicity, or increased for those with slow early response (SER) in order to improve disease control.

One approach to response-adapted therapy is to increase RT dose among those with incomplete responses to chemotherapy. For example, the DAL HD-90 and GPOH-HD 95 increased RT dose to 30–35 Gy among patients with post-chemotherapy residual imaging abnormalities >50 mL and/or of 25% of the initial tumor volume (Dorffel et al. 2003; Ruhl et al. 2001); these protocols also intensified chemotherapy among patients with disease deemed high risk at diagnosis. Long-term toxicities associated with this radiation dose in young children is a concern based on experiences in previous treatment eras, however, and specific data on this has not been provided. Another study titrating RT dose to chemotherapy response was reported by Hudson et al. on 159 children and adolescents with unfavorable HL (stage I and II with bulk, and/or "B" symptoms and all stage III and IV). Patients received three alternating cycles (total of six cycles) of VAMP/COP (vinblastine, doxorubicin, methotrexate, prednisone, cyclophosphamide, vincristine, procarbazine) chemotherapy followed by response-based IFRT: 15 Gy for those achieving CR after two cycles, and 25.5 Gy for those achieving a partial response, and to all sites of bulky disease. Five-year EFS and OS rates were 75.6% and 92.7%, respectively, which were below expectation, and the study was closed prematurely (Hudson et al. 2004). These findings suggest that RT intensification alone may be insufficient to offset a partial response to chemotherapy regimens that limit alkylator dose in high-risk patients.

Chemotherapy may also be intensified or reduced based on early response. Following three cycles of DBVE-PC chemotherapy (doxorubicin, bleomycin, vincristine, etoposide, cyclophosphamide, prednisone), patients on the POG 9425 study received 21 Gy regional RT after a RER, while those with SER received two more DBVE-PC prior to RT. Two-year EFS was 88.2%, with no statistical difference between early and slow responders (Schwartz et al. 2002). The CCG 59704 treated 99 children with advanced-stage HL with four cycles of dose escalated BEACOPP (bleomycin, etoposide, doxorubicin, cyclophosphamide, vincristine, procarbazine, prednisone) with rapid responders after two cycles of chemotherapy receiving an additional four cycles of COPP/ABV without RT (females) or two cycles of ABVD with IFRT (males). Slow responders received four cycles of BEACOPP and IFRT. This aggressive approach was found to be generally tolerable, although one treatment-related death from myelosuppression occurred. With a median follow-up of six months, one relapse was reported (Kelly et al. 2002). It is important to note that this regimen would be expected to compromise fertility in long-term survivors. Similarly, low-risk patients on POG 9426 received two cycles (for RER) or four cycles (for SER) of DBVE (doxorubicin, bleomycin, vincristine, etoposide) followed by RT with excellent EFS and OS (Tebbi et al. 2006). The French Society of Pediatric Oncology MDH90 treated 202 children with stage I or II HL with four cycles of VBVP (vinblastine, bleomycin, etoposide, and prednisone). Good responders received 20 Gy IFRT alone. Poor responders were given additional one to two cycles of OPPA chemotherapy and after a second evaluation received either 20 Gy IFRT (good responders at second evaluation) or 40 Gy IFRT (poor responders). Eighty-five percent were good responders to VBVP, and thereby were not exposed to alkylators or anthracycline. The 5-year OS and EFS were 97.5% and 91.1%, respectively (Landman-Parker et al. 2000). Again, the administration of 40 Gy would be expected to cause substantial morbidity across the spectrum of exposed normal tissues, as well as increase the risk for SC.

Taken together, these studies suggest that response-adapted therapy may be particularly useful in identifying patients with very favorable disease, who can be treated with abbreviated chemotherapy with limited exposure to anthracyclines and alkylating agents, and low-dose IFRT. These patients may also be good candidates for omission of RT altogether. Further, chemotherapy intensification may offset the adverse prognosis associated with SER, although confirmation of these findings is needed, and extent to which treatment needs to be intensified among slow responders remains uncertain.

The ongoing COG Intermediate-Risk HL study should clarify some of these issues. Patients with stage IA/IIA bulky disease, IB, IIB, IIIA, or IVA disease receive two cycles of ABVE-PC (doxorubicin, bleomycin, vincristine, etoposide, prednisone, cyclophosphamide) prior to response evaluation with CT imaging. Those with RER, and who go on to CR after an additional two cycles of the same chemotherapy, are randomized to 21 Gy IFRT or no additional treatment. Patients with SER to two cycles of chemotherapy are randomized to either standard therapy (an additional two cycles of ABVE-PC+21 Gy IFRT) or intensified therapy (standard therapy plus two additional cycles of DECA (dexamethasone, cytarabine, cisplatin) prior to IFRT). This trial will provide useful data regarding the selection of patients who may avoid RT, and the value of chemotherapy intensification among those with SER.

Most protocols employing response-adapted modifications of therapy evaluate response with CT scanning. There is an enlarging body of clinical studies demonstrating that FDG-Positron Emission Tomography (FDG-PET) following of the initial (one or two) chemotherapy cycles may help identify good-prognosis patients, and facilitate treatment intensification (Hutchings et al. 2006; Jhanwar and Straus 2006; Reinhardt et al. 2005). Whether RT can be omitted among patients with a negative PET scan after chemotherapy is unknown. One randomized study in adult patients with bulky HL demonstrated a 10% decrease in EFS when RT was omitted among patients with a normal FDG-PET scan following six cycles of VE-BEP (vinblastine, etoposide, bleomycin, epirubicin, prednisone) chemotherapy, compared to patients who subsequently received 32 Gy IFRT (Picardi et al. 2007). The issue is being investigated in European studies of adult HL.

7.2.5 Modern Radiation Therapy

One notable feature of observational studies that document increased risks of SC among children receiving RT for HL, is that the RT provided to patients in those studies is long outdated, and the estimated SC risks associated with their treatment is not likely applicable to patients receiving contemporary RT. For example, the Late Effects Study Group (Bhatia et al. 2003) analyzed patients treated from 1955–1986, prior to the widespread use of customized lung shielding, megavoltage linear accelerators, or CT-based imaged guided RT planning (Hoppe et al. 1994). Many patients would have received doses ≥50% higher than currently prescribed, using mantle and upper abdominal fields significantly larger than contemporary RT. Case-control data from a large international study suggest that SC risk is dose-dependent, with patients receiving <23 Gy mediastinal RT experiencing significantly lower risk of breast cancer than those receiving higher doses (Travis et al. 2005). Further, the transition from extended-field RT to IFRT significantly reduces the dose to breast and lung tissue (Koh et al. 2005), and has been predicted to result in a substantial reduction in SC risk (Hodgson et al. 2007). An illustrative example of this is shown in Fig. 7.1, demonstrating that the lower dose and smaller RT fields used with modern IFRT substantially reduce the exposure of normal tissues.

7.2.6 Involved Node Radiotherapy

Although restricting RT volumes to lymph node regions originally involved with disease (IFRT) significantly reduces normal tissue exposure while maintaining low relapse rates, many guidelines describing IFRT recommend treatment of nodal structures adjacent to initially enlarged nodes. In fact, the definitions of lymph nodes regions were initially based on anatomic or bony

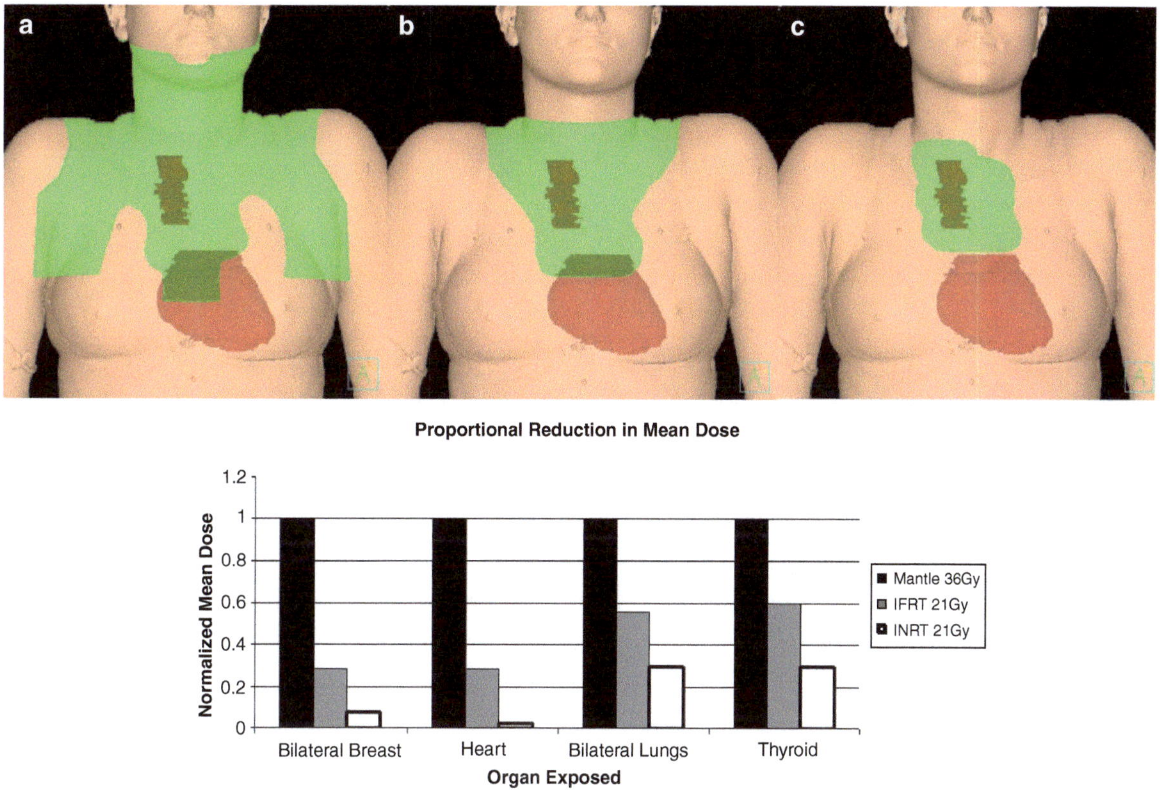

Fig. 7.1 (**a**) Surface renderings of CT-planning images demonstrating typical RT fields for (**a**) historic mantle RT, (**b**) contemporary involved-field RT (IFRT), and (**c**) involved node RT (INRT) for a patient with stage I disease involving the upper mediastinum. The post-chemotherapy volume of initially involved para-tracheal nodes is shown in *dark red*. The silhouette of the contoured cardiac volume is also shown. (**b**) Reduction in dose to breast, lung, heart, and thyroid for the female patient shown in (**a**). The prescribed dose for the mantle field is 36 Gy, comparable to (or less than) RT received by patients evaluated by the Late Effects Study Group. IFRT and INRT fields are prescribed 21 Gy in keeping with contemporary Children's Oncology Group protocols. The proportional reduction in normal tissue dose occurs as a result of the reduction in treated volume and dose with IFRT and INRT is shown

landmarks, and did not have the benefit of CT scanning to identify the location of nodes within lymphoid regions. For example, "standard" IFRT includes treatment of uninvolved hilar and subcarinal lymph nodes in cases with anterior mediastinal involvement, which exposes additional breast, lung, and cardiac tissue to radiation (Table 7.4). In this era of combined-modality therapy, protocol delineation of involved fields has been increasingly fluid and variable,

The premise of involved node radiotherapy (INRT) is that the effectiveness of RT could be maintained and the radiation dose to normal tissues reduced by further limiting the volume of treatment to the specific lymph nodes initially involved with disease (Girinsky et al. 2006), rather than the whole Kaplan lymph node regions (Kaplan and Rosenberg 1966). The concept is based on evidence that recurrence occurs most often in initially involved lymph nodes (Dhakal et al. 2009; Shahidi et al. 2006), suggesting that chemotherapy is adequate to treat disease contained within radiologically normal lymph nodes, while RT is needed only to treat sites of macroscopic enlargement. In contrast to conventional IFRT, uninvolved hila are not included in the CTV for mediastinal presentations, and the length of the treated volume is not routinely extended beyond 1 cm for the planning target volume (Fig. 7.1) (Girinsky et al. 2006). This approach has the potential to significantly reduce the irradiated volume of normal tissues compared to IFRT, and is being employed in ongoing EORTC-GELA and GHSG studies of adult HL.

Table 7.4 Involved-field radiation guidelines

Involved node(s)	Radiation field
Unilateral neck	Unilateral neck + ipsilateral supraclavicular
Supraclavicular	Supraclavicular + mid/low neck + infraclavicular[a]
Axilla	Axilla ± infraclavicular/ supraclavicular
Mediastinum	Mediastinum + hila + infraclavicular/supraclavicular[b]
Hila	Hila ± mediastinum
Spleen	Spleen ± adjacent para-aortics
Para-aortics	Para-aortics ± spleen
Iliac	Iliacs + inguinal/femoral

[a] Upper neck region not treated if supraclavicular involvement is extension of the mediastinal disease

[b] Clinical target volume (CTV) encompasses post-chemotherapy mediastinal width laterally and pre-chemotherapy extent in superior-inferior direction

7.2.7 RT Volumes for Advanced-Stage Disease

In most pediatric protocols employing RT for advanced-stage disease, RT volumes encompassed all initially involved nodal sites of disease, above and below the diaphragm. The GPOH-HD-95 protocol treated patients with lung metastases with 12 Gy to the involved lung(s) unless a CR occurred with two cycles of chemotherapy. Similarly, the CCG 5942 protocol treated the involved lungs to 10.5 Gy. Whole lung RT is used in the ongoing COG trial for intermediate-risk HL for patients with pulmonary or extensive pleural involvement.

Whole lung fields treat a significant volume of normal tissue, and it is not clear the therapeutic ratio of whole lung RT is favorable. Similarly, the benefit of irradiating an uninvolved lymph node region that bridges two affected sites is not clear, although such treatment can include a significant volume of normal tissue. This emphasizes the importance of analyzing patterns of failure in this disease, in order to reduce the radiation dose to normal tissues while maintaining efficacy (Constine et al. 2005). Future studies will determine if restricting RT to areas of initial bulk disease (generally defined as 5 cm or more at the time of disease presentation), or post-chemotherapy residual disease (generally defined as 2 cm or more, or residual PET avidity), is an effective approach in children with advanced-stage HL.

7.3 Future

Improving treatment for children with HL is challenging due to the success of current therapy. Refinement of risk categories, and response-based treatment strategies, should allow continued reduction in therapy-induced toxicity for favorable patients, and better disease control for unfavorable patients.

Refining the role of RT in such trials will continue to be a critical objective. The full extent to which contemporary low-dose IFRT will reduce late effects compared to full-dose extended-field RT is not established, although growth and functional impairment is substantially reduced. Technical innovations in RT delivery and imaging provide the foundation for future advances, potentially allowing further reduction in the volume of normal tissue treated, while preserving the proven efficacy of RT in the management of HL.

References

Adams MJ, Lipsitz SR, Colan SD et al (2004) Cardiovascular status in long-term survivors of Hodgkin's disease treated with chest radiotherapy. J Clin Oncol 22:3139–3148

Aleman BM, Raemaekers JM, Tirelli U et al (2003a) Involved-field radiotherapy for advanced Hodgkin's lymphoma. N Engl J Med 348:2396–2406

Aleman BM, van den Belt-Dusebout AW, Klokman WJ et al (2003b) Long-term cause-specific mortality of patients treated for Hodgkin's disease. J Clin Oncol 21:3431–3439

Alm El-Din MA, Hughes KS, Finkelstein DM et al (2009) Breast cancer after treatment of Hodgkin's lymphoma: risk factors that really matter. Int J Radiat Oncol Biol Phys 73:69–74

Bader SB, Weinstein H, Mauch P et al (1993) Pediatric stage IV Hodgkin disease. Long-term survival. Cancer 72:249–255

Bayle-Weisgerber C, Lemercier N, Teillet F et al (1984) Hodgkin's disease in children. Results of therapy in a mixed group of 178 clinical and pathologically staged patients over 13 years. Cancer 54:215–222

Bhatia S, Yasui Y, Robison LL et al (2003) High risk of subsequent neoplasms continues with extended follow-up of childhood Hodgkin's disease: report from the Late Effects Study Group. J Clin Oncol 21:4386–4394

Bonadonna G, Valagussa P, Santoro A (1985) Prognosis of bulky Hodgkin's disease treated with chemotherapy alone or combined with radiotherapy. Cancer Surv 4:439–458

Bramswig JH, Heimes U, Heiermann E et al (1990) The effects of different cumulative doses of chemotherapy on testicular function. Results in 75 patients treated for Hodgkin's disease during childhood or adolescence. Cancer 65:1298–1302

Catane R, Schwade JG, Turrisi AT III et al (1979) Pulmonary toxicity after radiation and bleomycin: a review. Int J Radiat Oncol Biol Phys 5:1513–1518

Constine LS, Donaldson SS, McDougall IR et al (1984) Thyroid dysfunction after radiotherapy in children with Hodgkin's disease. Cancer 53:878–883

Constine LS, Marcus R, Chauvenet A et al (2005) Patterns of failure after response-based, dose-dense therapy for intermediate/high risk peciatric Hodgkin's disease (POG 9425). Int J Radiat Oncol Biol Phys 63:S21–S22

Constine LS, Tarbell N, Hudson MM et al (2008) Subsequent malignancies in children treated for Hodgkin's disease: associations with gender and radiation dose. Int J Radiat Oncol Biol Phys 72:24–33

Dhakal S, Biswas T, Liesveld JL et al (2009) Patterns and timing of initial relapse in patients subsequently undergoing transplantation for Hodgkin's lymphoma. Int J Radiat Oncol Biol Phys 75:188–192

Donaldson SS (1981) Hodgkin's disease: treatment with low dose radiation and chemotherapy. Front Radiat Ther Oncol 16:122–133

Donaldson SS, Kaplan HS (1982) Complications of treatment of Hodgkin's disease in children. Cancer Treat Rep 66:977–989

Donaldson SS, Glatstein E, Rosenberg SA et al (1976) Pediatric hodgkin's disease. II. Results of therapy. Cancer 37:2436–2447

Donaldson SS, Hudson MM, Lamborn KR et al (2002) VAMP and low-dose, involved-field radiation for children and adolescents with favorable, early-stage Hodgkin's disease: results of a prospective clinical trial. J Clin Oncol 20:3081–3087

Dorffel W, Luders H, Ruhl U et al (2003) Preliminary results of the multicenter trial GPOH-HD 95 for the treatment of Hodgkin's disease in children and adolescents: analysis and outlook. Klin Pädiatr 215:139–145

Friedmann AM, Hudson MM, Weinstein HJ et al (2002) Treatment of unfavorable childhood Hodgkin's disease with VEPA and low-dose, involved-field radiation. J Clin Oncol 20:3088–3094

Fryer CJ, Hutchinson RJ, Krailo M et al (1990) Efficacy and toxicity of 12 courses of ABVD chemotherapy followed by low-dose regional radiation in advanced Hodgkin's disease in children: a report from the Children's Cancer Study Group. J Clin Oncol 8:1971–1980

Gehan EA, Sullivan MP, Fuller LM et al (1990) The intergroup Hodgkin's disease in children. A study of stages I and II. Cancer 65:1429–1437

Girinsky T, van der Maazen R, Specht L et al (2006) Involved-node radiotherapy (INRT) in patients with early Hodgkin lymphoma: concepts and guidelines. Radiother Oncol 79:270–277

Gobbi PG, Cavalli C, Gendarini A et al (1985) Reevaluation of prognostic significance of symptoms in Hodgkin's disease. Cancer 56:2874–2880

Hancock SL, Tucker MA, Hoppe RT (1993) Factors affecting late mortality from heart disease after treatment of Hodgkin's disease. JAMA 270:1949–1955

Hasenclever D, Diehl V (1998) A prognostic score for advanced Hodgkin's disease. International Prognostic Factors Project on advanced Hodgkin's disease. N Engl J Med 339:1506–1514

Hodgson DC, Zhang-Salomons J, Rothwell D et al (2003) Evolution of treatment for Hodgkin's disease: a population-based study of radiation therapy use and outcome. Clin Oncol (R Coll Radiol) 15:255–263

Hodgson DC, Koh ES, Tran TH et al (2007) Individualized estimates of second cancer risks after contemporary radiation therapy for Hodgkin lymphoma. Cancer 110:2576–2586

Hoppe RT, Hanlon AL, Hanks GE et al (1994) Progress in the treatment of Hodgkin's disease in the United States, 1973 versus 1983. The Patterns of Care Study. Cancer 74:3198–3203

Hudson MM, Greenwald C, Thompson E et al (1993) Efficacy and toxicity of multiagent chemotherapy and low-dose involved-field radiotherapy in children and adolescents with Hodgkin's disease. J Clin Oncol 11:100–108

Hudson MM, Krasin M, Link MP et al (2004) Risk-adapted, combined-modality therapy with VAMP/COP and response-based, involved-field radiation for unfavorable pediatric Hodgkin's disease. J Clin Oncol 22:4541–4550

Hull MC, Morris CG, Pepine CJ et al (2003) Valvular dysfunction and carotid, subclavian, and coronary artery disease in survivors of hodgkin lymphoma treated with radiation therapy. JAMA 290:2831–2837

Hunger SP, Link MP, Donaldson SS (1994) ABVD/MOPP and low-dose involved-field radiotherapy in pediatric Hodgkin's disease: the Stanford experience. J Clin Oncol 12:2160–2166

Hutchings M, Loft A, Hansen M et al (2006) FDG-PET after two cycles of chemotherapy predicts treatment failure and progression-free survival in Hodgkin lymphoma. Blood 107:52–59

Hutchinson RJ, Fryer CJ, Davis PC et al (1998) MOPP or radiation in addition to ABVD in the treatment of pathologically staged advanced Hodgkin's disease in children: results of the Children's Cancer Group Phase III Trial. J Clin Oncol 16:897–906

Jhanwar YS, Straus DJ (2006) The role of PET in lymphoma. J Nucl Med 47:1326–1334

Kaplan HS, Rosenberg SA (1966) The treatment of Hodgkin's disease. Med Clin N Am 50:1591–1610

Kelly KM, Hutchinson RJ, Sposto R et al (2002) Feasibility of upfront dose-intensive chemotherapy in children with advanced-stage Hodgkin's lymphoma: preliminary results from the Children's Cancer Group Study CCG-59704. Ann Oncol 13(Suppl 1):107–111

Koh E, Tran T, Heydarian M et al (2005) A dosimetric study of mantle versus involved-field radiotherapy for Hodgkin's lymphoma: implications for second cancer risk and cardiac toxicity. Int J Radiat Oncol Biol Phys 63:S422–S423

Kremer LC, van Dalen EC, Offringa M et al (2001) Anthracycline-induced clinical heart failure in a cohort of 607 children: long-term follow-up study. J Clin Oncol 19:191–196

Kremer LC, van Dalen EC, Offringa M et al (2002) Frequency and risk factors of anthracycline-induced clinical heart failure in children: a systematic review. Ann Oncol 13:503–512

Kung FH, Schwartz CL, Ferree CR et al (2006) POG 8625: a randomized trial comparing chemotherapy with chemoradiotherapy for children and adolescents with Stages I, IIA, IIIA1 Hodgkin Disease: a report from the Children's Oncology Group. J Pediatr Hematol Oncol 28:362–368

Landman-Parker J, Pacquement H, Leblanc T et al (2000) Localized childhood Hodgkin's disease: response-adapted chemotherapy with etoposide, bleomycin, vinblastine, and prednisone before low-dose radiation therapy-results of the French Society of Pediatric Oncology Study MDH90. J Clin Oncol 18:1500–1507

Lipshultz SE, Colan SD, Gelber RD et al (1991) Late cardiac effects of doxorubicin therapy for acute lymphoblastic leukemia in childhood. N Engl J Med 324:808–815

Lipshultz SE, Lipsitz SR, Mone SM et al (1995) Female sex and drug dose as risk factors for late cardiotoxic effects of doxorubicin therapy for childhood cancer. N Engl J Med 332:1738–1743

Maity A, Goldwein JW, Lange B et al (1992) Mediastinal masses in children with Hodgkin's disease. An analysis of the Children's Hospital of Philadelphia and the Hospital of the University of Pennsylvania experience. Cancer 69:2755–2760

Marina NM, Greenwald CA, Fairclough DL et al (1995) Serial pulmonary function studies in children treated for newly diagnosed Hodgkin's disease with mantle radiotherapy plus cycles of cyclophosphamide, vincristine, and procarbazine alternating with cycles of doxorubicin, bleomycin, vinblastine, and dacarbazine. Cancer 75:1706–1711

Mauch P, Goodman R, Rosenthal DS et al (1979) An evaluation of total nodal irradiation as treatment for stage III A Hodgkin's disease. Cancer 43:1255–1261

Mauch PM, Weinstein H, Botnick L et al (1983) An evaluation of long-term survival and treatment complications in children with Hodgkin's disease. Cancer 51:925–932

Metayer C, Lynch CF, Clarke EA et al (2000) Second cancers among long-term survivors of Hodgkin's disease diagnosed in childhood and adolescence. J Clin Oncol 18:2435–2443

Nachman JB, Sposto R, Herzog P et al (2002) Randomized comparison of low-dose involved-field radiotherapy and no radiotherapy for children with Hodgkin's disease who achieve a complete response to chemotherapy. J Clin Oncol 20:3765–3771

Oberlin O, Leverger G, Pacquement H et al (1992) Low-dose radiation therapy and reduced chemotherapy in childhood Hodgkin's disease: the experience of the French Society of Pediatric Oncology. J Clin Oncol 10:1602–1608

Ortin TT, Shostak CA, Donaldson SS (1990) Gonadal status and reproductive function following treatment for Hodgkin's disease in childhood: the Stanford experience. Int J Radiat Oncol Biol Phys 19:873–880

Picardi M, De Renzo A, Pane F et al (2007) Randomized comparison of consolidation radiation versus observation in bulky Hodgkin's lymphoma with post-chemotherapy negative positron emission tomography scans. Leuk Lymphoma 48:1721–1727

Pihkala J, Saarinen UM, Lundstrom U et al (1996) Myocardial function in children and adolescents after therapy with anthracyclines and chest irradiation. Eur J Cancer 32A:97–103

Polliack A (1995) Late therapy-induced cardiac and pulmonary complications in cured patients with Hodgkin's disease treated with conventional combination chemo-radiotherapy. Leuk Lymphoma 15(Suppl 1):7–10

Reinhardt MJ, Herkel C, Altehoefer C et al (2005) Computed tomography and 18F-FDG positron emission tomography for therapy control of Hodgkin's and non-Hodgkin's lymphoma patients: when do we really need FDG-PET? Ann Oncol 16:1524–1529

Ruhl U, Albrecht M, Dieckmann K et al (2001) Response-adapted radiotherapy in the treatment of pediatric Hodgkin's disease: an interim report at 5 years of the German GPOH-HD 95 trial. Int J Radiat Oncol Biol Phys 51:1209–1218

Ruhl U, Albrecht MR, Lueders H et al (2004) The German multinational GPOH-HD 95 trial: treatment results and analysis of failures in pediatric Hodgkins disease using combination chemotherapy with and without radiation. Int J Radiat Oncol Biol Phys 60:S131

Sackmann-Muriel F, Bonesana AC, Pavlovsky S et al (1981) Hodgkin's disease in childhood: therapy results in Argentina. Am J Pediatr Hematol Oncol 3:247–254

Schellong G, Potter R, Bramswig J et al (1999) High cure rates and reduced long-term toxicity in pediatric Hodgkin's disease: the German-Austrian multicenter trial DAL-HD-90. The German-Austrian Pediatric Hodgkin's Disease Study Group. J Clin Oncol 17:3736–3744

Schonfeld SJ, Gilbert ES, Dores GM et al (2006) Acute myeloid leukemia following Hodgkin lymphoma: a population-based study of 35, 511 patients. J Natl Cancer Inst 98:215–218

Schwartz CL, Constine LS, London W et al (2002) POG 9425: response-based, intensively timed therapy for intermediate/high stage (IS/HS) pediatric Hodgkin's disease. Proc Am Soc Clin Oncol 21:389a

Shahidi M, Kamangari N, Ashley S et al (2006) Site of relapse after chemotherapy alone for stage I and II Hodgkin's disease. Radiother Oncol 78:1–5

Sklar C, Whitton J, Mertens A et al (2000) Abnormalities of the thyroid in survivors of Hodgkin's disease: data from the Childhood Cancer Survivor Study. J Clin Endocrinol Metab 85:3227–3232

Smith RS, Chen Q, Hudson MM et al (2003) Prognostic factors for children with Hodgkin's disease treated with combined-modality therapy. J Clin Oncol 21:2026–2033

Specht L (1996) Prognostic factors in Hodgkin's disease. Semin Radiat Oncol 6:146–161

Swerdlow AJ, Barber JA, Hudson GV et al (2000) Risk of second malignancy after Hodgkin's disease in a collaborative British cohort: The relation to age at treatment. J Clin Oncol 18:498–509

Tebbi CK, Mendenhall N, London WB et al (2006) Treatment of stage I, IIA, IIIA1 pediatric Hodgkin disease with doxorubicin, bleomycin, vincristine and etoposide (DBVE) and radiation: a Pediatric Oncology Group (POG) study. Pediatr Blood Cancer 46:198–202

Travis LB, Gospodarowicz M, Curtis RE et al (2002) Lung cancer following chemotherapy and radiotherapy for Hodgkin's disease. J Natl Cancer Inst 94:182–192

Travis LB, Hill D, Dores GM et al (2005) Cumulative absolute breast cancer risk for young women treated for Hodgkin lymphoma. J Natl Cancer Inst 97:1428–1437

van den Berg H, Furstner F, van den BC et al (2004) Decreasing the number of MOPP courses reduces gonadal damage in survivors of childhood Hodgkin disease. Pediatr Blood Cancer 42:210–215

Villani F, Viviani S, Bonfante V et al (2000) Late pulmonary effects in favorable stage I and IIA Hodgkin's disease treated with radiotherapy alone. Am J Clin Oncol 23:18–21

Weiner MA, Leventhal BG, Marcus R et al (1991) Intensive chemotherapy and low-dose radiotherapy for the treatment of advanced-stage Hodgkin's disease in pediatric patients: a Pediatric Oncology Group study. J Clin Oncol 9:1591–1598

Weiner MA, Leventhal B, Brecher ML et al (1997) Randomized study of intensive MOPP-ABVD with or without low-dose total- nodal radiation therapy in the treatment of stages IIB, IIIA2, IIIB, and IV Hodgkin's disease in pediatric patients: a Pediatric Oncology Group study. J Clin Oncol 15:2769–2779

The Role of Imaging in Radiotherapy for Hodgkin Lymphoma

8

Martin Hutchings, Anne Kiil Berthelsen, and Sally F. Barrington

Contents

M. Hutchings (✉)
Dept. of Oncology and Haematology, The Finsen Centre, Rigshospitalet, Copenhagen University Hospital, 9 Blegdamsvej, 2100 Copenhagen, Denmark
e-mail: hutchings@dadlnet.dk

A.K. Berthelsen
Dept. of Radiation Oncology & PET Centre, Rigshospitalet, Copenhagen University Hospital, 9 Blegdamsvej, 2100 Copenhagen, Denamark
e-mail: anne.kiil.berthelsen@rh.regionh.dk

S.F. Barrington
The PET Imaging Centre, Guy's and St. Thomas' Hospital, Lambeth Palace Road, London SE1 7EH, UK
e-mail: sally.barrington@kcl.ac.uk

8.1 Introduction

Over the last 3 decades, radiotherapy for Hodgkin lymphoma (HL) has changed from extended-field radiotherapy (mantle field, inverted Y field) and subtotal nodal irradiation, encompassing all or almost all lymphoid tissue, to involved-field radiotherapy, where only the initially involved lymph node regions with or without adjacent regions are irradiated (Aleman et al. 2003a; Bonadonna et al. 2004; Specht et al. 1998). More recently, many groups have introduced involved-node radiotherapy where the planning target volume (PTV) is limited to the initially involved structures plus a margin of 1–2 cm (Girinsky et al. 2006b). This evolution has been driven by the wish to avoid the excessive treatment-related morbidity and mortality of large radiation fields and doses, which unfortunately has been observed in several large cohorts (Aleman et al. 2003b; Specht et al. 1998). However, the significant reduction of the irradiated volumes would not have been safe without the important development in imaging methods which has taken place in the same period. In the 1980s, lymphangiography and staging laparotomy were made redundant by computerised tomography (CT). Gallium scans proved to have a high sensitivity for staging of HL, but this method has been replaced by the even more sensitive and quicker imaging modality of positron emission tomography using the tracer fluorodeoxyglucose (FDG-PET), subsequently referred to as PET (Friedberg et al. 2004; Kostakoglu et al. 2002; Paul 1987; Wirth et al. 2002). Dual-modality PET/CT is the most accurate imaging method so far for determination of disease extent in HL (Hutchings et al. 2006a). Examples of PET/CT scans showing uptake in different anatomical disease

L. Specht and J. Yahalom (eds.), *Radiotherapy for Hodgkin Lymphoma*,
DOI: 10.1007/978-3-540-78944-4_8, © Springer-Verlag Berlin Heidelberg 2011

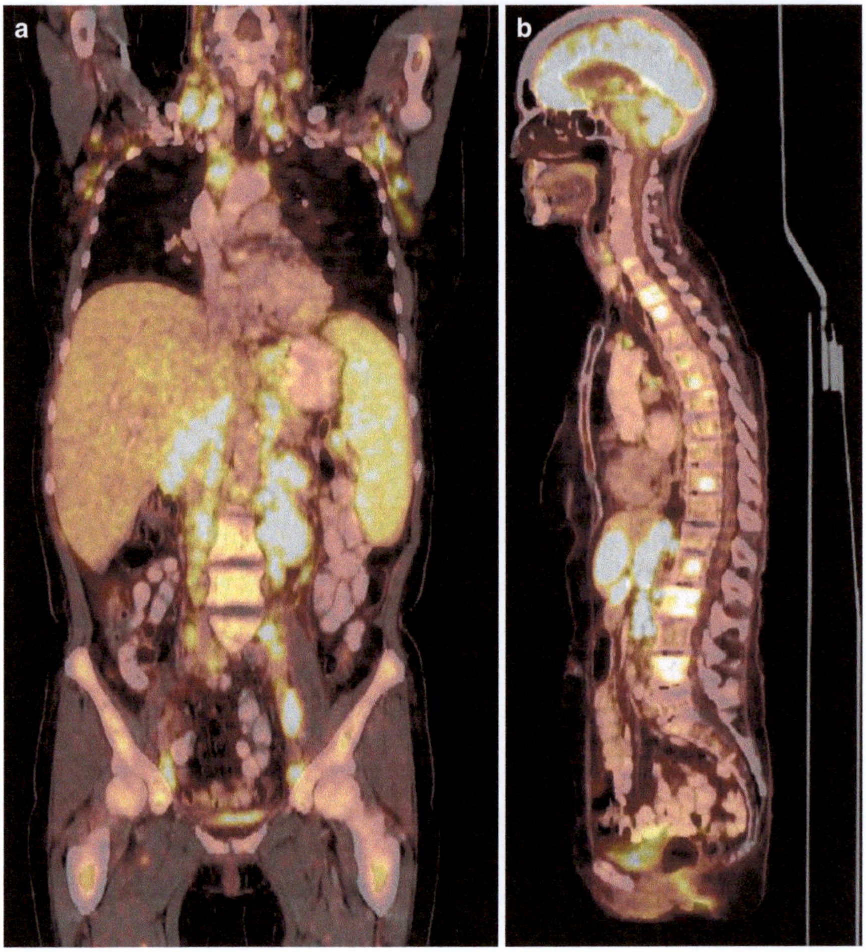

Fig. 8.1 Examples of FDG uptake in advanced-stage Hodgkin lymphoma. Panel A shows a coronal section of a PET/CT scan of a patient with involvement of several lymph node regions and the spleen, while panel B shows a sagittal section of a patient with abdominal lymph node and bone marrow involvement

localisations are shown in Fig. 8.1. Other imaging methods are valuable for certain indications. Magnetic resonance imaging (MRI) is comparable to CT in accuracy and has the advantage of excellent soft-tissue contrast and lack of exposure to ionising radiation (Bendini et al. 1996; Gossmann et al. 2005; Tomura et al. 1998). The disadvantages are higher costs and longer acquisition times. While conventional MRI detection relies on relatively insensitive size criteria, lymphotropic MRI contrast agents have shown promising results in the detection of minimal nodal involvement (Gossmann et al. 2005). However, in most centres, MRI is still reserved for imaging of suspected bone and central nervous system involvement, which is relatively rare in HL. Ultrasound imaging is a valuable tool for characterisation of peripheral glands and abdominal involvement, but rarely adds to the value of CT in HL staging, except when used to investigate testicular and breast involvement (Castroagudin et al. 2007; Gerrits et al. 1994; Liu et al. 2006). Furthermore, the information from a staging ultrasonic scan is difficult to use for subsequent radiotherapy planning. At present, CT and PET/CT are the cornerstone imaging methods in HL. This chapter will focus on the role of these methods, not only in the radiotherapy planning, but also on their role and potential in the selection of HL patients for radiotherapy.

8.2 CT and PET/CT in the Selection of Patients for Radiotherapy

8.2.1 Pre-chemotherapy Selection at Staging

In general terms, localised HL is treated with a brief course of chemotherapy followed by radiotherapy to all the initially involved sites of disease, while in advanced-stage HL, radiotherapy is given to initial sites of bulky disease and to residual masses in patients who achieve a partial remission (PR) after chemotherapy. A CT or PET/CT scan is the mainstay of HL staging. Along with physical examination and the presence or absence of B-symptoms (fever, night sweats and weight loss), the staging scan is the main determinant of clinical stage, and hence crucial for the selection of patients for the different radiotherapeutic strategies.

While CT was introduced to the management of lymphomas on the basis of little scientific evidence, PET and PET/CT have been investigated thoroughly since the mid-1990s (Hutchings et al. 2004). PET has very high sensitivity for nodal staging and is especially sensitive in the detection of peripheral and thoracic lymph nodes, where the sensitivity of PET seems to be higher than the sensitivity of CT, even when CT is combined with other conventional methods (Bangerter et al. 1998; Jerusalem et al. 2001; Rigacci et al. 2007; Weihrauch et al. 2002). Though the available data are limited, the sensitivity of PET tends to be higher than the sensitivity of conventional methods for detecting extranodal disease, both in the bone marrow and in other organs (Carr et al. 1998; Pakos et al. 2005). Studies looking specifically at the value of PET/CT as compared with CT and/or PET found PET/CT to be more accurate for staging than both PET and CT, with an equal sensitivity and a better specificity (Allen-Auerbach et al. 2004; Hutchings et al. 2006a). PET/CT has fewer false-positive findings than PET alone, especially in the deep nodal regions of the abdomen and the mediastinum, a fact probably owed to the improved distinction between malignant and non-malignant FDG uptake (e.g. intestinal uptake, brown fat, muscle uptake). Although PET/CT has less of a tendency towards upstaging of patients than PET alone, and although PET/CT correctly downstages a fraction of patients compared with both CT and PET, PET/CT still results in upward-stage migration for 10–20% of patients, some of whom move from early to advanced stage. Since early and advanced-stage HL patients are treated very differently, the tendency towards upward-stage migration is important. As early-stage HL patients have an excellent prognosis and carry a high risk of treatment-related late morbidity and mortality, important ongoing efforts aim to reduce the toxicity of treatment without impairing efficacy. PET/CT should support rather than oppose this effort and should thus ideally be used for staging of HL when accompanied by steps to reduce the intensity of chemo- and/or radiotherapy to early-stage patients in general.

8.2.2 Post-Chemotherapy Evaluation

As stated above, patients with advanced-stage HL are commonly offered radiotherapy to initial sites of bulky disease and to residual masses in case of PR after chemotherapy. Until recently, post-chemotherapy evaluation was performed according to the International Workshop Criteria (IWC) for NHL and Cotswolds Criteria for HL. These criteria were based mainly on morphological criteria with a reduction in tumour size on CT being the most important factor (Cheson et al. 1999; Lister et al. 1989).

After completion of chemotherapy for HL, CT scans will often reveal residual masses. It is very difficult with CT to assess whether these represent viable lymphoma or fibrotic tissue. To perform a biopsy on all lesions would be impractical, and even if undertaken would be inaccurate as residual masses may contain a mixture of fibrosis and viable lymphoma cells, and hence a number of false-negative results would be expected due to sampling error. A large number of studies have shown a consistently high negative predictive value (NPV) for post-treatment PET in HL patients (De Wit et al. 2001; Dittmann et al. 2001; Guay et al. 2003; Jerusalem et al. 1999; Lang et al. 2001; Mikhaeel et al. 2000; Rahmouni et al. 2005; Spaepen et al. 2001). Based on this body of evidence, the International Workshop Criteria and Cotswolds Criteria were revised. According to the new criteria, patients with a PET-negative residual mass are in CR and therefore not candidates for consolidation radiotherapy (Cheson et al. 2007; Juweid et al. 2007). Hopefully, the number of false-negatives according to the new response criteria will be much smaller than the number of false-positives according to the old ones, thus sparing a significant number of patients from unnecessary treatment with no or only very few extra relapses.

The new response criteria if widely adopted are likely to significantly influence the pattern of referral of HL patients for consolidation radiotherapy, but the criteria are not as yet supported by substantial amounts of clinical data. An Italian analysis gave cause for some concern, as 160 patients with bulky HL and a negative post-treatment PET were randomised to receive radiotherapy to the original bulky site or no further treatment. At 18 months of follow-up, 14% of patients in the "no further treatment" arm had relapsed versus only 2.5% in the radiotherapy arm (Picardi et al. 2007). On the contrary, the interim analysis of the German HD15 study showed a 94% NPV of post-chemotherapy PET for patients who received no radiotherapy despite having at least one residual mass of more than 2.5 cm, indicating that radiotherapy can be safely omitted in advanced-stage HL patients who are PET-negative after the end of chemotherapy (Kobe et al. 2008).

8.2.3 Early Treatment Monitoring and Risk-Adapted Treatment Selection

Tumour response is the most important surrogate for other measures of clinical benefit from the treatment of HL, such as progression-free and overall survival. Early prediction of response to therapy could enable patients with a good response to be treated less intensively, thus reducing their risk of long-term toxicity, and patients with a poor response to be switched sooner to treatment regimens that would improve the likelihood and duration of remission. This concept of risk-adapted therapy is being increasingly recognised as a way to achieve higher cure rates with lower or equal risk of treatment-related morbidity and mortality. As with post-treatment evaluation, conventional methods for treatment response monitoring are based on morphological criteria, and a reduction in tumour size on CT is the most important determinant (Armitage et al. 1986; Gupta et al. 1999; Rankin 2003). However, this is not an accurate predictor of outcome, possibly because the malignant cells in HL make up only a small fraction of the tumour volume (Canellos 1988). Furthermore, the shrinkage of the tumour takes time and thus cannot form the basis for adjustment of therapy until late during treatment. PET enables early evaluation of metabolic changes rather than the morphological changes of the lymphoma that occur later during therapy. Several studies have shown that responders and non-responders can be accurately identified by PET after only 1–3 chemotherapy cycles, and that early interim PET is a reliable surrogate for progression-free survival (Gallamini et al. 2006; 2007; Hutchings et al. 2005; 2006b; Zinzani et al. 2006). However, there is yet no evidence that patients benefit from having treatment adapted according to the results of early PET. At the time of writing, a number of trials are addressing this issue in early-stage HL. The UK's NCRI Lymphoma Clinical Studies Group PET trial as well as the EORTC/GELA H10 protocols investigate the consequences of omitting radiotherapy in early PET-negative early-stage HL patients. Provided these and other similar trials turn out in favour of PET-response adapted therapy, they will have an important impact on the role of radiotherapy in HL, as 75–80% of all early-stage patients are expected to be PET-negative after two cycles of chemotherapy (Radford et al. 2007).

8.3 CT and PET/CT for Radiotherapy Planning in HL

8.3.1 Current Concepts and Guidelines

Radiotherapy for HL has changed from extended fields developed for single modality treatment to more and more conformal fields designed for combined-modality treatment, encompassing only the initially macroscopically involved regions or nodes in early-stage disease and residual masses after chemotherapy in advanced disease (Girinsky et al. 2006a; b; Specht et al. 1998; Yahalom 2005). These changes were made possible by the introduction of CT and advanced 3-D planning and have led to dramatic reductions in the volume of normal tissue being irradiated in most HL patients, most certainly reducing the risk of serious late effects. However, with increasing conformality of radiotherapy for lymphomas, the risk of geographical misses will also increase. Hence, the timing as well as the anatomical and diagnostic accuracy of the imaging procedures used for treatment planning are essential. The use of respiratory gating, image-guided radiotherapy and intensity-modulated radiotherapy in HL are being investigated in specialised centres. Such techniques are likely to further increase the demand for accurate lymphoma imaging.

Accurate determination of the extent of disease at diagnosis (pre-chemotherapy) and at radiotherapy planning (post-chemotherapy) is critical. CT scans are employed for treatment planning for delineation purposes, but also because the CT numbers are correlated with the electron density of the corresponding tissues at each voxel relative to the electron density of water. The information from the planning CT scan can therefore be employed by the dose-planning algorithm for calculation of the absorption and scattering of the radiation in the tissues. The delineation of the lymphoma volume must be based on the best diagnostic information available of both anatomy and physiology of the disease (Gregoire 2004; Jarritt et al. 2006). As PET adds to the accuracy for staging of HL, it is by implication also recommended in defining the initially involved regions intended to be irradiated in patients with early-stage disease. Therefore, treatment planning using a combined PET/CT with diagnostic quality CT is preferable (Berthelsen et al. 2007).

In the primary treatment of early-stage HL, chemotherapy is usually the initial treatment followed by radiotherapy. In this situation the initial lymphoma volume seen on the pre-chemotherapy PET/CT scan must be contoured on the planning PET/CT or CT performed after chemotherapy, where the lymphoma may no longer be visible. The goal is to contour the tissue volume that contained the lymphoma tissue before chemotherapy, i.e. the tissue volume with a high risk of harbouring residual tumour cells. In order to use staging PET/CT for radiotherapy planning, the images must be spatially fused with the planning CT or PET/CT data set. For this purpose, pre-chemotherapy PET/CT images should ideally be acquired with the patient in the treatment position, with a flat-bed insert, with the use of appropriate immobilisation devices, and using skin position markers visible on the CT images. A multidisciplinary imaging team including the radiation oncologist needs to be involved upfront before chemotherapy is given, in order to best achieve this goal and ensure that clinical examinations and imaging studies necessary for later treatment planning are carried out appropriately. When contouring the pre-chemotherapy lymphoma volume the radiation oncologist is guided by the fused pre-chemotherapy images with regard to the initial location and extent of the disease. However, normal structures that have been displaced by enlarged lymph nodes should not be included in the target volume. Therefore, the radiation oncologist will have to modify the fused image of the pre-chemotherapy tumour volume on the planning CT to make allowances for the shrinkage of tissues during chemotherapy (Girinsky et al. 2006b). Figure 8.2 shows the steps involved in the target volume definition for a patient with early-stage HL treated initially with brief chemotherapy. On the other hand, if extranodal tissue, e.g. lung, was initially infiltrated by lymphoma, then this tissue volume should be included in the target volume if the entire initial tumour volume is the target, even if the tissue is no longer macroscopically involved after chemotherapy.

Although virtually all HL masses are PET-positive, it is not uncommon to see variable parts of clearly involved volumes that are abnormal on CT despite being PET-negative. This has led to the suggested concept of 'dose-painting', where different radiotherapy doses would be delivered according to different levels of metabolic activity. This concept has not been proven of any value in clinical practice. Girinsky et al. showed that in early-stage HL on average only 25% of the lymphoma volumes were FDG avid (Girinsky et al. 2007). In this study an automated segmentation method was used based on fixed thresholds originally developed for head and neck cancer. Other methods of qualitative evaluation or quantitative segmentation may yield different percentages of FDG avid volumes. Interestingly, the PET-positive and PET-negative lymphoma masses regressed equally during chemotherapy. Although non-malignant reactive parts of the lymph node masses may also shrink during chemotherapy, this indicates that both PET-positive and PET-negative lymphoma contain active lymphoma tissue, and thus argues against the concept of dose-painting.

In advanced disease, radiotherapy is used less frequently and usually only to residual disease and/or to sites of bulky disease at staging. In this situation PET may help in discriminating between a residual mass with viable lymphoma cells and a residual mass consisting only of fibrotic tissue. This is the background for the revised response criteria as described above, according to which radiotherapy should only be given to post-chemotherapy PET-positive patients. However, as PET cannot detect microscopic disease it is still not clear whether the target volume for irradiation in this situation should be only PET-positive lesions or whether it should also include CT-positive but PET-negative areas.

8.3.2 Clinical Data on CT and PET in HL Radiotherapy

Only limited clinical data are available regarding the value of CT and the addition of PET in target definition for the planning of radiotherapy for HL (Specht 2007; van Baardwijk et al. 2006). The impact of CT on modern HL radiotherapy techniques has not been studied, as CT was introduced at a time when extended-field irradiation was still predominant. However, CT is not an objective and uniform measure of lymphoma

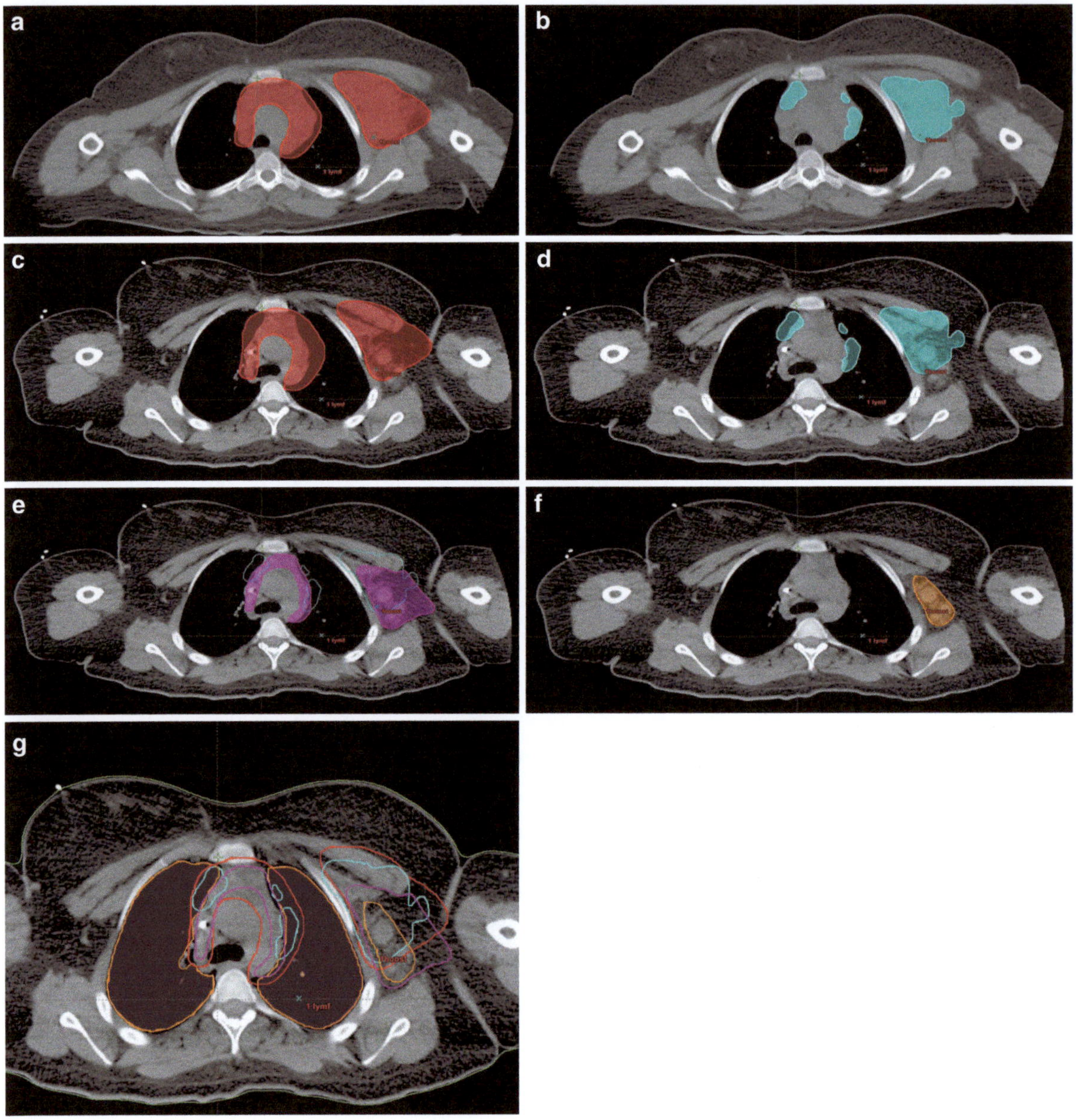

Fig. 8.2 Example of PET/CT based radiotherapy for early-stage Hodgkin lymphoma. Staging PET/CT is performed with a flat-top bed and with the patient in a position as similar as possible to the later treatment position. The CT images of the pre-chemotherapy PET/CT are used to delineate the involved masses as determined by morphology on CT (panel A, *red*) and by FDG uptake (panel B, *blue*). After completion of chemotherapy, the initial PET/CT is co-registered with the planning CT and the lymphoma contours are imported to the planning CT images (panels C and D). The involved volume (panel E, *purple*) is defined using information from both PET and CT at staging, taking into account tumour shrinkage and other anatomical changes. This volume encompasses all of the initially involved tissue volume while still respecting normal structures such as lungs, thoracic and axillary wall and mediastinal normal structures. The boost volume is defined using information from the planning (post-chemotherapy) CT or PET/CT scan, and encompasses the residual tumour masses (panel F, orange). All volumes are shown in panel G.Accurate determination of the disease extent allows for small margins to define the clinical target volume (CTV). Likewise, the margins defining the planning treatment volume (PTV) are kept to a minimum using very careful positioning and modern position tracking with on-board imaging or cone-beam CT. CTV and PTV are not shown in the figure

involvement. Vorwerk et al. investigated different size criteria for CT evaluation of pathological lymph nodes in HL and found that the choice of CT reading criteria has profound influence on both staging, treatment strategy and the size/number of involved radiotherapy fields (Vorwerk et al. 2008). Likewise, where extended-field irradiation is still used the impact of PET is not expected to be very large, since additional involvement found on PET will often be included in the large treatment fields anyway (Dizendorf et al. 2003; Lee et al. 2004). But with modern and more conformal radiotherapy PET results in significant changes (Girinsky et al. 2007; Hutchings et al. 2007; Krasin et al. 2004). In a prospective study by Hutchings and co-workers, 30 patients with early-stage Hodgkin lymphoma had involved-field radiotherapy planned with and without the information of the pre-chemotherapy FDG-PET scan. The radiation fields would have been changed by FDG-PET in 10 cases; in seven cases the irradiated volume would have increased, in two cases it would have decreased, and in one case radiotherapy would have been omitted altogether because the FDG-PET scan showed more advanced disease (Hutchings et al. 2007). Girinsky et al. investigated the impact of PET on radiation fields in 30 patients treated according to the EORTC involved-node radiotherapy guidelines (Girinsky et al. 2006b). They found a significant effect on the delineation in 36% of the patients (Girinsky et al. 2007). Despite the body of evidence showing the significant impact of PET/CT on treatment volumes in HL radiotherapy planning, there is as yet no evidence of the impact on patient outcome.

8.4 Conclusion

PET/CT has replaced CT as the state-of-the-art imaging method in HL staging. This gives a higher sensitivity and a better staging accuracy and also results in a tendency towards upward-stage migration. This means that some patients, who would previously have been given combined modality treatment, are now offered chemotherapy, either alone or with subsequent radiotherapy only to residual masses. PET/CT after completion of chemotherapy has been incorporated into the revised response criteria. However, it is not clear whether the PET status should influence which patients are given consolidation and boost radiotherapy to residual masses. A number of studies are underway that examine the role of early interim PET/CT in the selection of good-prognosis early-stage patients who may be cured by a brief course of chemotherapy without radiotherapy.

When incorporated into the existing treatment guidelines, PET/CT will result in larger radiotherapy fields for early-stage HL patients. However, this patient group is characterised by an excellent survival and a high risk of treatment-related morbidity and mortality. Thus, larger radiotherapy fields are not appropriate for early-stage patients in general. The increased staging accuracy brought about by PET/CT, and the more precise delineation of the involved lymph nodes, should be used to allow for more patient-tailored and less-toxic therapy, aiming to treat only the initially involved lymph nodes. There is yet no data to show an impact on patient outcome, neither from the use of PET/CT in the selection of HL patients for radiotherapy, nor from the use of PET/CT in the radiotherapy planning.

References

Aleman BM, Raemaekers JM, Tirelli U et al (2003a) Involved-field radiotherapy for advanced Hodgkin's lymphoma. N Engl J Med 348:2396–2406

Aleman BM, van den Belt-Dusebout AW, Klokman WJ et al (2003b) Long-term cause-specific mortality of patients treated for Hodgkin's disease. J Clin Oncol 21:3431–3439

Allen-Auerbach M, Quon A, Weber WA et al (2004) Comparison between 2-deoxy-2-[18F]fluoro-D-glucose positron emission tomography and positron emission tomography/computed tomography hardware fusion for staging of patients with lymphoma. Mol Imaging Biol 6:411–416

Armitage JO, Weisenburger DD, Hutchins M et al (1986) Chemotherapy for diffuse large-cell lymphoma – rapidly responding patients have more durable remissions. J Clin Oncol 4:160–164

Bangerter M, Moog F, Buchmann I et al (1998) Whole-body 2-[18F]-fluoro-2-deoxy-D-glucose positron emission tomography (FDG-PET) for accurate staging of Hodgkin's disease. Ann Oncol 9:1117–1122

Bendini M, Zuiani C, Bazzocchi M et al (1996) Magnetic resonance imaging and 67Ga scan versus computed tomography in the staging and in the monitoring of mediastinal malignant lymphoma: a prospective pilot study. Magma 4:213–224

Berthelsen AK, Dobbs J, Kjellen E et al (2007) What's new in target volume definition for radiologists in ICRU Report 71? How can the ICRU volume definitions be integrated in clinical practice? Cancer Imaging 7:104–116

Bonadonna G, Bonfante V, Viviani S et al (2004) ABVD plus subtotal nodal versus involved-field radiotherapy in early-stage Hodgkin's disease: long-term results. J Clin Oncol 22:2835–2841

Canellos GP (1988) Residual mass in lymphoma may not be residual disease. J Clin Oncol 6:931–933

Carr R, Barrington SF, Madan B et al (1998) Detection of lymphoma in bone marrow by whole-body positron emission tomography. Blood 91:3340–3346

Castroagudin JF, Molina E, Abdulkader I et al (2007) Sonographic features of liver involvement by lymphoma. J Ultrasound Med 26:791–796

Cheson BD, Horning SJ, Coiffier B et al (1999) Report of an international workshop to standardize response criteria for non-Hodgkin's lymphomas. NCI Sponsored International Working Group. J Clin Oncol 17:1244–1253

Cheson BD, Pfistner B, Juweid ME et al (2007) Revised response criteria for malignant lymphoma. J Clin Oncol 25:579–586

De Wit M, Bohuslavizki KH, Buchert R et al (2001) 18FDG-PET following treatment as valid predictor for disease-free survival in Hodgkin's lymphoma. Ann Oncol 12:29–37

Dittmann H, Sokler M, Kollmannsberger C et al (2001) Comparison of 18FDG-PET with CT scans in the evaluation of patients with residual and recurrent Hodgkin's lymphoma. Oncol Rep 8:1393–1399

Dizendorf EV, Baumert BG, von Schulthess GK et al (2003) Impact of whole-body 18F-FDG PET on staging and managing patients for radiation therapy. J Nucl Med 44:24–29

Friedberg JW, Fischman A, Neuberg D et al (2004) FDG-PET is superior to gallium scintigraphy in staging and more sensitive in the follow-up of patients with de novo hodgkin lymphoma: a blinded comparison. Leuk Lymphoma 45:85–92

Gallamini A, Rigacci L, Merli F et al (2006) The predictive value of positron emission tomography scanning performed after two courses of standard therapy on treatment outcome in advanced stage Hodgkin's disease. Haematologica 91: 475–481

Gallamini A, Hutchings M, Rigacci L et al (2007) Early interim 2-[18F]fluoro-2-deoxy-D-glucose positron emission tomography is prognostically superior to international prognostic score in advanced-stage Hodgkin's lymphoma: a report from a joint Italian-Danish study. J Clin Oncol 25: 3746–3752

Gerrits CJ, van OH, van LK et al (1994) Ultrasound examination of pathological cervical lymph nodes in patients with non-Hodgkin's lymphoma and Hodgkin's disease. Br J Haematol 88:626–628

Girinsky T, Pichenot C, Beaudre A et al (2006a) Is intensity-modulated radiotherapy better than conventional radiation treatment and three-dimensional conformal radiotherapy for mediastinal masses in patients with Hodgkin's disease, and is there a role for beam orientation optimization and dose constraints assigned to virtual volumes? Int J Radiat Oncol Biol Phys 64:218–226

Girinsky T, van der Maazen R, Specht L et al (2006b) Involved-node radiotherapy (INRT) in patients with early Hodgkin lymphoma: concepts and guidelines. Radiother Oncol 79: 270–277

Girinsky T, Ghalibafian M, Bonniaud G et al (2007) Is FDG-PET scan in patients with early stage Hodgkin lymphoma of any value in the implementation of the involved-node radiotherapy concept and dose painting? Radiother Oncol 85:178–186

Gossmann A, Eich HT, Engert A et al (2005) CT and MR imaging in Hodgkin's disease – present and future. Eur J Haematol Suppl 83–89

Gregoire V (2004) Is there any future in radiotherapy planning without the use of PET: unraveling the myth. Radiother Oncol 73:261–263

Guay C, Lepine M, Verreault J et al (2003) Prognostic value of PET using 18F-FDG in Hodgkin's disease for posttreatment evaluation. J Nucl Med 44:1225–1231

Gupta RK, Gospodarowicz MK, Lister TA (1999) Clinical evaluation and staging. In: Mauch P, Armitage JO, Diehl V et al (eds) Hodgkin's disease. Lippincott Williams and Wilkins, Philadelphia

Hutchings M, Eigtved AI, Specht L (2004) FDG-PET in the clinical management of Hodgkin lymphoma. Crit Rev Oncol Hematol 52:19–32

Hutchings M, Mikhaeel NG, Fields PA et al (2005) Prognostic value of interim FDG-PET after two or three cycles of chemotherapy in Hodgkin lymphoma. Ann Oncol 16:1160–1168

Hutchings M, Loft A, Hansen M et al (2006a) Positron emission tomography with or without computed tomography in the primary staging of Hodgkin's lymphoma. Haematologica 91:482–489

Hutchings M, Loft A, Hansen M et al (2006b) FDG-PET after two cycles of chemotherapy predicts treatment failure and progression-free survival in Hodgkin lymphoma. Blood 107:52–59

Hutchings M, Loft A, Hansen M et al (2007) Clinical impact of FDG-PET/CT in the planning of radiotherapy for early-stage Hodgkin lymphoma. Eur J Haematol 78:206–212

Jarritt PH, Carson KJ, Hounsell AR et al (2006) The role of PET/CT scanning in radiotherapy planning. Br J Radiol 79(Spec No 1):S27–S35

Jerusalem G, Beguin Y, Fassotte MF et al (1999) Whole-body positron emission tomography using 18F-fluorodeoxyglucose for posttreatment evaluation in Hodgkin's disease and non-Hodgkin's lymphoma has higher diagnostic and prognostic value than classical computed tomography scan imaging. Blood 94:429–433

Jerusalem G, Beguin Y, Fassotte MF et al (2001) Whole-body positron emission tomography using 18F-fluorodeoxyglucose compared to standard procedures for staging patients with Hodgkin's disease. Haematologica 86:266–273

Juweid ME, Stroobants S, Hoekstra OS et al (2007) Use of positron emission tomography for response assessment of lymphoma: consensus of the Imaging Subcommittee of International Harmonization Project in Lymphoma. J Clin Oncol 25:571–578

Kobe C, Dietlein M, Franklin J et al (2008) Positron emission tomography has a high negative predictive value for progression or early relapse for patients with residual disease after first-line chemotherapy in advanced-stage Hodgkin lymphoma. Blood 112:3989–3994

Kostakoglu L, Leonard JP, Kuji I et al (2002) Comparison of fluorine-18 fluorodeoxyglucose positron emission tomography and Ga-67 scintigraphy in evaluation of lymphoma. Cancer 94:879–888

Krasin MJ, Hudson MM, Kaste SC (2004) Positron emission tomography in pediatric radiation oncology: integration in the treatment-planning process. Pediatr Radiol 34:214–221

Lang O, Bihl H, Hultenschmidt B et al (2001) Clinical relevance of positron emission tomography (PET) in treatment control and relapse of Hodgkin's disease. Strahlenther Onkol 177: 138–144

Lee YK, Cook G, Flower MA et al (2004) Addition of 18F-FDG-PET scans to radiotherapy planning of thoracic lymphoma. Radiother Oncol 73:277–283

Lister TA, Crowther D, Sutcliffe SB et al (1989) Report of a committee convened to discuss the evaluation and staging of patients with Hodgkin's disease: Cotswolds meeting. J Clin Oncol 7:1630–1636

Liu KL, Chang CC, Huang KH et al (2006) Imaging diagnosis of testicular lymphoma. Abdom Imaging 31:610–612

Mikhaeel NG, Timothy AR, Hain SF et al (2000) 18-FDG-PET for the assessment of residual masses on CT following treatment of lymphomas. Ann Oncol 11(Suppl 1):147–150

Pakos EE, Fotopoulos AD, Ioannidis JP (2005) 18F-FDG PET for evaluation of bone marrow infiltration in staging of lymphoma: a meta-analysis. J Nucl Med 46:958–963

Paul R (1987) Comparison of fluorine-18-2-fluorodeoxyglucose and gallium-67 citrate imaging for detection of lymphoma. J Nucl Med 28:288–292

Picardi M, De Renzo A, Pane F et al (2007) Randomized comparison of consolidation radiation versus observation in bulky Hodgkin's lymphoma with post-chemotherapy negative positron emission tomography scans. Leuk Lymphoma 48:1721–1727

Radford JA, Barrington SF, O'Doherty MJ et al (2007) Interim results of a UK NCRI randomised trial comparing involved field radiotherapy with no further treatment after 3 cycles ABVD and a negative PET scan in clinical stages IA/IIA Hodgkin lymphoma. Haematologica 92(suppl 5):32

Rahmouni A, Luciani A, Itti E (2005) Quantitative CT analysis for assessing response in lymphoma (Cheson's criteria). Cancer Imaging 5(Spec No A):S102–S106

Rankin SC (2003) Assessment of response to therapy using conventional imaging. Eur J Nucl Med Mol Imaging 30(Suppl 1):S56–S64

Rigacci L, Vitolo U, Nassi L et al (2007) Positron emission tomography in the staging of patients with Hodgkin's lymphoma. A prospective multicentric study by the Intergruppo Italiano Linfomi. Ann Hematol 86:897–903

Spaepen K, Stroobants S, Dupont P et al (2001) Can positron emission tomography with [(18)F]-fluorodeoxyglucose after first-line treatment distinguish Hodgkin's disease patients who need additional therapy from others in whom additional therapy would mean avoidable toxicity? Br J Haematol 115:272–278

Specht L (2007) 2-[18F]fluoro-2-deoxyglucose positron-emission tomography in staging, response evaluation, and treatment planning of lymphomas. Semin Radiat Oncol 17: 190–197

Specht L, Gray RG, Clarke MJ et al (1998) Influence of more extensive radiotherapy and adjuvant chemotherapy on long-term outcome of early-stage Hodgkin's disease: a meta-analysis of 23 randomized trials involving 3,888 patients. International Hodgkin's Disease Collaborative Group. J Clin Oncol 16:830–843

Tomura N, Hirano H, Sashi R et al (1998) Comparison of MR imaging and CT in discriminating tumor infiltration of bone and bone marrow in the skull base. Comput Med Imaging Graph 22:41–51

van Baardwijk A, Baumert BG, Bosmans G et al (2006) The current status of FDG-PET in tumour volume definition in radiotherapy treatment planning. Cancer Treat Rev 32: 245–260

Vorwerk H, Obenauer S, Schmidberger H et al (2008) The significance of a uniform definition of pathological lymph nodes in Hodgkin lymphoma: impact of different thresholds for positive lymph nodes in CT imaging on staging and therapy. Radiother Oncol 87:74–81

Weihrauch MR, Re D, Bischoff S et al (2002) Whole-body positron emission tomography using 18F-fluorodeoxyglucose for initial staging of patients with Hodgkin's disease. Ann Hematol 81:20–25

Wirth A, Seymour JF, Hicks RJ et al (2002) Fluorine-18 fluorodeoxyglucose positron emission tomography, gallium-67 scintigraphy, and conventional staging for Hodgkin's disease and non-Hodgkin's lymphoma. Am J Med 112:262–268

Yahalom J (2005) Transformation in the use of radiation therapy of Hodgkin lymphoma: new concepts and indications lead to modern field design and are assisted by PET imaging and intensity modulated radiation therapy (IMRT). Eur J Haematol 75(suppl 66):90–97

Zinzani PL, Tani M, Fanti S et al (2006) Early positron emission tomography (PET) restaging: a predictive final response in Hodgkin's disease patients. Ann Oncol 17:1296–1300

Target Definitions for Hodgkin Lymphoma: The Involved Node Radiation Field Concept

9

Theodore Girinsky, Mithra Ghalibafian, and Lena Specht

Contents

T. Girinsky (✉)
Dept. of Radiation Oncology, Institut Gustave-Roussy, 39 Rue Camille Desmoulins, 94805 Villejuif Cedex, France
e-mail: girinsky@igr.fr

M. Ghalibafian
Dept. of Radiation Oncology, Mahak Hospital, Tehran, Iran

L. Specht
Depts. of Oncology and Haematology, The Finsen Centre, Rigshospitalet, University of Copenhagen, 9 Blegdamsvej, 2100 Copenhagen, Denmark
e-mail: specht@dadlnet.dk

9.1 Introduction

The involved node radiation (INRT) field concept was developed approximately 10 years ago when two fundamental facts became acknowledged. The first was the deleterious effect of large radiation fields and high radiation doses in terms of late complications (cardiovascular and second cancers) (Aleman et al. 2003; Bhatia et al. 1996; Hancock et al. 1993; Mauch 1995; Ng et al. 2002; van Leeuwen et al. 2003). The second was that the effectiveness of the new chemotherapy regimens was being persistently demonstrated (Bonadonna et al. 2004). Nevertheless, local relapses continued to be a major cause of treatment failure in patients treated with chemotherapy alone (Biti et al. 1992; Longo et al. 1991; Pavlovsky et al. 1988).

The basic assumption was that local relapses would occur preferentially, if not exclusively, in the initially involved nodes. This hypothesis was supported by Shahidi et al. who demonstrated that in patients with early-stage Hodgkin lymphoma (HL) treated with chemotherapy alone 83% of recurrences occurred in initially involved nodes, and in 45% it was the sole site of recurrence (Shahidi et al. 2006).

We also assumed that adding a small amount of radiation (in terms of total dose and field size) to fewer cycles of less toxic chemotherapy regimens would improve outcome of combined modality therapies (Donaldson et al. 2007; Landman-Parker et al. 2000). We reasoned that this strategy would result in a reduction in the incidence of late complications caused by either radiation and/or chemotherapy.

The new concept with regard to radiotherapy for HL means that only the initially involved lymph nodes should be irradiated. This implies that the initially

L. Specht and J. Yahalom (eds.), *Radiotherapy for Hodgkin Lymphoma*,
DOI: 10.1007/978-3-540-78944-4_9, © Springer-Verlag Berlin Heidelberg 2011

involved lymph nodes should first be accurately identified (Girinsky et al. 2008). Hence, the involved nodes delineated on the CT scan performed before chemotherapy should be correctly and precisely applied to post-chemotherapy CT scans (Girinsky et al. 2006).

This new concept, which will be described below, may possibly represent an (unavoidable) intermediary step between the former involved field concept and the next possible foreseeable concept of delivering radiation to post-chemotherapy lymph node remnants alone.

As radiation fields become smaller, the complexity of devising them and consequently the risk of errors may increase considerably. To minimize the risk of mistakes, stringent imaging acquisition and contouring methods are mandatory.

9.2 Imaging Procedure Guidelines for the Assessment of Initially Involved Lymph Nodes and the Design of Involved Node Radiation Fields

As mentioned above, implementing stringent imaging procedures is essential to obtain accurate co-registrations of pre- and post-chemotherapy scans. Imaging should be performed on patients in the treatment position and the use of i.v. contrast should be mandatory. Before chemotherapy an FDG-PET/CT scan should be performed. After chemotherapy the usual CT simulation should be carried out.

The procedure commonly employed in centers using the INRT concept is as follows:

- A pre-chemotherapy PET/CT is performed (usually as part of the staging procedure) with i.v. contrast and with the patient in a position suited for later radiotherapy. If the quality of the CT scan of the PET/CT is unsatisfactory, an additional separate CT scan can be performed before chemotherapy (always in the treatment position). It is noteworthy that PET/CT scans performed with i.v. contrast exhibit only minimal differences in terms of SUV (standardized uptake value) from PET/CT scans performed without contrast, and that the contrast has no impact on the clinical diagnostic interpretation (Berthelsen et al. 2005). Performing the CT scan with i.v. contrast is critical as lymph node involvement can be extremely difficult to assess without it. A lymph node can be mistaken for a muscle, blood vessel or even a cardiac cavity (see Fig. 9.1).
- A post-chemotherapy planning CT is performed as usual with the patient immobilized in the same position as for the pre-chemotherapy PET/CT.
- The pre-chemotherapy PET/CT is co-registered with the post-chemotherapy planning CT. Figures 9.2–9.4 demonstrate the need to perform these imaging procedures on patients in the treatment position in order to obtain good co-registration images, as deformable co-registration procedures are not yet generally available for routine use. Proper co-registration of all imaging procedures not only allows one to take full advantage of the information provided by the PET scan, but also permits accurate assessment of lymph node shrinkage or disappearance on the post-chemotherapy CT simulation. Both the information provided by the pre-chemotherapy FDG-PET and the post-chemotherapy CT simulation are crucial for the radiotherapy planning. Moreover, the information on lymph node shrinkage may be used as surrogate proof of initial histological involvement.

9.3 Assessment and Delineation of Initially Involved Lymph Nodes

9.3.1 Introduction

Simple and practical guidelines are required so that the new concept of radiation fields can be adequately implemented in daily clinical practice and so that lymph node involvement can be accurately diagnosed. Indeed, the current definitions of lymph node involvement cannot be used reliably. If a threshold of 1–1.5 cm in the longest diameter were used (Cheson et al. 1999, 2007; Lister et al. 1989), all visible lymph nodes on each CT scan slice would have to be measured and this would be too time consuming. It could also lead to incorrect assumptions about lymph node involvement for to two main reasons. First, in HL a change in lymph node architecture caused by HL involvement does not necessarily lead to a corresponding change in lymph node size (Castellino et al. 1984; Guermazi 2001;

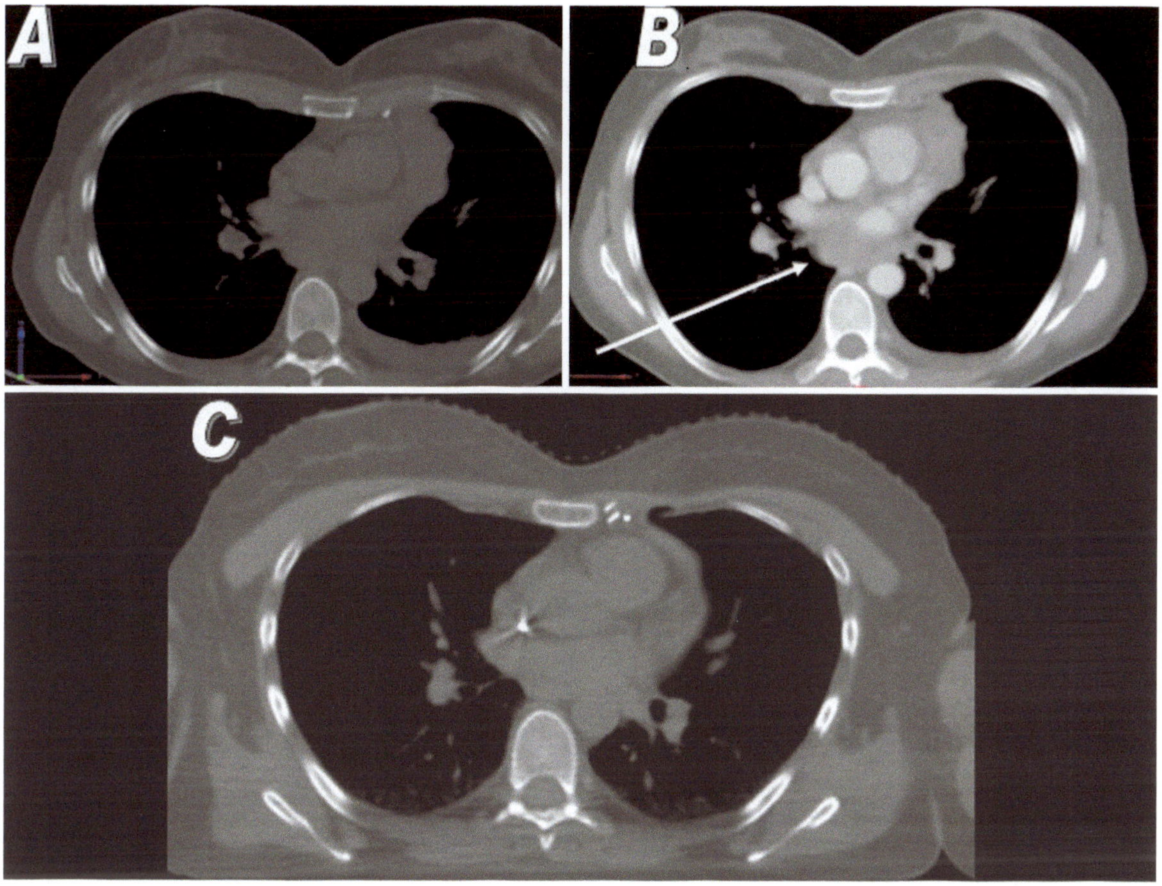

Fig. 9.1 (**a**) Chest CT scan without i.v. contrast. (**b**) Chest CT scan with i.v. contrast revealing a subcarinal mass that could have been mistaken for the left auricle. (**c**) CT simulation performed after chemotherapy

Hanna et al. 1993). Examples of this are shown in Figs. 9.5–9.8, demonstrating initial involvement of small lymph nodes. Second, on transverse CT scan slices, the size criterion is even less reliable because lymph nodes are cross sectioned in various directions. Today, the assessment of initially involved lymph nodes and the delineation of involved node radiation fields can be achieved with great accuracy. This is partly due to the introduction and commercialization of PET/CT scanners allowing proper fusion between morphological and metabolic imaging modalities. Metabolic imaging is particularly useful in HL as lymph node involvement can in some cases be demonstrated by morphological criteria exclusively through a change in architecture visible only on lymphography (Castellino et al. 1984; Guermazi 2001; Hanna et al. 1993). The diagnostic usefulness of the PET scan was demonstrated by Vallete et al., showing a close correlation between FDG-PET and lymphography in patients with negative CT scans of the infradiaphragmatic area (Valette et al. 2007). However, it must be stressed that FDG-PET should only be used for diagnostic purposes (Girinsky et al. 2007; Hutchings et al. 2007; Specht 2007). Contouring should not be performed using FDG-PET alone for three main reasons. First, large tumor masses can exhibit heterogeneous FDG avidity (see Fig. 9.9). Second, FDG-avid areas may not be lymph nodes (see Fig. 9.9). Third, some involved lymph nodes may exhibit low or no FDG avidity (see Figs. 9.6 and 9.7). This phenomenon has been demonstrated in HL (Girinsky et al. 2007), and it was also proven true in a recent meta-analysis in patients with head and neck cancers (Kyzas et al. 2008). The assistance of a radiologist and a nuclear medicine physician in the contouring of involved lymph nodes is highly advisable whenever possible.

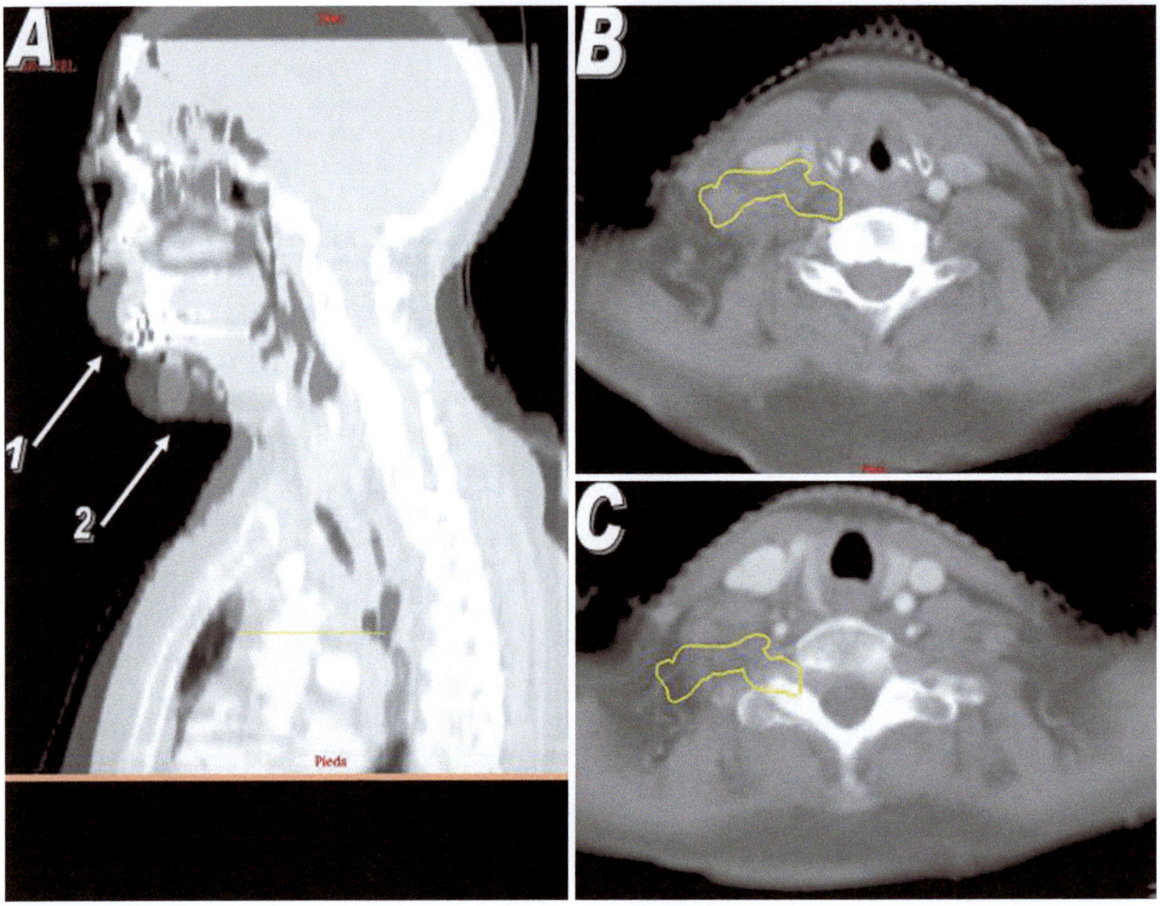

Fig. 9.2 (**a**) Co-registration of pre- and post-chemotherapy CT scans: arrow #1 shows the position of the chin on the pre-chemotherapy CT scan and arrow #2 its position on the post-chemotherapy CT scan. (**b**) Delineation of involved lymph nodes on the pre-chemotherapy CT scan (*yellow outline*). (**c**) The superimposition of lymph node contouring on the post-chemotherapy CT scan is obviously wrongly located because of different treatment positions shown in A

However, it is recommended that the radiation oncologist seeks to improve his or her own expertise.

9.3.2 Assessment of Initially Involved Lymph Nodes

Two prerequisites are essential for proper assessment of lymph node involvement. First, all patients should have pre- and post-chemotherapy cervical, thoracic, abdominal and pelvic CT scans (axillary lymph node areas should be clearly visible on thoracic CT scans). Second, the assessment of initial lymph node involvement should be carried out with full knowledge of the natural history of the disease (e.g., natural disease spread to local adjacent areas, multiple small lymph nodes adjacent to a grossly involved area).

9.3.2.1 Stepwise Assessment of Lymph Node Involvement

A meticulous analysis of all imaging procedures should be carried out using a stepwise approach. From an efficiency point of view, it is highly advisable to assess initially involved lymph nodes and delineate the involved node fields on the same day (less time consuming and greater precision). This becomes absolutely indispensable when co-registration of various imaging procedures is unsatisfactory (likely to occur if patients were not placed in the treatment position).

First, the analysis of the pre-chemotherapy CT scan should be considered as a preliminary evaluation of the initially involved lymph nodes.

Second, these preliminary findings are complemented with FDG-PET metabolic information. Examples obtained from various cancer centers in

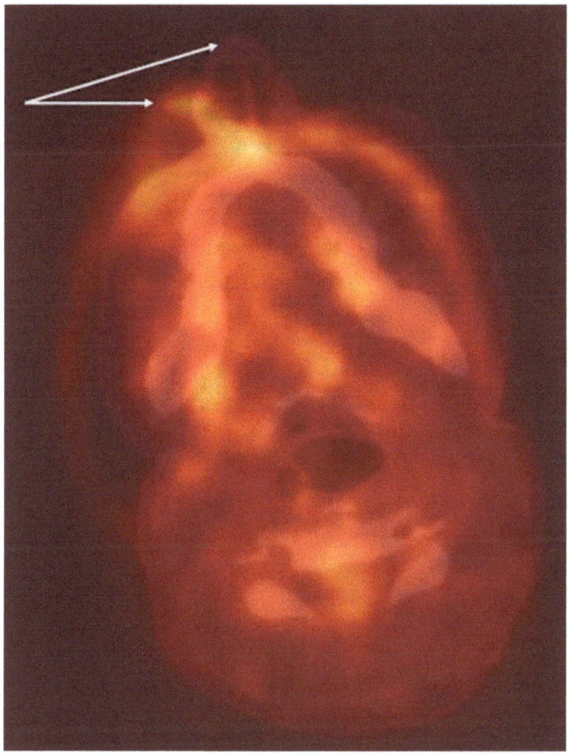

Fig. 9.3 A PET/CT carried out on a patient who was not in the treatment position. Adequate scan fusion is impossible with such imaging procedures which thus preclude an accurate detection of initially involved lymph nodes

France indicated that, in most cases, pre-chemotherapy PET/CT scans were not acquired with i.v. contrast. Under such circumstances, a meticulous analysis of the FDG-PET becomes invaluable and usually provides additional data.

After these two steps, a "pre-chemotherapy assessment" of the initially involved nodes is submitted.

The third and final step is the comparison of the pre-chemotherapy CT with the CT simulation performed after chemotherapy. The disappearance or shrinkage of the "proposed" initially involved lymph nodes can be considered as proof of initial involvement.

We will not discuss obvious unilateral or bilateral lymph node involvement, which is beyond the scope of this chapter. We will however provide examples and clues which could facilitate the detection of inconspicuous involved lymph nodes.

9.3.2.2 The Pre-Chemotherapy Assessment

Asymmetry on the pre-chemotherapy CT and/or PET scan is extremely useful, especially when imaging procedures were performed without IV contrast.

- First proposition based on the analysis of the CT scan

Slight asymmetries in cervical, axillary, hilar and internal mammary lymph node areas may be detected (see Fig. 9.10). In general, an asymmetry on CT scan slices should be considered as an indication of possible lymph node involvement.

- Second proposition based on the analysis of FDG-PET and CT scan.

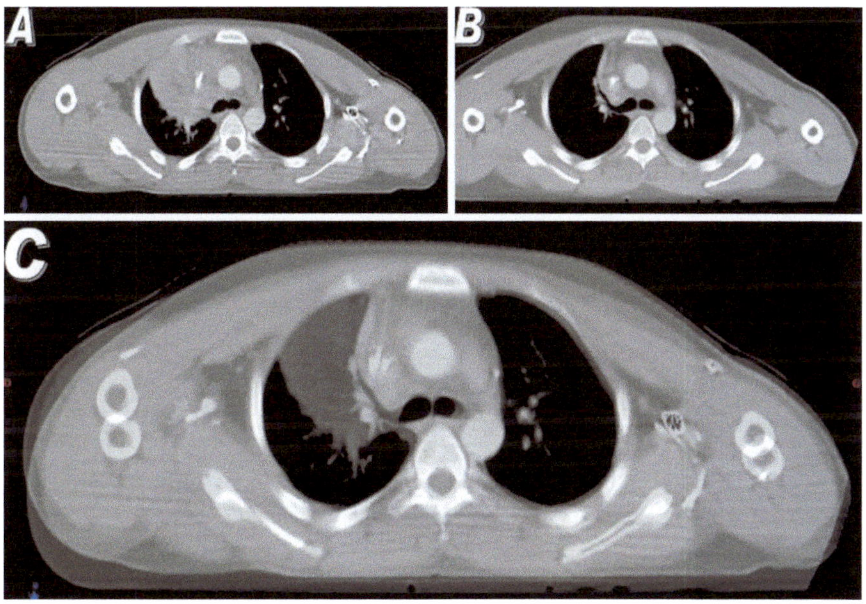

Fig. 9.4 Example of excellent co-registration in a patient in the right treatment position during the pre- and post-chemotherapy CT scan. (**a**) Axial CT scan before chemotherapy. (**b**) Axial CT scan after chemotherapy. (**c**) Fusion image showing tumor regression after chemotherapy

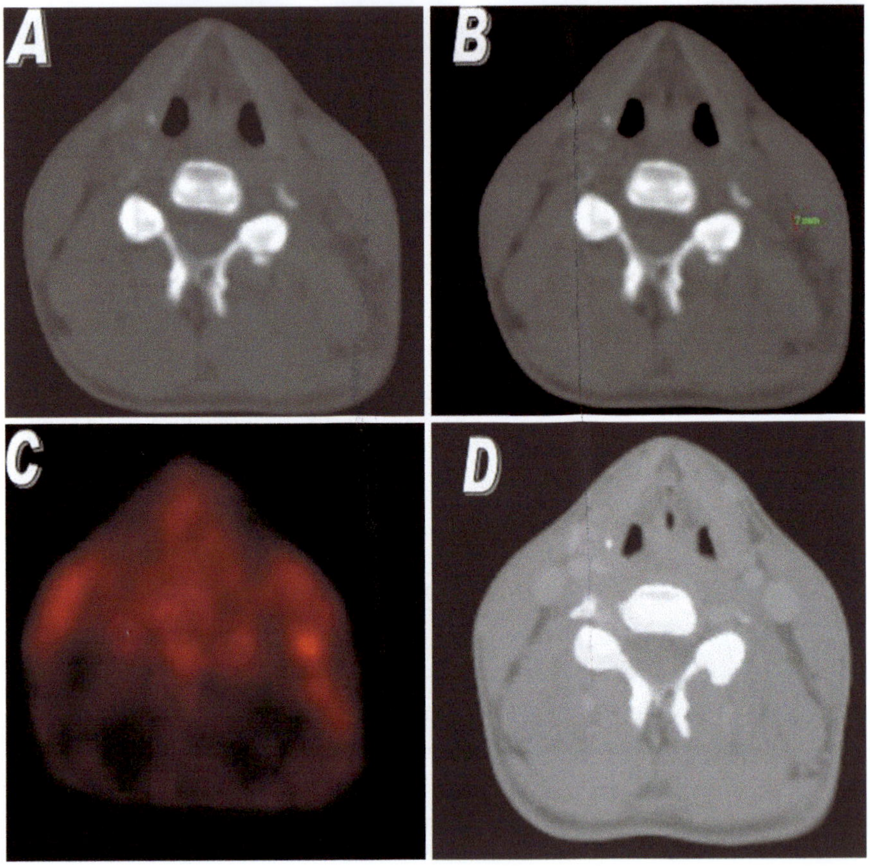

Fig. 9.5 (**a**) Small lymph nodes in the left cervical area on a pre-chemotherapy CT scan. (**b**) Measurement of the larger lymph node (7 mm in its largest diameter). (**c**) Fusion of the pre-chemotherapy CT and PET scan. (**d**) Left cervical area on a post-chemotherapy CT scan (CT simulation).

The FDG-PET analysis may reinforce previous findings on CT (see Fig. 9.11). A careful and precise analysis of FDG-PET may even provide additional information (see Fig. 9.11b and d). An important point should be underlined. In our experience, even faint FDG avidity could signal lymph node involvement. The faint signal is probably emanating from a small number of cells. In all cases, the suspected lymph node on the pre-chemotherapy CT scan should be compared with the corresponding one on the post-chemotherapy CT scan.

In some cases, FDG-PET analysis does not support the previous CT findings (see Figs. 9.6d–g and 9.12). In a few cases, the analysis of the PET scan casts doubts on earlier CT findings because there is no PET avidity in that area. The final decision then will mainly rely on the CT scan analysis performed after chemotherapy (false FDG-PET negative in Fig. 9.6, true FDG-PET negative in Fig. 9.12).

The FDG-PET analysis may provide additional information. In most cases, detecting initially involved lymph nodes can be extremely difficult if imaging procedures were carried out without i.v. contrast. In those cases, FDG-PET could be extremely useful because of its ability to detect involved lymph nodes which were otherwise overlooked. In some reports, FDG-PET allowed the detection of overlooked lymph nodes in 25–36% of the patients (Girinsky et al. 2007; Hutchings et al. 2007; Specht 2007). FDG-PET can provide strong additional information but in a few cases, it simply adds further clues to those seen on the pre-chemotherapy CT scan (see Figs. 9.5, 9.6a, b, 9.7, and 9.13g, h). In this case, further suspicion should be verified with the post-chemotherapy CT scan. Strong additional data are displayed in Figs. 9.13 (cervical areas), 9.14 (axillary areas), 9.15 and 9.16 (mediastinal areas), 9.17 (thoracic wall), and 9.18 (internal mammary and infradiaphragmatic lymph node areas).

- Synopsis of the analysis of the pre-chemotherapy imaging procedures.

In most cases, the first proposition based on CT is further reinforced by the PET scan analysis. However, in

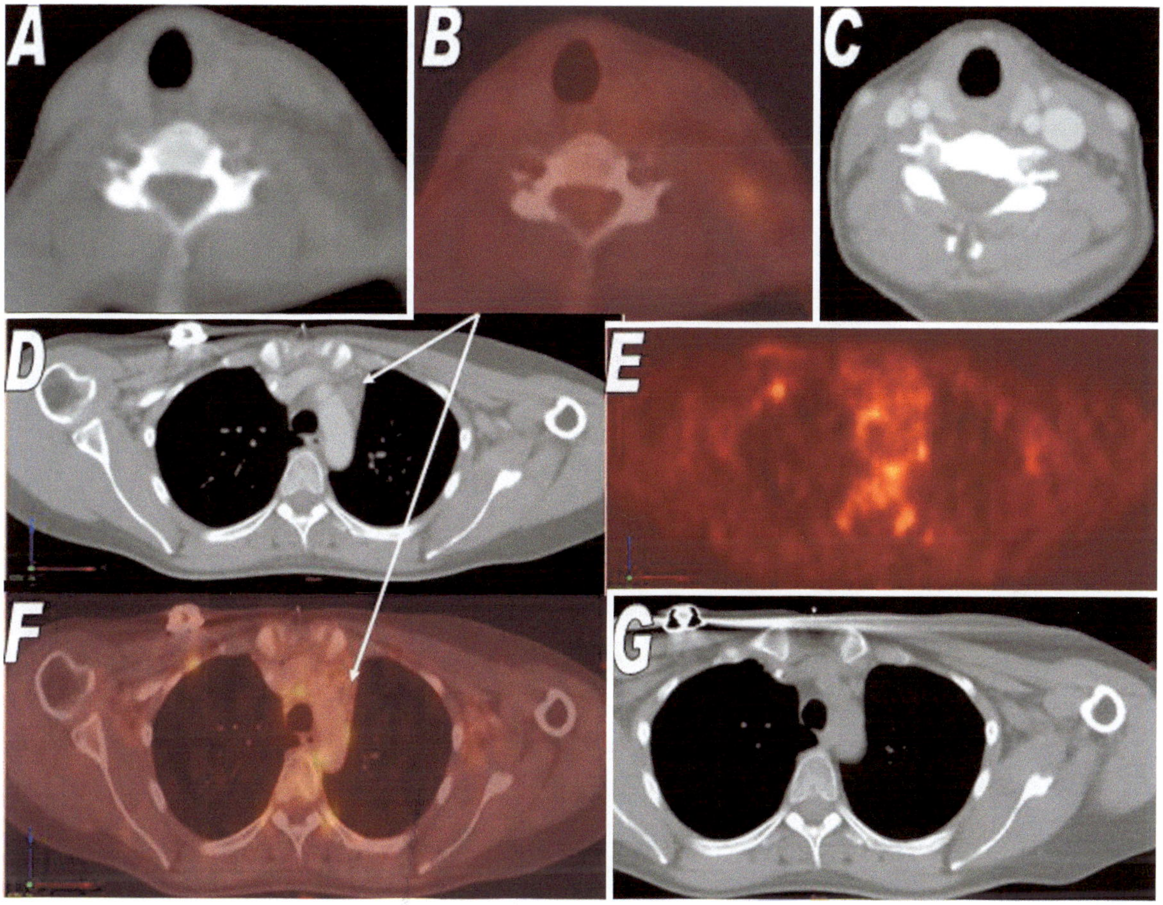

Fig. 9.6 (**a**) Left cervical area with a few small lymph nodes. (**b**) Faint FDG avidity in the left cervical area. (**c**) Left cervical area on a post-chemotherapy CT scan showing almost complete remission. (**d**) Small mediastinal lymph node abutting the aortic arch on a pre-chemotherapy CT scan. (**e**) Absence of lymph node FDG avidity. (**f**) Absence of lymph node FDG avidity on the PET/CT fusion. (**g**) Mediastinal area on a post-chemotherapy CT scan showing a decrease in size of the lymph node

a few cases, radiation oncologists might be faced with conflicting data between these two pre-chemotherapy imaging procedures. In the latter case, the final decision as to whether lymph nodes are involved or not, relies on a comparison with the post-chemotherapy CT scan. Complete remission or a decrease in the size of lymph nodes can be considered tantamount to surrogate proof of initial involvement.

9.3.2.3 Final Conclusion Based on the Analysis of Post-Chemotherapy CT Scans

Figures 9.5–9.8 show that initially small and more or less FDG-avid lymph nodes decreased in size or were in complete remission after chemotherapy. These findings indicate that all lymph nodes were initially involved and that they should all be included in the INRT fields. Interestingly, Fig. 9.6d–g show that a non-FDG-avid mediastinal lymph node shrank significantly after chemotherapy and therefore should be irradiated. On the other hand, Fig. 9.9 shows that although there were two highly FDG-avid areas in the mediastinum (c and d) the pre-chemotherapy CT scan did not depict obvious lymph node involvement. The post-chemotherapy CT scan confirmed the absence of any change in that area which should therefore not be irradiated. Figure 9.19 shows that the possible lymph node involvement seen on the pre-chemotherapy CT and PET scans (Figs. 9.10 and 9.11) had actually disappeared or regressed, and consequently it should be included in the INRT fields.

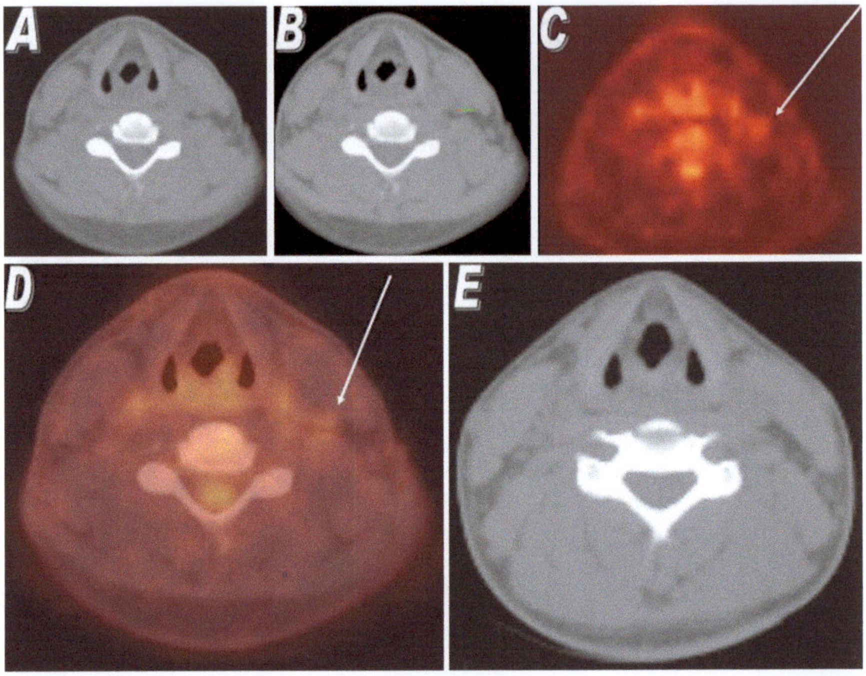

Fig. 9.7 (**a**) Small left cervical node abutting the jugular vein. (**b**) Lymph node largest diameter = 8.5 mm. (**c**) Slight asymmetry on the FDG-PET in the left cervical area. (**d**) Fusion of the CT and FDG-PET showing faint FDG avidity of the lymph node. (**e**) Left cervical area on the post-chemotherapy CT simulation

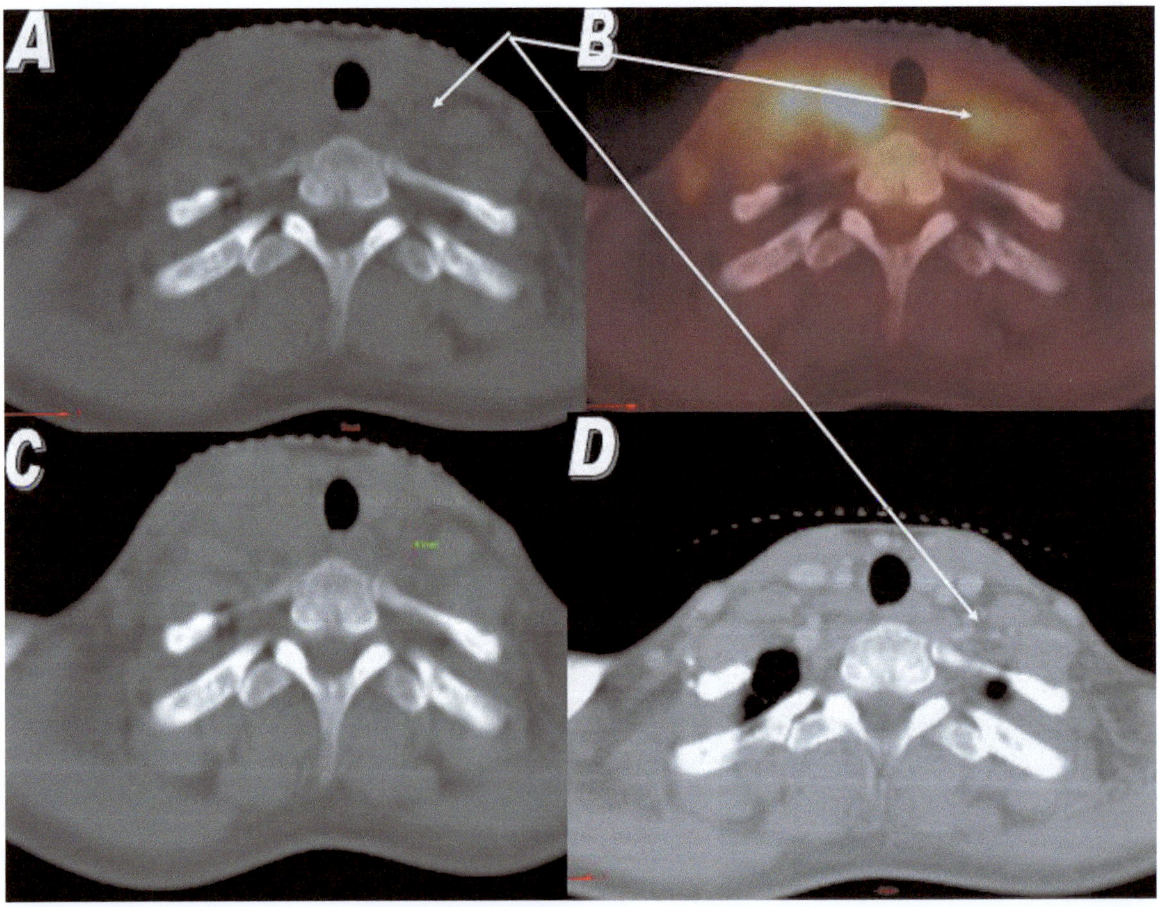

Fig. 9.8 (**a**) Small left cervical node abutting the anterior scalene muscle. (**b**) Lymph node largest diameter = 9.5 mm. (**c**) Low FDG avidity of the lymph node. (**d**) Left cervical area after chemotherapy on the CT simulation

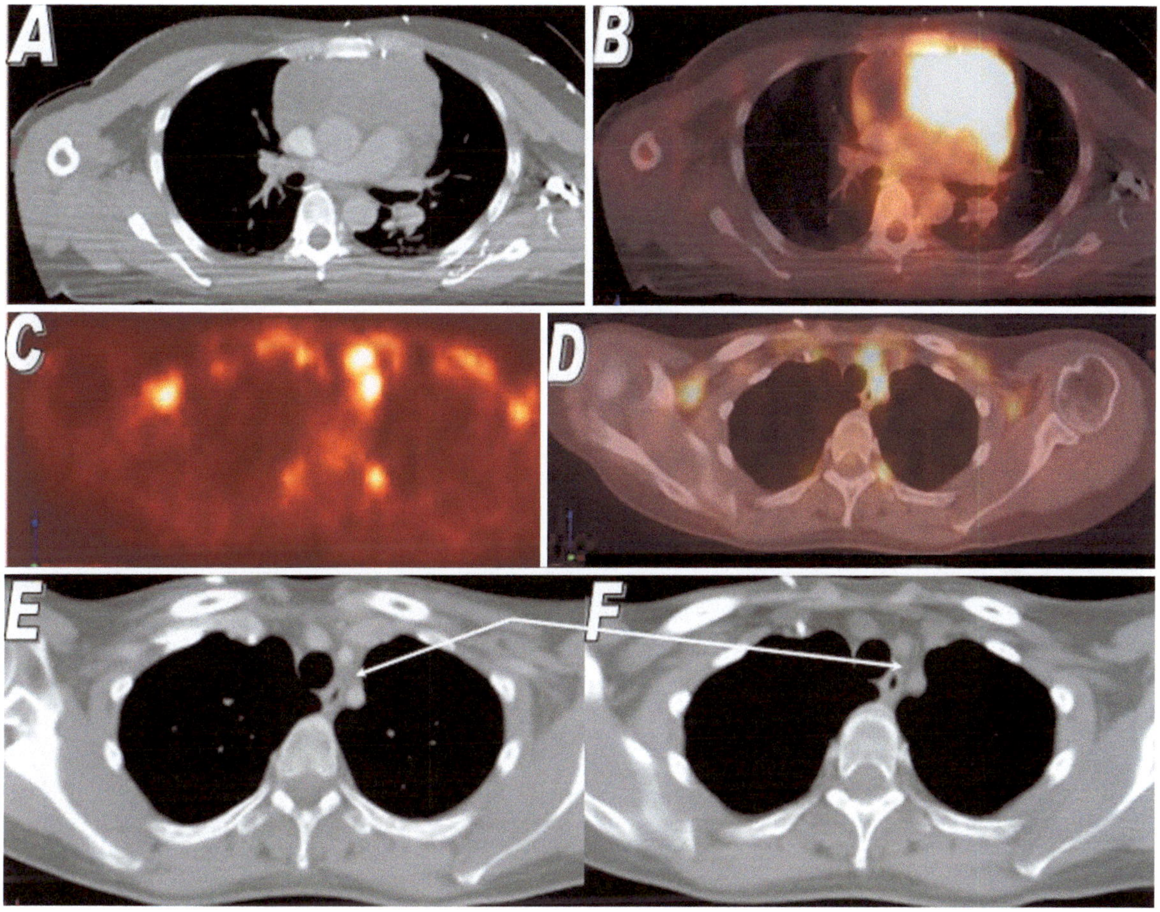

Fig. 9.9 (**a**) A large mediastinal mass on the pre-chemotherapy CT scan. (**b**) Fusion of the CT and FDG-PET showing heterogeneous FDG-avid mass. (**c**) FDG-PET of the upper part of the mediastinum before chemotherapy. (**d**) Fusion of the CT and FDG-PET showing brown fat avidity of the axillary areas as well as two highly FDG-avid areas in the mediastinum. (**e**) Normal upper mediastinum on a CT scan before chemotherapy. (**f**) Upper mediastinum on a CT simulation with no change after chemotherapy

Figures 9.20–9.23 show that the additional information provided by PET (Figs. 9.13–9.16, respectively) was correct as all the overlooked lymph nodes on CT scan images are in complete remission or CRu (unconfirmed complete remission). The lymph nodes were therefore initially involved and should be included in the INRT fields.

Figure 9.24 shows complete remission of initial thoracic wall involvement (Fig. 9.17). That part of the thoracic wall should therefore be included in the INRT fields with adequate radiation coverage. Figure 9.25 shows a complete remission status of the initially involved internal mammary nodes (Fig. 9.18).

9.3.2.4 Conclusions

A precise and stepwise analysis of all pre- and post-chemotherapy images allows accurate assessment of initially involved lymph nodes. Such steps are absolutely essential when planning proper INRT.

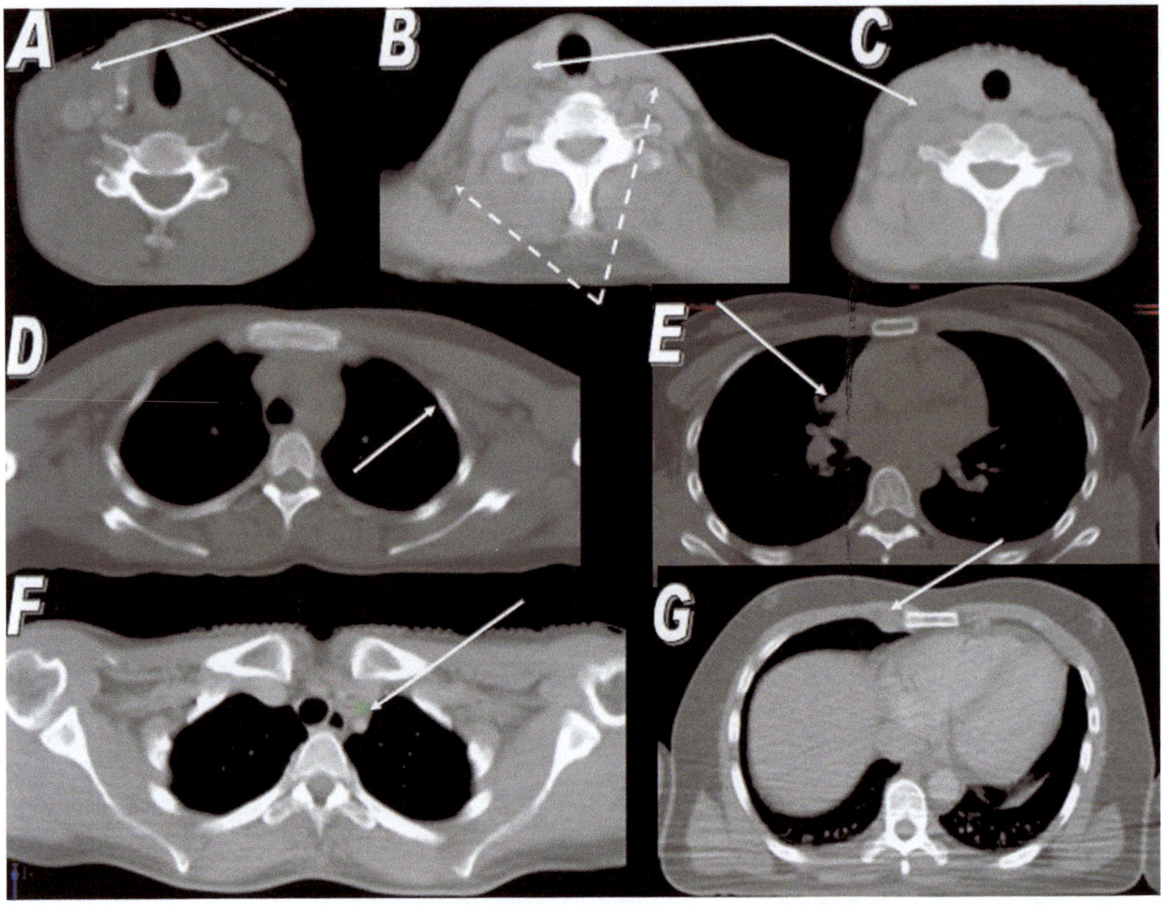

Fig. 9.10 (**a**) Enlargement of the sternocleiodomastoid muscle without clearly visible lymph nodes. (**b, c**) Slight asymmetry in the right cervical area. (**d**) Asymmetry between axillary areas looking slightly abnormal on the left. (**e**) Slight abnormality located close to the superior vena cava. (**f**) Small left paratracheal mediastinal lymph node (9.4 mm). (**g**) Right internal mammary region looks asymmetrical compared to the other side

9.4 Delineation of Involved Node Fields

9.4.1 General Guidelines

A few essential guidelines for delineating INRT fields should be strictly applied. As mentioned above, the correct delineation and implementation of involved node fields relies on contrast-enhanced imaging procedures performed with the patient in the treatment position. These procedures allow properly co-registered images and accurately delineated involved node radiation fields.

9.4.1.1 Pre-Chemotherapy Contouring

Pre-chemotherapy contouring is based on the informa tion assembled from FDG-PET and CT which was described in the previous paragraph. Contouring on the pre-chemotherapy CT scan outlines the area where all initially involved nodes are located. There are three simple reasons underlying such contouring. First, it would be impossible, tedious and also too time consuming to contour each involved lymph node. Second, it would be unwise to assume that the exact position of the initially involved lymph node could be accurately reproduced on a CT scan performed a few months after

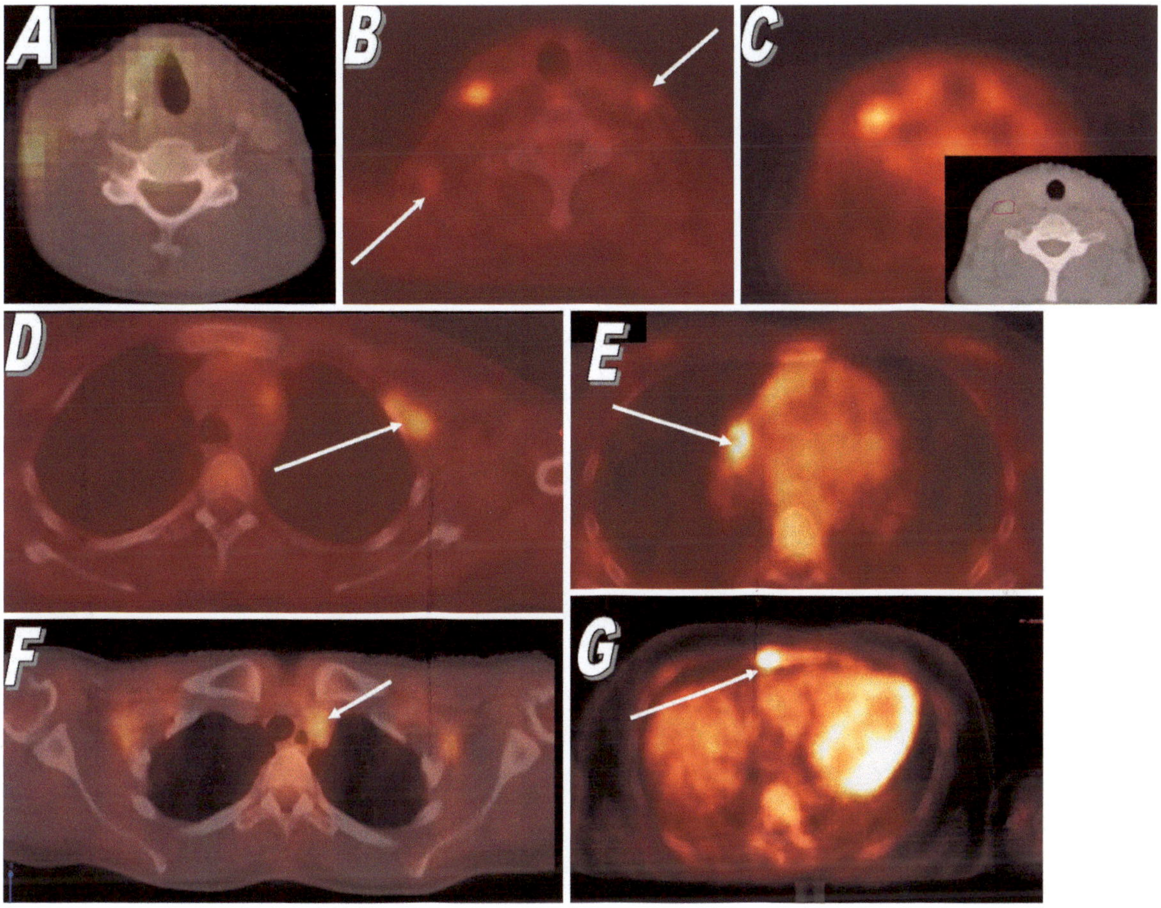

Fig. 9.11 (**a**) FDG-avid area in the right cervical area by the sternocleidomastoid muscle. (**b**) FDG avidity of the posteriorly located lymph node. In addition, a possible FDG-avid area abutting the trapezius muscle in the left cervical area and an additional area in the right cervical area (*dotted lines* on Figure 9.10). (**c**) The small abnormality in the left cervical area is FDG avid. (**d**) The left axillary area shows two FDG-avid abnormalities. In addition, there is a small faintly FDG-avid lymph node in the mediastinum. (**e**) The area above the right hilum is FDG avid suggesting the presence of an involved lymph node. (**f**) The small lymph node exhibits high FDG avidity. (**g**) The right internal mammary area is FDG avid confirming its involvement

chemotherapy. Third, it would also be unwise to presuppose that irradiation would be precisely delivered to those precisely delineated lymph nodes during each fraction of fractionated radiotherapy.

9.4.1.2 Post-Chemotherapy Contouring

Post-chemotherapy contouring readjusts the superimposed pre-chemotherapy outline according to the normal structures in the vicinity. Normal structures that were displaced by the initially enlarged lymph nodes or tumor masses should not be included in the irradiated volume. Also, whenever possible, cervical blood vessels should be protected (e.g., when initially involved lymph nodes were at a distance from them).

9.4.2 Specific Guidelines

9.4.2.1 Introduction

The remission status after chemotherapy should at least for the time being be exclusively verified on CT scans for each initially involved lymph node. Complete

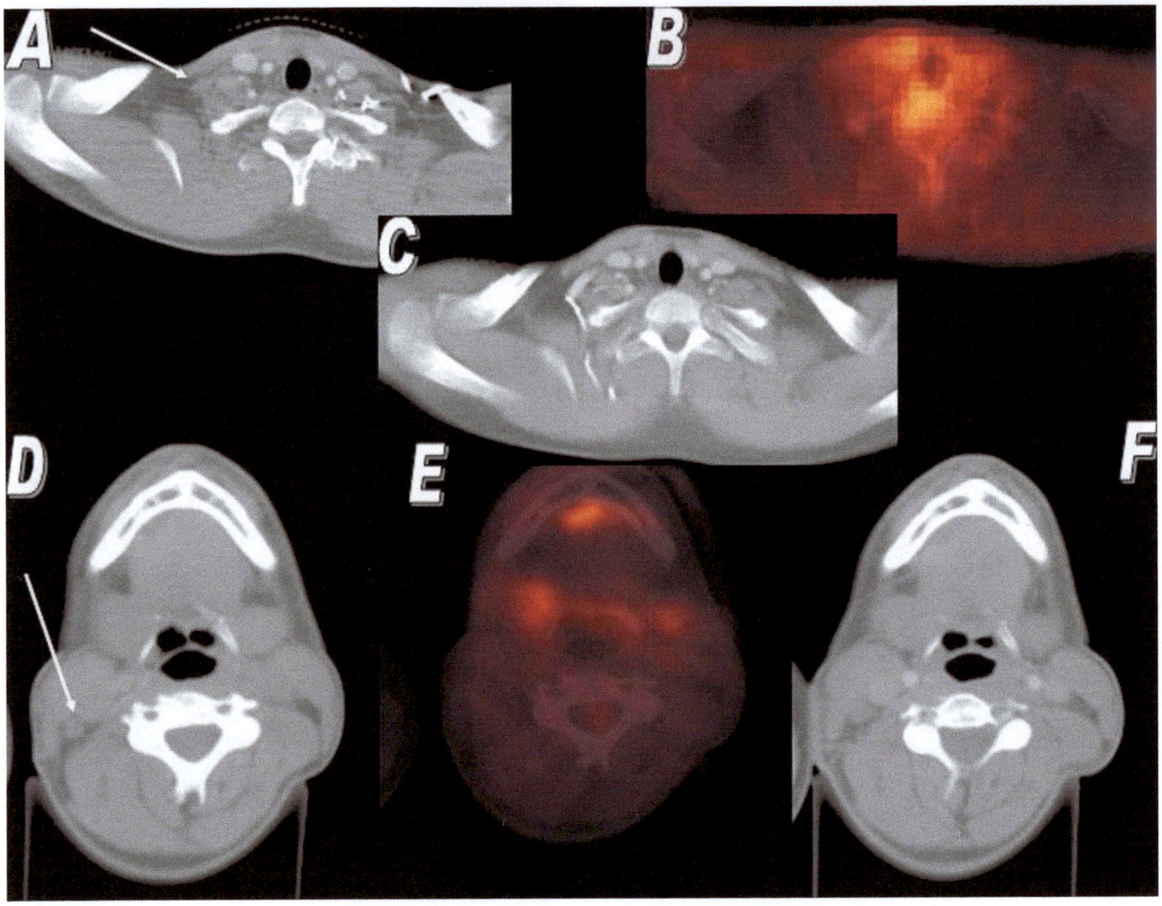

Fig. 9.12 (**a**) The right cervical area looks suspicious (two possible lymph nodes). (**b**) The analysis of the PET scan does not show any FDG avidity in the area. (**c**) The final proof is provided by the post-chemotherapy CT scan showing a blood vessel. (**d**) A suspicious lymph node in the right cervical area. (**e**) FDG-PET shows no FDG avidity. (**f**) The post-chemotherapy CT scan demonstrates no change in the lymph node size

remission (CR) is defined as the complete disappearance of clinically and/or radiologically detectable disease. A complete remission unconfirmed (Cru) is defined as at least a 75% decrease in tumor size. A partial response (PR) is at least a 50% decrease in tumor size. Failure is less than a 50% decrease or any increase in tumor size (Cheson et al. 1999).

Assessing remission on CT alone was decided many years ago by the EORTC lymphoma group when we embarked upon the involved node radiation field concept. The rationale was based mostly on two facts. First, at that time, data on the possible use of FDG-PET for assessing the remission status were scant. Second, in order to properly appraise the value of the new INRT concept, it was not advisable to modify any other previous criteria or treatment parameters (e.g., the definition of the remission status or the radiation dose given to patients in CR, CRu or PR). In addition, with FDG-PET there is still wide variability between readers and equipment, leading to a risk of false positive or negative results. If response criteria and radiation doses change in the next few years, the guidelines will have to be slightly modified.

9.4.2.2 Initially Involved Lymph Nodes in CR or CRu

- General rules

In case of CR or CRu, a clinical target volume (CTV) should be determined. Conceptually, the CTV is the

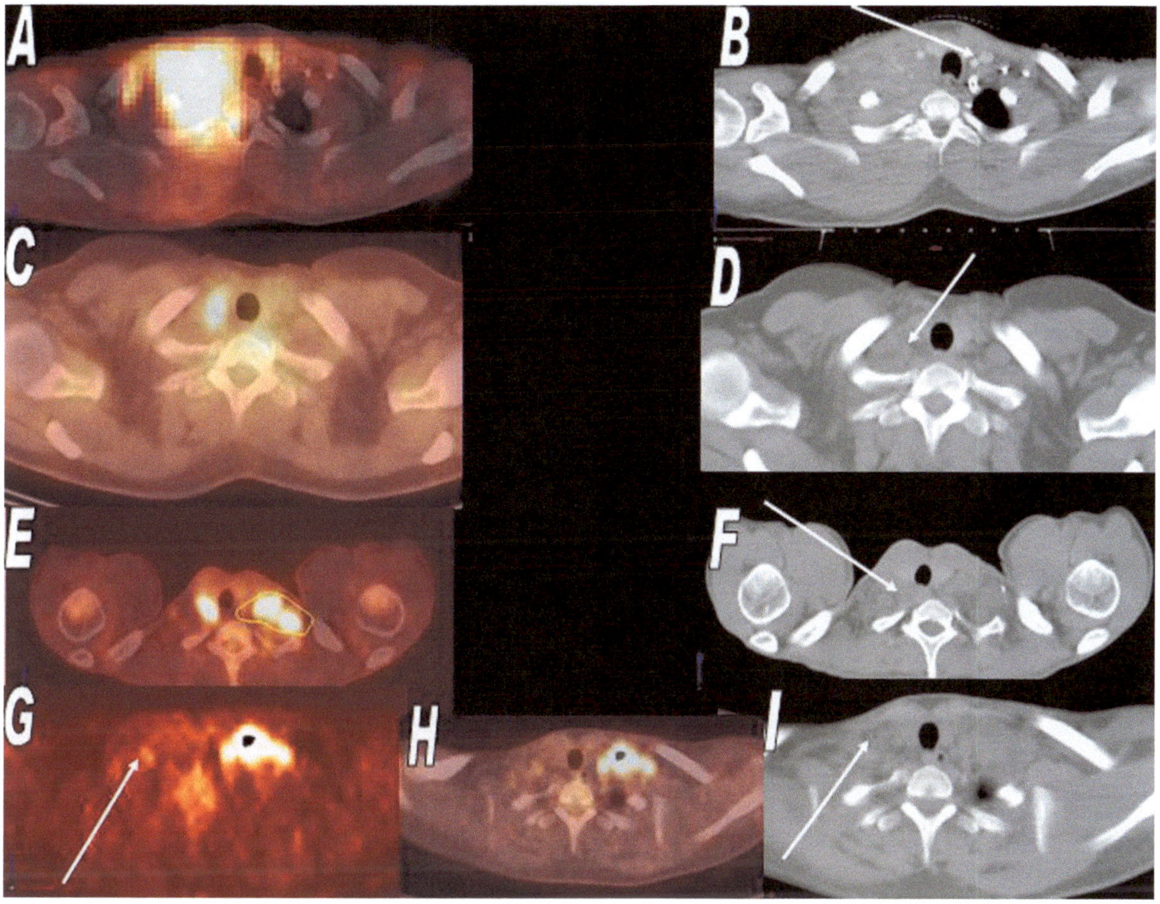

Fig. 9.13 (**a**) PET/CT fusion of a supraclavicular area showing an additional left paratracheal lymph node that is difficult to visualize on the CT scan (**b**). (**c**) Right FDG-avid supraclavicular lymph node barely visible on the CT scan (**d**). (**e**) PET/CT fusion depicting a lymph node in the right cervical area that is difficult to visualize on the CT scan (**f**). (**g**) Possible additional right cervical node on FDG-PET and PET/CT fusion (**h**). (**i**) CT scan axial slice of the area

initial volume of each lymph node before chemotherapy. As described in the previous paragraph, from a practical point of view, the CTV is the addition of all areas where involved lymph nodes were initially located.

The planning target volume (PTV) is the CTV with a margin that takes into account organ movements and set-up variations. In most cases a 1 cm isotropic margin is sufficient.

- Cervical and axillary lymph node areas

Figure 9.26 shows a left cervical area (a) with multiple small lymph nodes. Contouring outlines the whole left cervical area (b). Additional contouring (d) is added as a result of the data provided by FDG-PET (c). Figure 9.27 shows the reasoning behind the design of the final involved node radiation field. The superimposed pre-chemotherapy contours were corrected to conform to the post-chemotherapy anatomy and to avoid pointless irradiation of normal tissues. The final CTV is thus obtained. The same reasoning and methodology apply to the axillary areas.

- Mediastinal area

A few guidelines can be added for the design of mediastinal involved node fields. First, the length of the

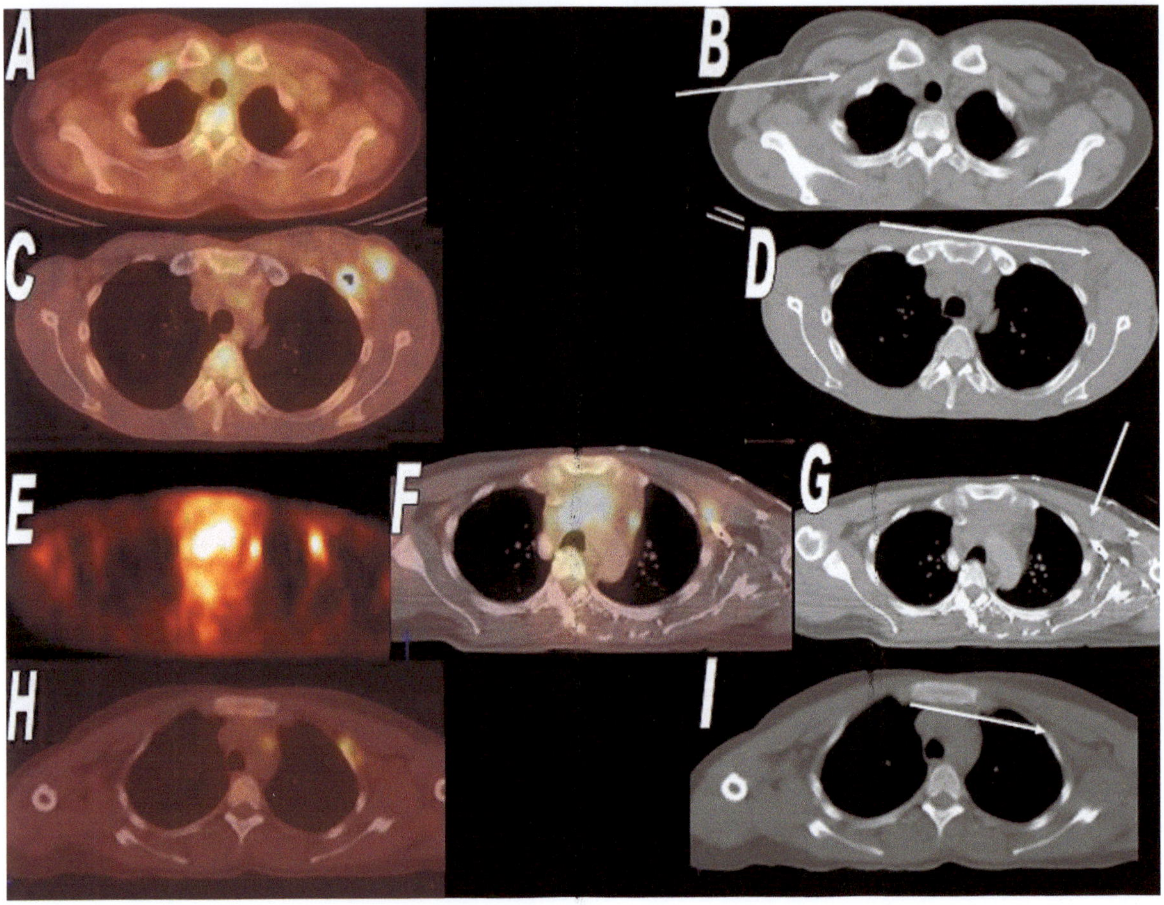

Fig. 9.14 (**a**) FDG-avid area under the pectoralis minor muscle (indicated by an arrow on Figure (**b**)). (**c**) Two FDG-avid areas in the left axilla depicting axillary lymph nodes which could be missed (**d**). (**e, f**) Unexpected FDG-avid area in the left axilla pinpointing a small axillary lymph node located under the pectoralis minor muscle (**g**). (**h**) Small FDG-avid area in the left axilla associated with a small lymph node (**i**)

CTV is the length of the mediastinal mass *before* chemotherapy, and its width is that of the mediastinal mass *after* chemotherapy. Second, in case of a CR, the CTV should not exceed the lateral outline of the normal mediastinum. Third, whenever possible, the origin of the coronaries as well as the cardiac cavities should be excluded from the CTV (e.g., in cases of complete remission or excellent regression of a tumor mass which was initially impinging on those two former organs at risk (see Fig. 9.28]). Figure 9.29 shows a first proposition based on the pre-chemotherapy CT scan (b), then the pre chemotherapy synopsis (d) based on the additional data provided by FDG-PET. The analysis of the post-chemotherapy CT scan corroborates the pre-chemotherapy synopsis as initially involved lymph nodes have either decreased or are in CR. The CTV is then based on previous contourings (e), and the final proposal for the CTV is shown in (f).

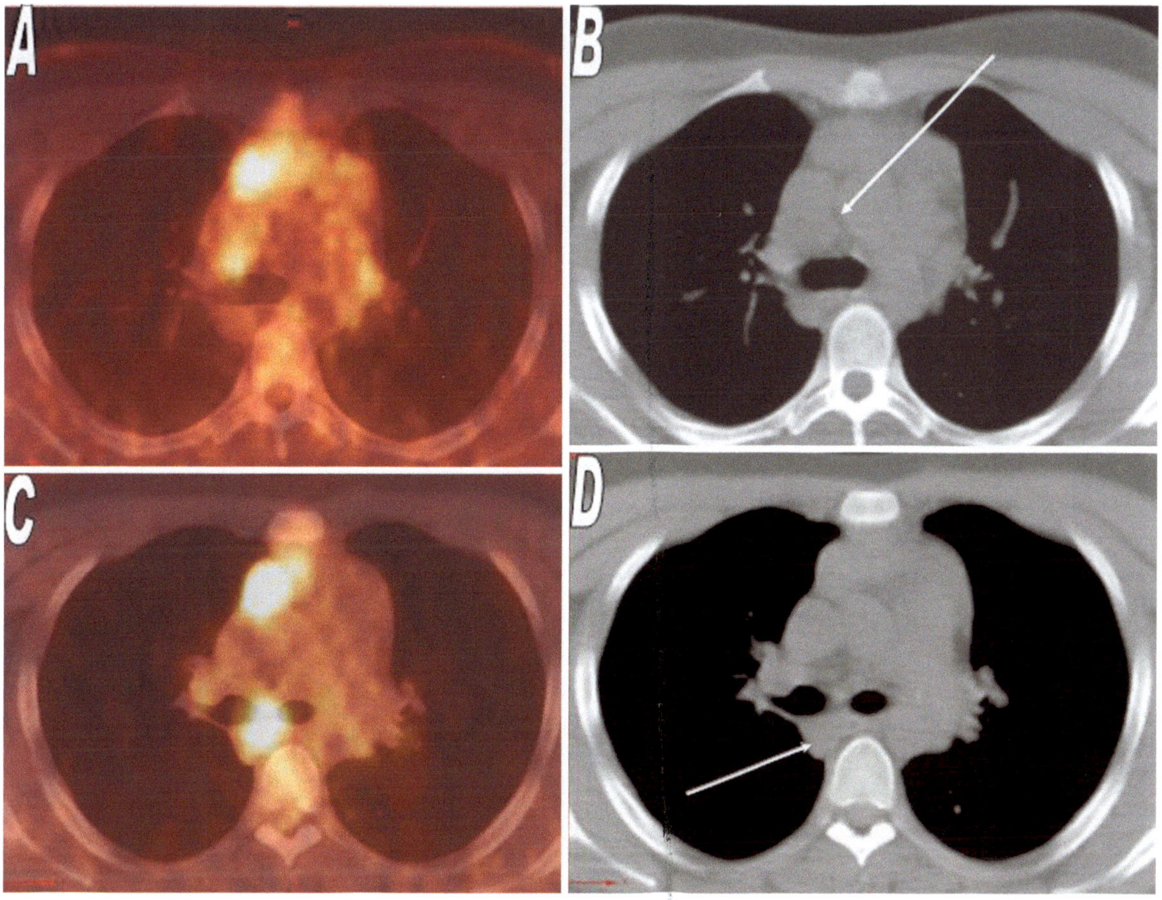

Fig. 9.15 (**a**) FDG-avid lymph node under the superior vena cava, that is difficult to visualize on the CT scan slice without IV contrast (**b**). (**c**) FDG-avid area revealing a subcarinal lymph node that could have been overlooked (**d**)

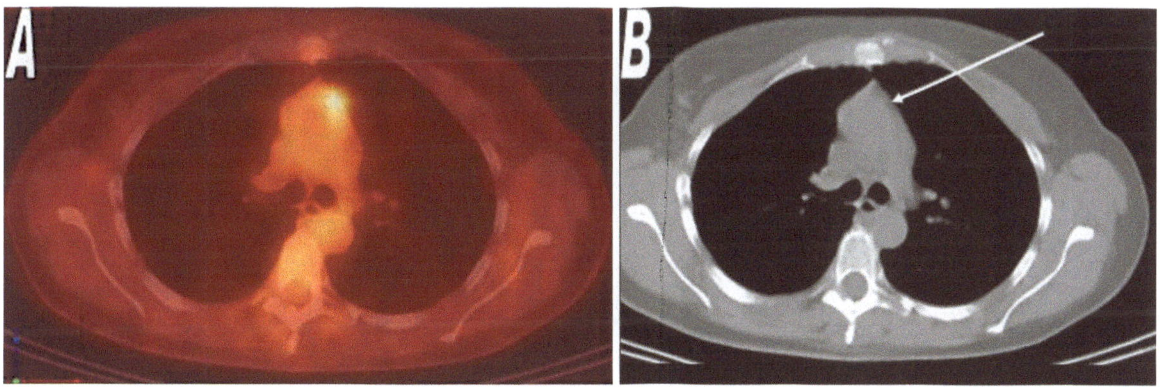

Fig. 9.16 (**a**) Small FDG-avid area revealing a barely visible lymph node in the thymic area (**b**). (**c**) Low FDG avidity revealing a small left hilar lymph node (**d**)

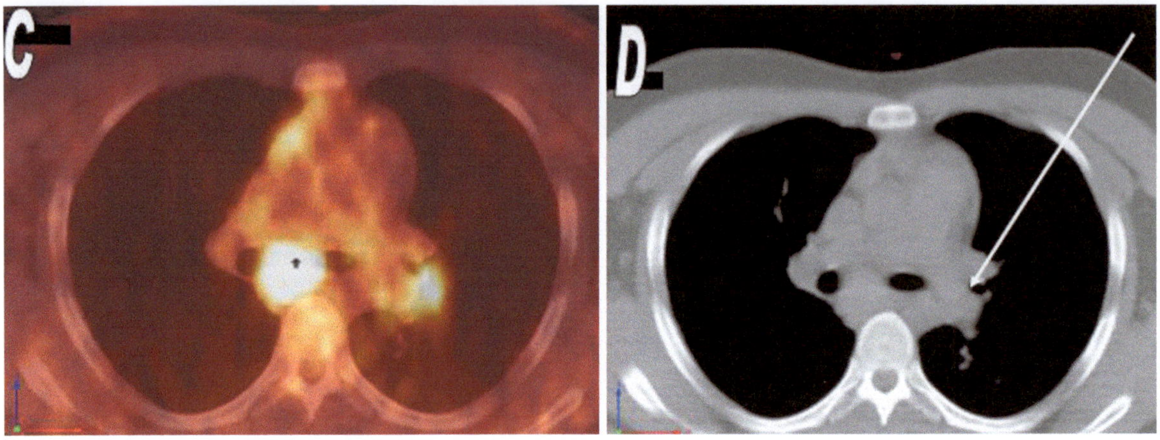

Fig. 9.16 (continued)

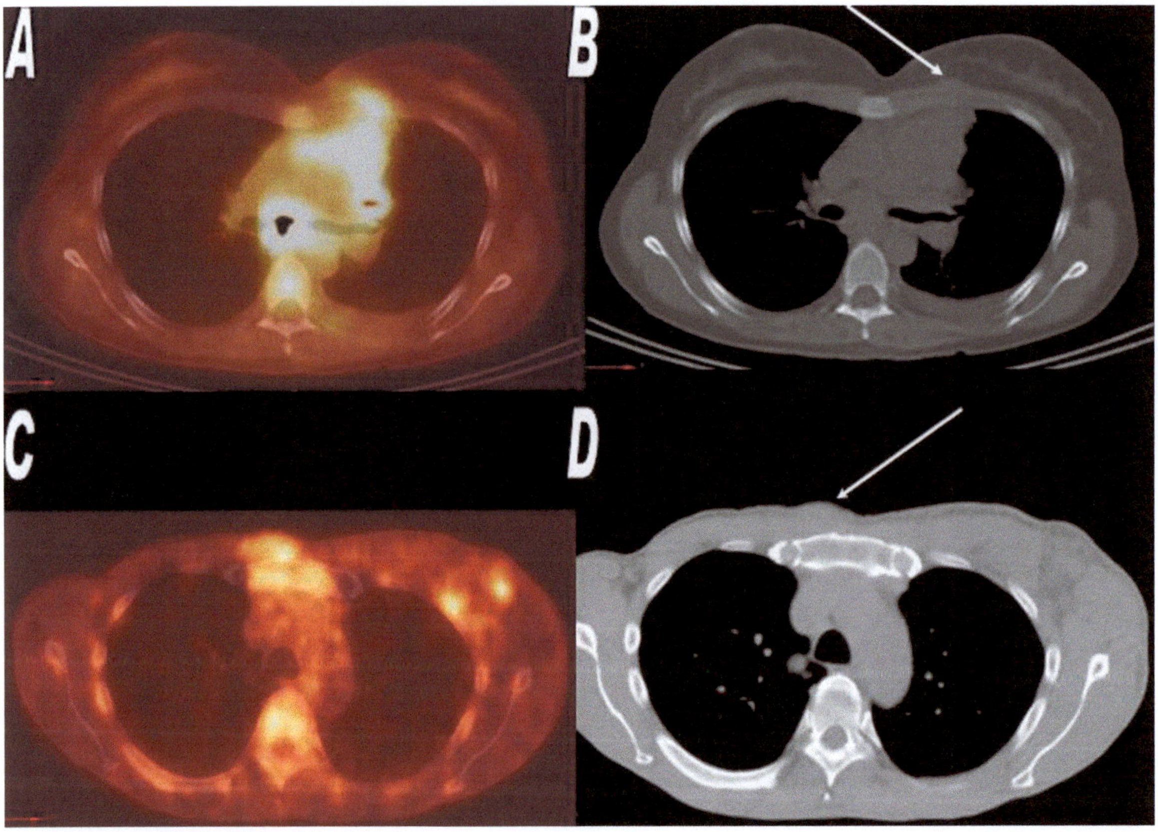

Fig. 9.17 (**a**) FDG-avid area in the left pectoralis major muscle revealing discreet left asymmetry of the thoracic wall (**b**). (**c**) FDG-avid area in the right pectoralis major muscle revealing discreet asymmetry on the CT scan (**d**).

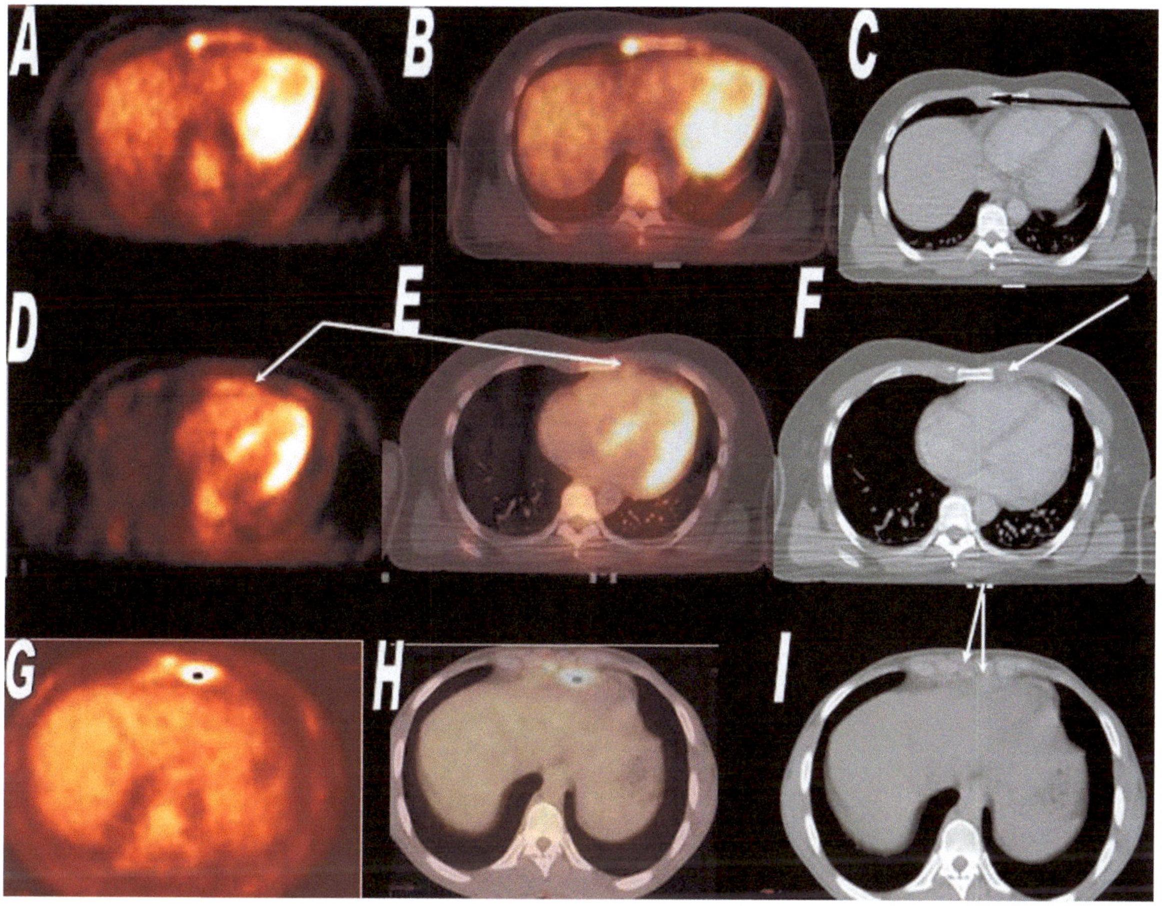

Fig. 9.18 (**a, b**) Right FDG-avid internal mammary area on PET and on the fused images. (**c**) Obvious right internal mammary lymph node involvement on the pre-chemotherapy CT scan. (**d, e**) Faint FDG avidity in the left internal mammary area. (**f**) Discreet anomaly in the left internal mammary area. (**g, h**) Two FDG-avid spots in the falciform ligament area. (**i**) Two small lymph nodes are visible on CT scan

9.4.2.3 Initially Involved Lymph Nodes in PR

- General rules

From a pragmatic point of view, the CTV should be contoured first followed by the GTV(s) which is (are) the initially lymph nodes in PR. Two PTVs are generated. First, PTV1 which is the CTV including the GTV with a 1 cm isotropic margin to take into account organ and set-up variations. Second, PTV2 which is the GTV alone with a 1 cm isotropic margin.

- Cervical and axillary lymph node areas

Figures 9.30 and 9.31 show the stepwise approach which allows one to determine the CTV and the GTV. The CTV was outlined using the method described earlier in the previous paragraph. The GTV outlines lymph nodes deemed in PR.

- Mediastinal lymph nodes

An identical stepwise approach is used to contour the mediastinal CTV and GTV as shown in Fig. 9.32.

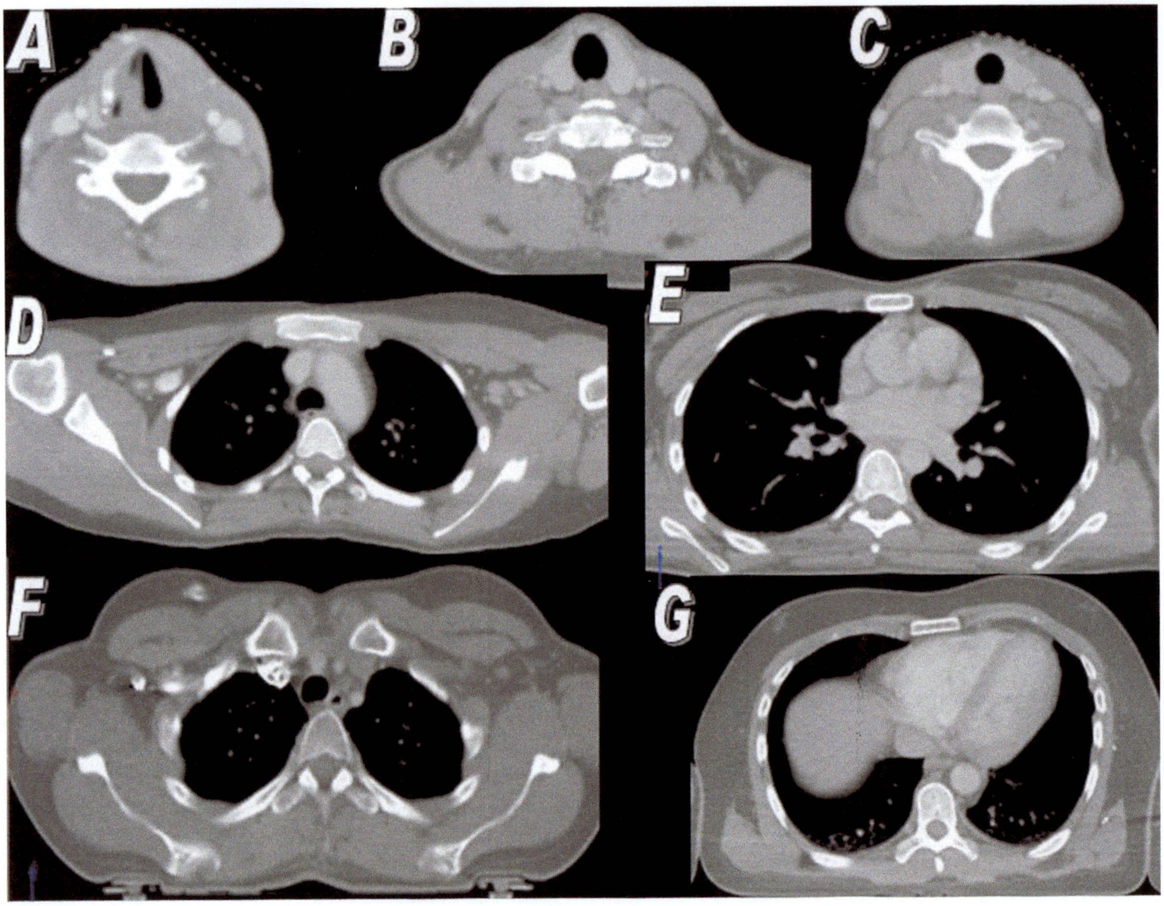

Fig. 9.19 Post-chemotherapy CT scans acquired prior to radiation therapy. They depict complete remission or a decrease in size of initially involved nodes, seen in Figures 9.10 and 9.11

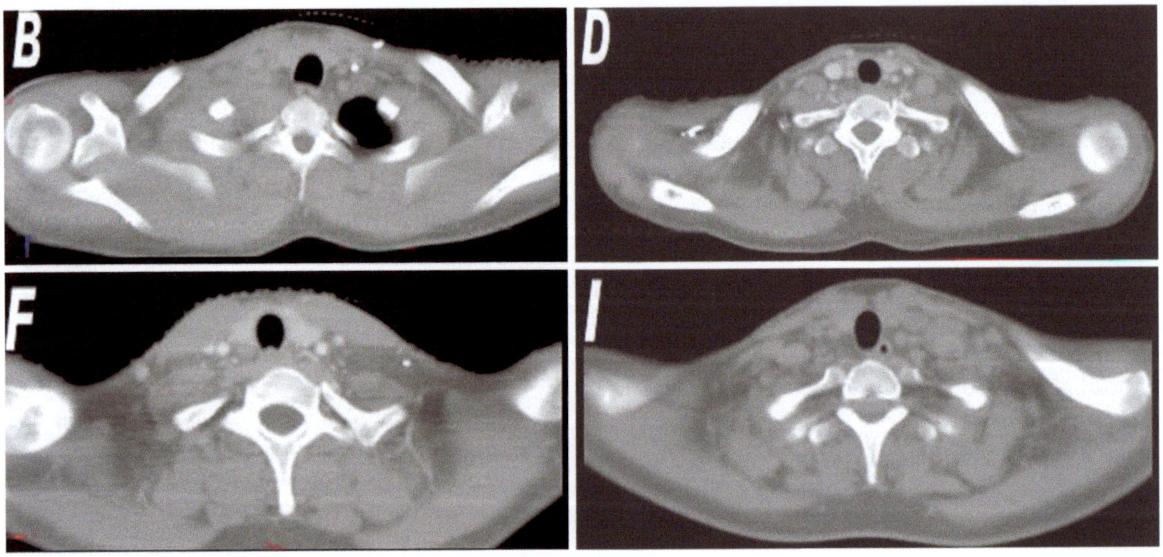

Fig. 9.20 CT scan axial slices of cervical and supraclavicular areas acquired after chemotherapy where additional information was provided by FDG-PET (see Figure 9.13)

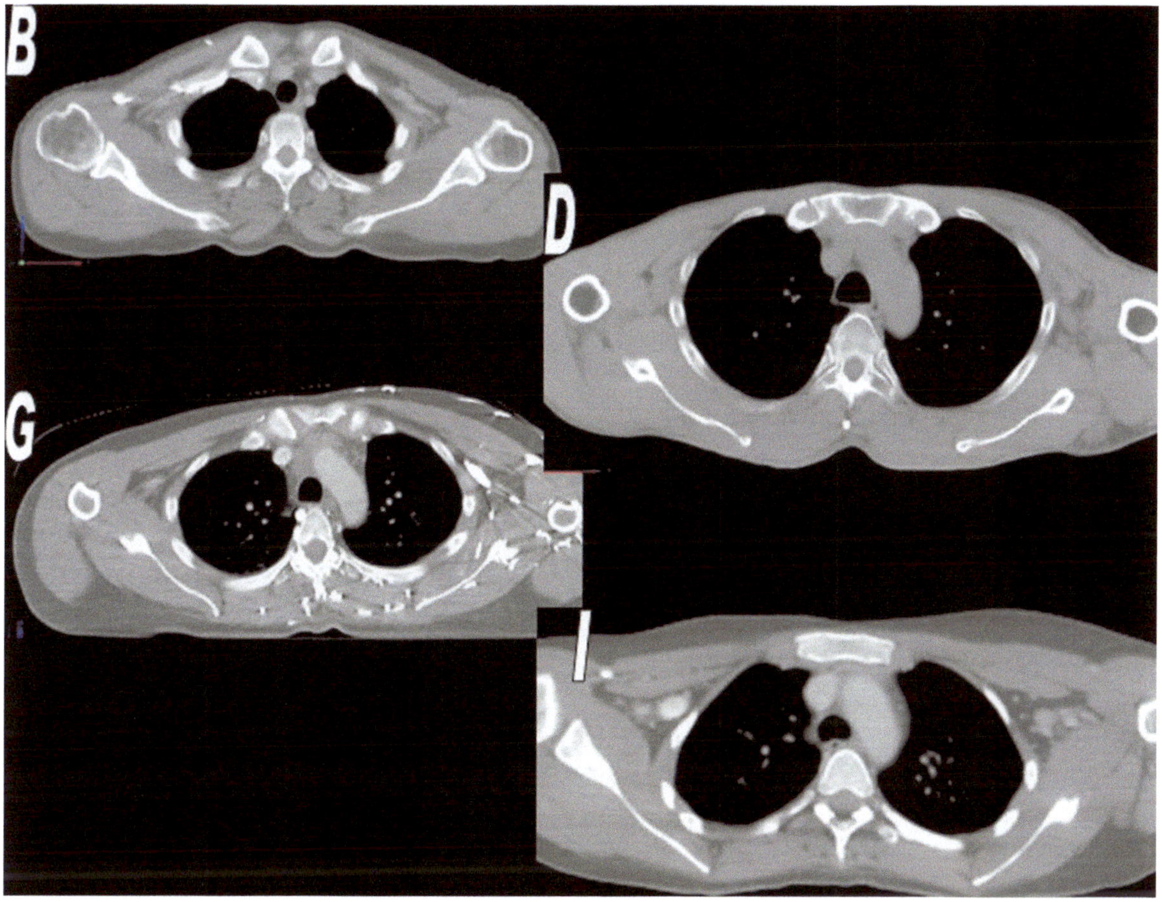

Fig. 9.21 CT scan axial slices of axillary areas acquired after chemotherapy where additional information was provided by FDG-PET (Figure 9.14). All areas displayed lymph node regression or complete remission

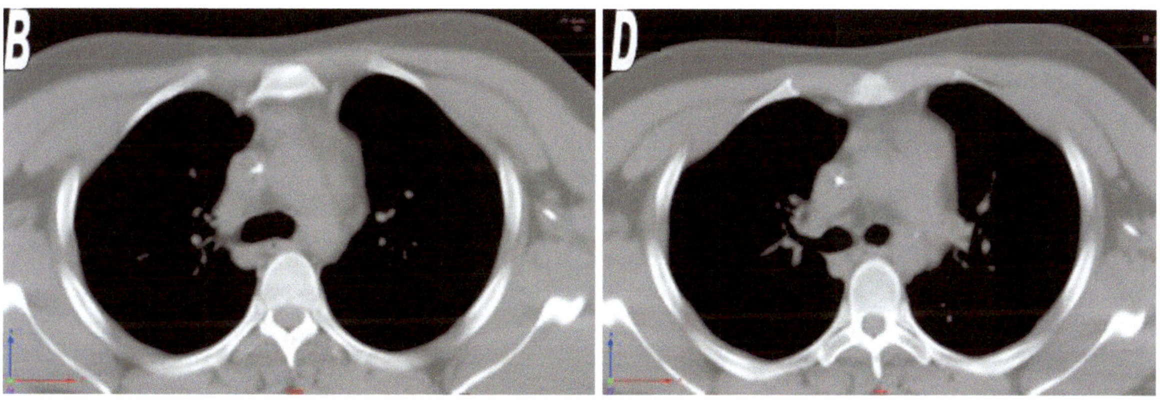

Fig. 9.22 Mediastinal CT scan axial slices acquired after chemotherapy where additional information was provided by FDG-PET (Figure 9.15). All areas displayed lymph node regression or complete remission

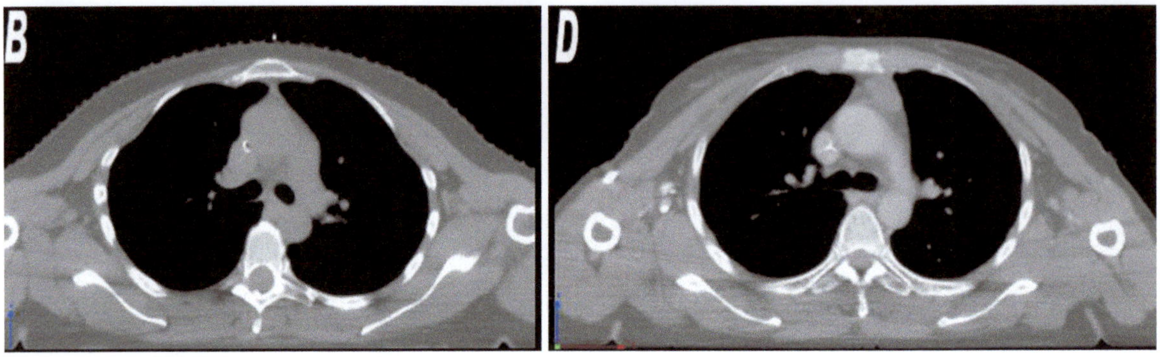

Fig. 9.23 Mediastinal CT scan axial slices acquired after chemotherapy where additional information was provided by FDG-PET (Figure 9.16). All areas displayed lymph node regression or complete remission

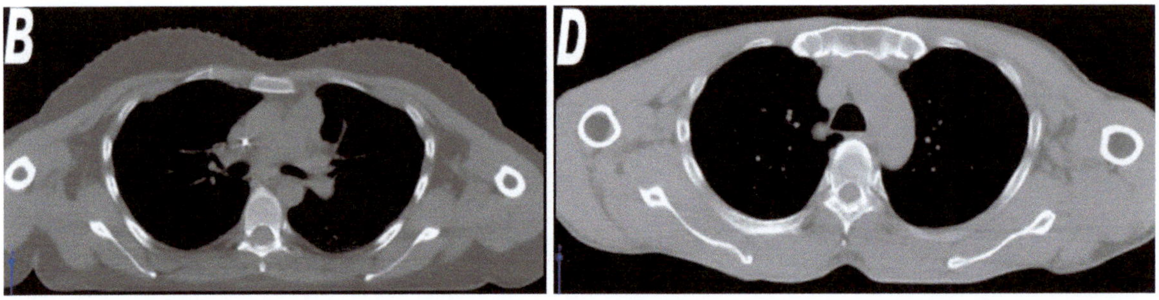

Fig. 9.24 Mediastinal CT scan axial slices acquired after chemotherapy where FDG-PET provided additional information on chest involvement (Figure 9.17). Initially involved areas display complete remission

9.5 Treatment and Dose Prescription

The dose should be specified according to ICRU 50/62 recommendations which do not yet, however, include specific criteria for the treatment of initially involved volumes after chemotherapy (ICRU 1993, 1999). In most cases, only one PTV will be required (all involved lymph nodes are included in the same radiation field). The ICRU reference point should then be located in the center or the central part of the PTV and when possible at the intersection of the beam axes. As, a certain degree of heterogeneity is expected, the entire PTV should receive a dose between 95% and 107% (i.e., the PTV should at least be included within the 95% isodose line). In rare cases, there may be one or more additional PTVs. In such cases, all PTVs should be included within their own 95% isodose line. If initially involved lymph nodes were far from each other (extremely rare situation in Hodgkin lymphoma), then separate fields should be devised.

The use of modern radiation techniques such as 3D-conformal radiotherapy (Fig. 9.33), intensity modulated radiotherapy or respiratory-gated radiotherapy is strongly recommended, notably in case of mediastinal

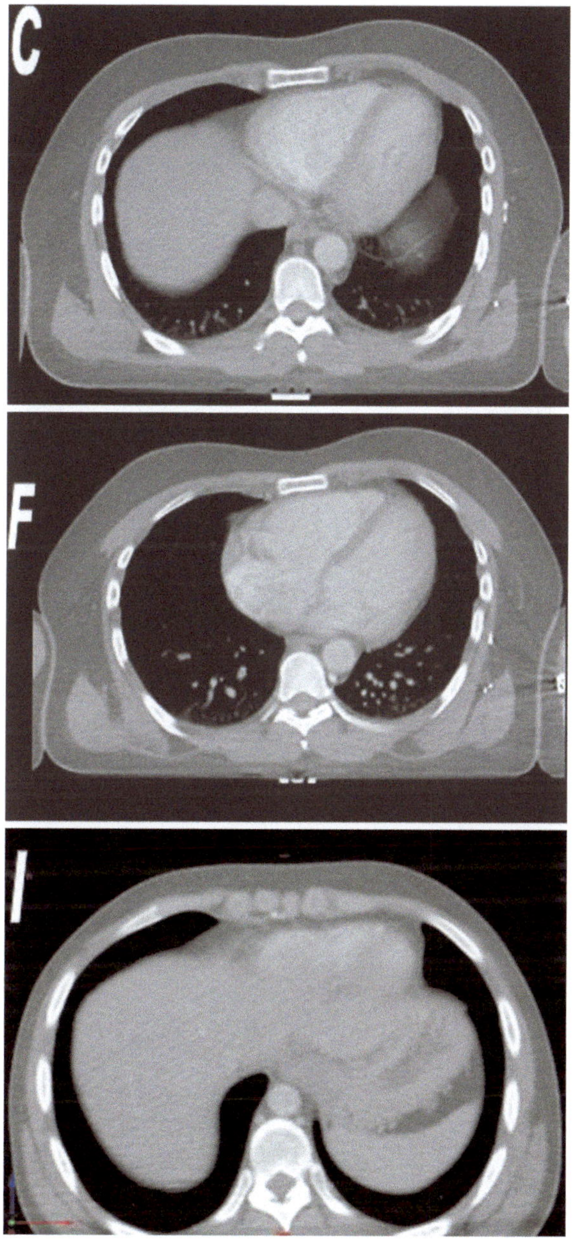

Fig. 9.25 CT scan axial slices of the lower mediastinum and the upper part of the abdomen acquired after chemotherapy where FDG-PET provided additional information (Figure 9.18). All areas display complete remission

involvement, in order to optimize the concept of INRT and reduce the amount of radiation delivered to normal tissues (Figs. 9.34c and d, 9.35). However, the final choice will be left to the discretion of the physician. Radiation treatments should be delivered using five fractions of 1.8–2 Gy per week. Portal imaging of all fields should be performed consecutively, within the first 2 days of treatment and once a week thereafter. Daily portal controls are recommended, whenever feasible.

Radiation doses are beyond the scope of this chapter and will not be discussed.

9.6 Quality Assurance Programs

The INRT field is a concept requiring precision and accuracy. A few mandatory measures are prerequisites to the successful implementation of this concept. First, radiation oncologists should attend training workshops where methods for assessing initially involved nodes and designing involved node fields are explained. Second, retrospective quality assurance meetings (monthly or every 3 months) should be organized with all the participating radiation oncologists (DICOM and DICOM-RT data saved on a CD-rom). However, the most efficient way to guarantee high-quality treatments is through a prospective web-based quality assurance program. Such a program interconnecting all major cancer centers is now operational in France (Figs. 9.36 and 9.37) and is expected to be expanded to all EORTC-GELA participating centers. As shown in Figs. 9.38 and 9.39 the design of the CTV varied slightly between the local treatment center and the "reference" center. A consensus bridging various differences in the design of CTVs was obtained through a phone call. We strongly believe that such a network will allow the delivery of high quality and homogeneous radiation treatments to patients with Hodgkin lymphoma.

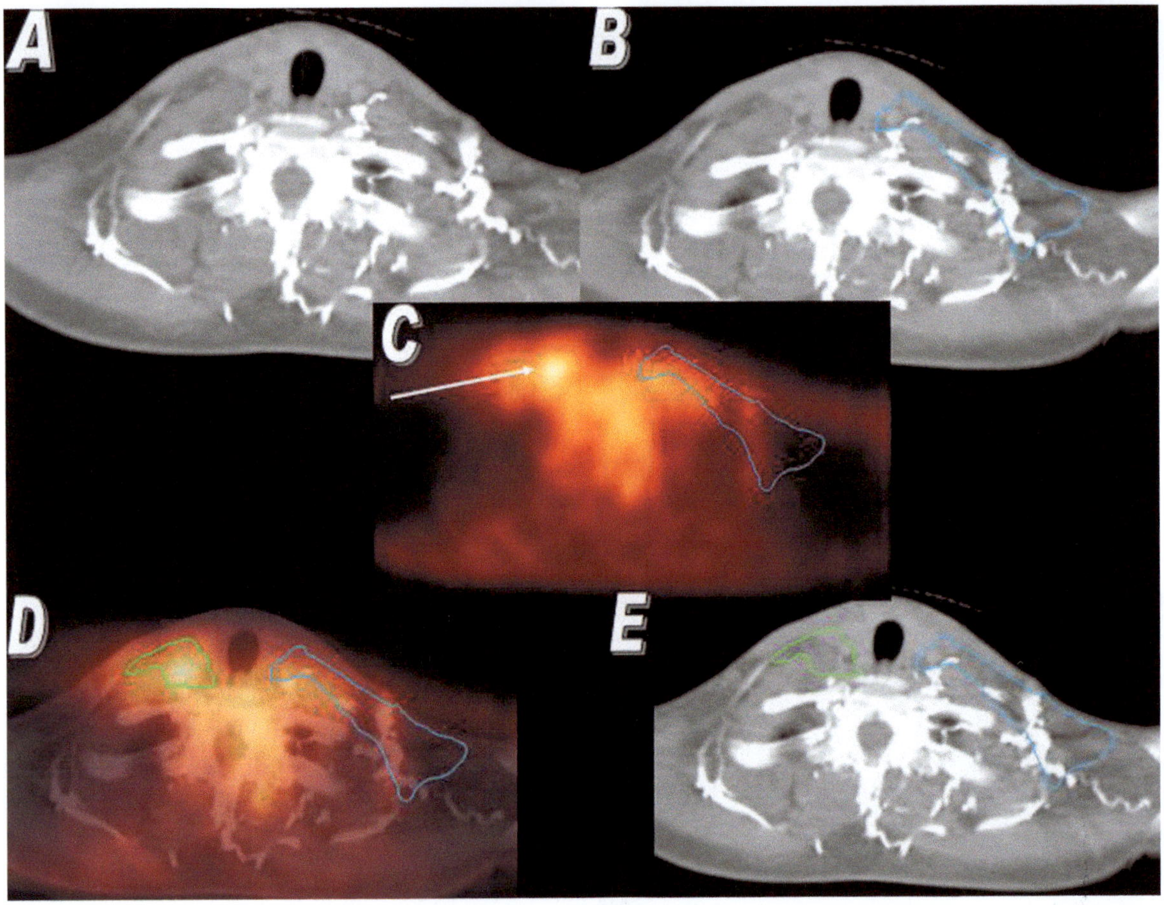

Fig. 9.26 (**a**) Pre-chemotherapy CT scan of the cervical area. (**b**) Contouring of the left cervical area. (**c**) FDG avidity in the right cervical area. (**d**) Additional contouring based on PET data. (**e**) Final contouring on the pre-chemotherapy CT scan

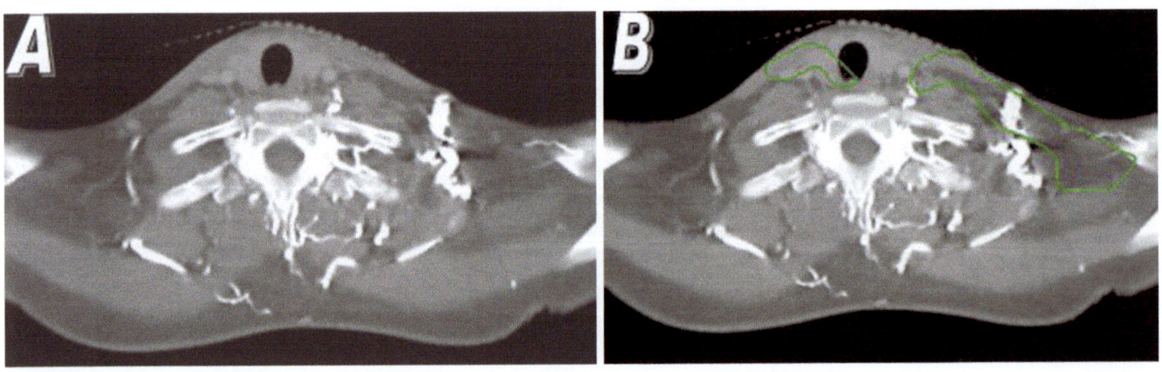

Fig. 9.27 (**a**) Post-chemotherapy CT simulation. (**b**) Superimposition of the pre-chemotherapy contourings (*green color*). (**c**) Pre- and post-chemotherapy (*purple color*) contourings. (**d**) Final proposal for the cervical CTV (*purple color*)

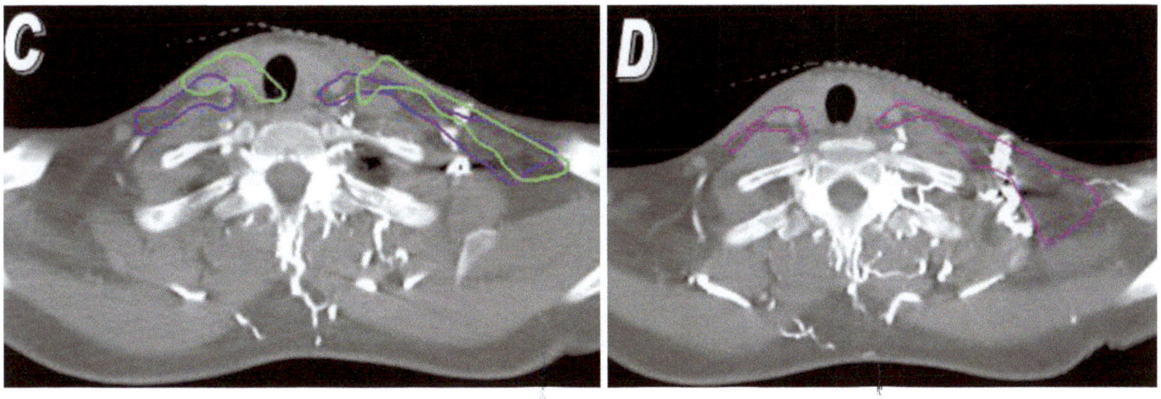

Fig.9.27 (continued)

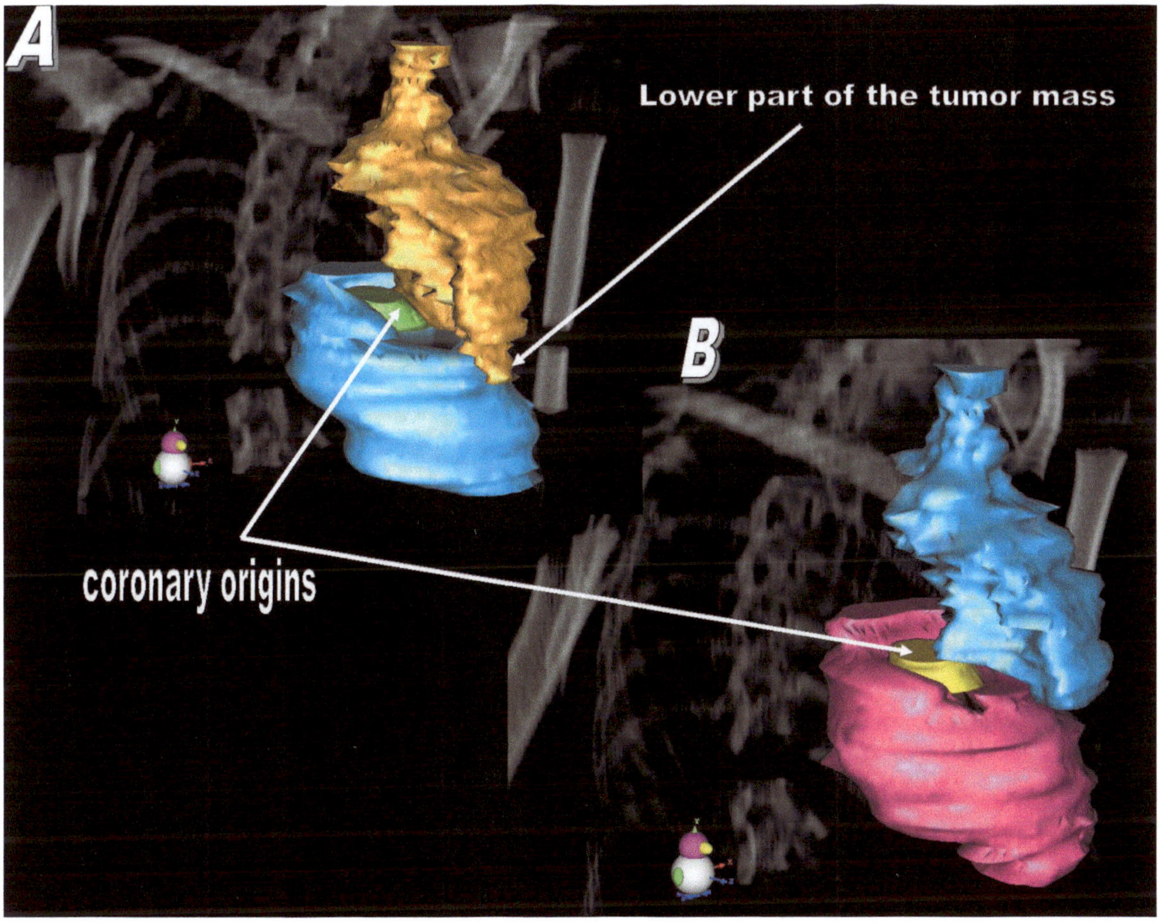

Fig. 9.28 (**a**) The 3D initial tumor volume (*yellow color* outlined on the CT scan before chemotherapy). (**b**) The 3D clinical target volume outlined on CT after chemotherapy (the *arrow* indicates the part of the tumor which regressed completely after chemotherapy and which is not included in the CTV)

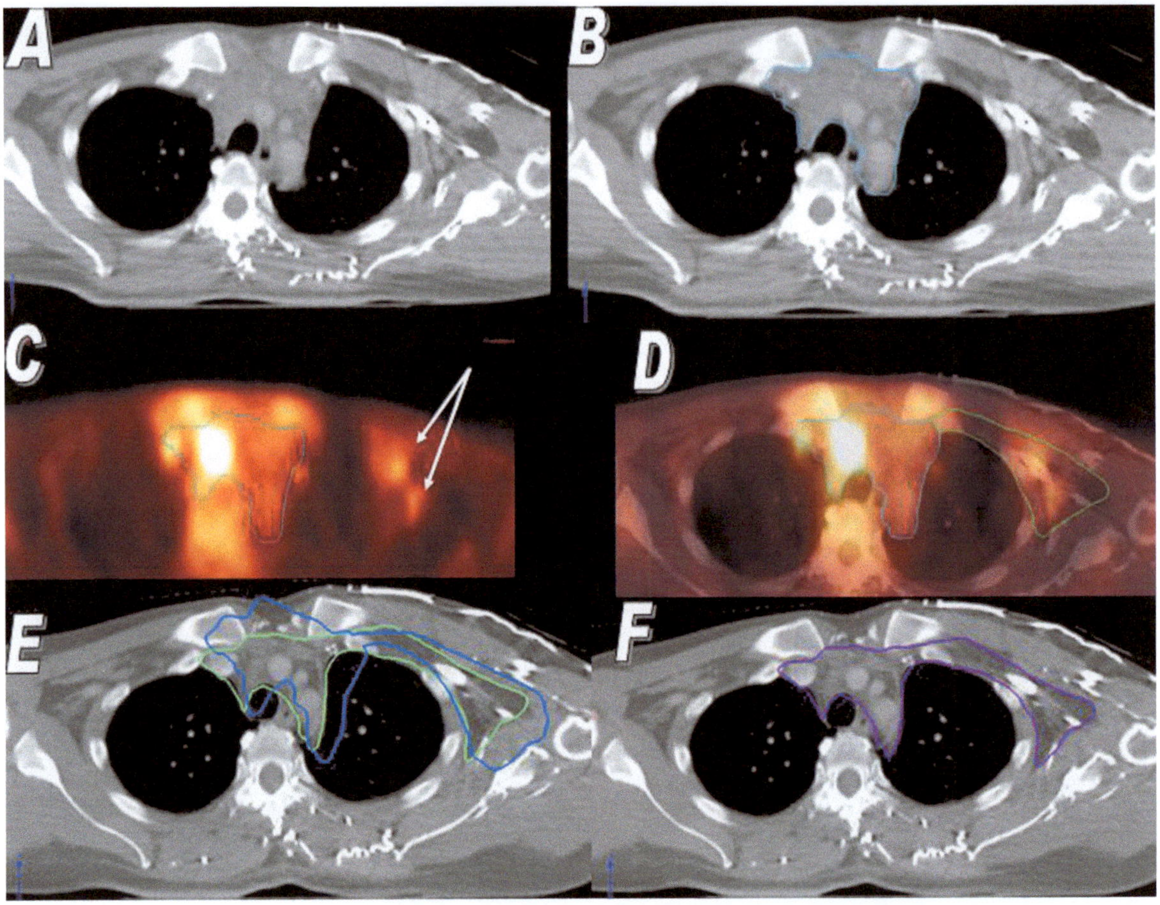

Fig. 9.29 (**a**) Pre-chemotherapy mediastinal CT scan. (**b**) Contouring of the mediastinal tumor mass (*blue color*). (**c**) FDG-PET provides additional information on axillary lymph nodes. (**d**) Fusion of PET and CT with additional contouring of the axillary area (*green color*). (**e**) Pre- (*blue color*) and post-chemotherapy (*green color*) contourings on the post-chemotherapy CT scan (**f**) Final proposal for the CTV

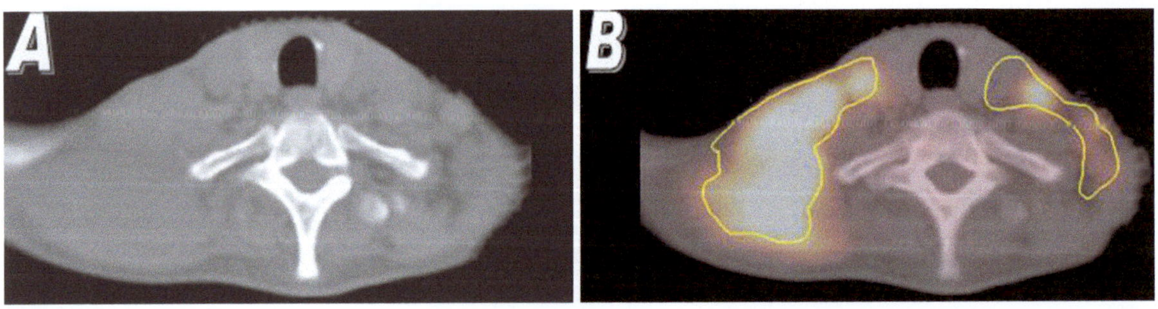

Fig. 9.30 (**a**) Cervical CT scan prior to chemotherapy. (**b**) GTV outlined on the FDG-PET/CT fusion. (**c**) Cervical CT scan after chemotherapy. (**d**) Clinical target volume (CTV) (*green color*). (**e**) Gross tumor volume (GTV) (*orange and red colors*)

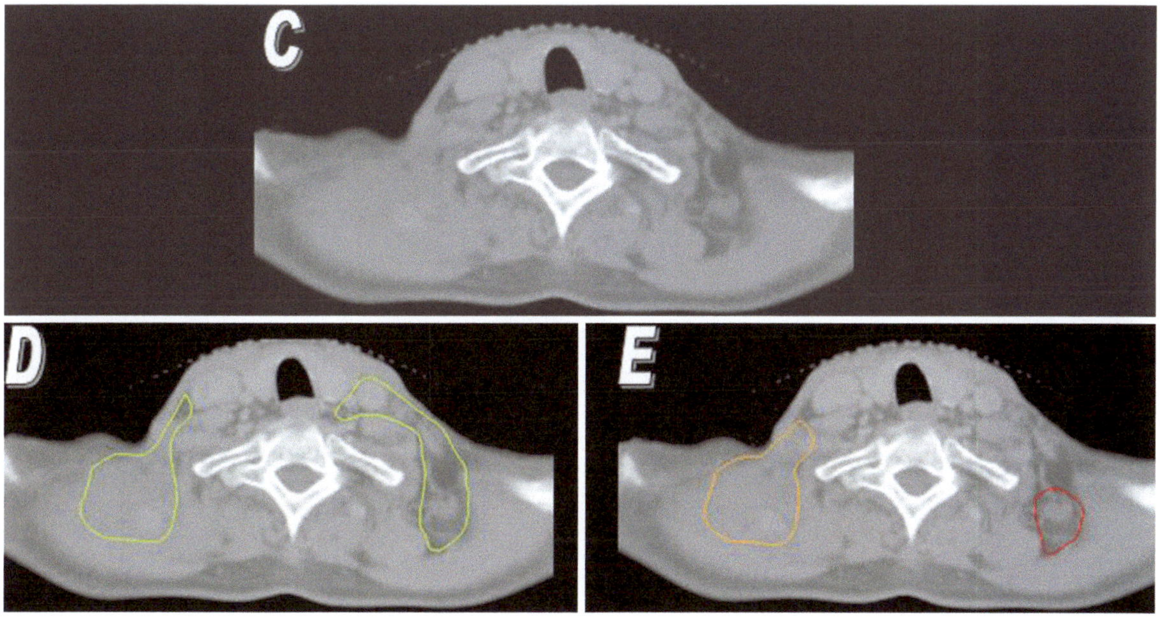

Fig.9.30 (continued)

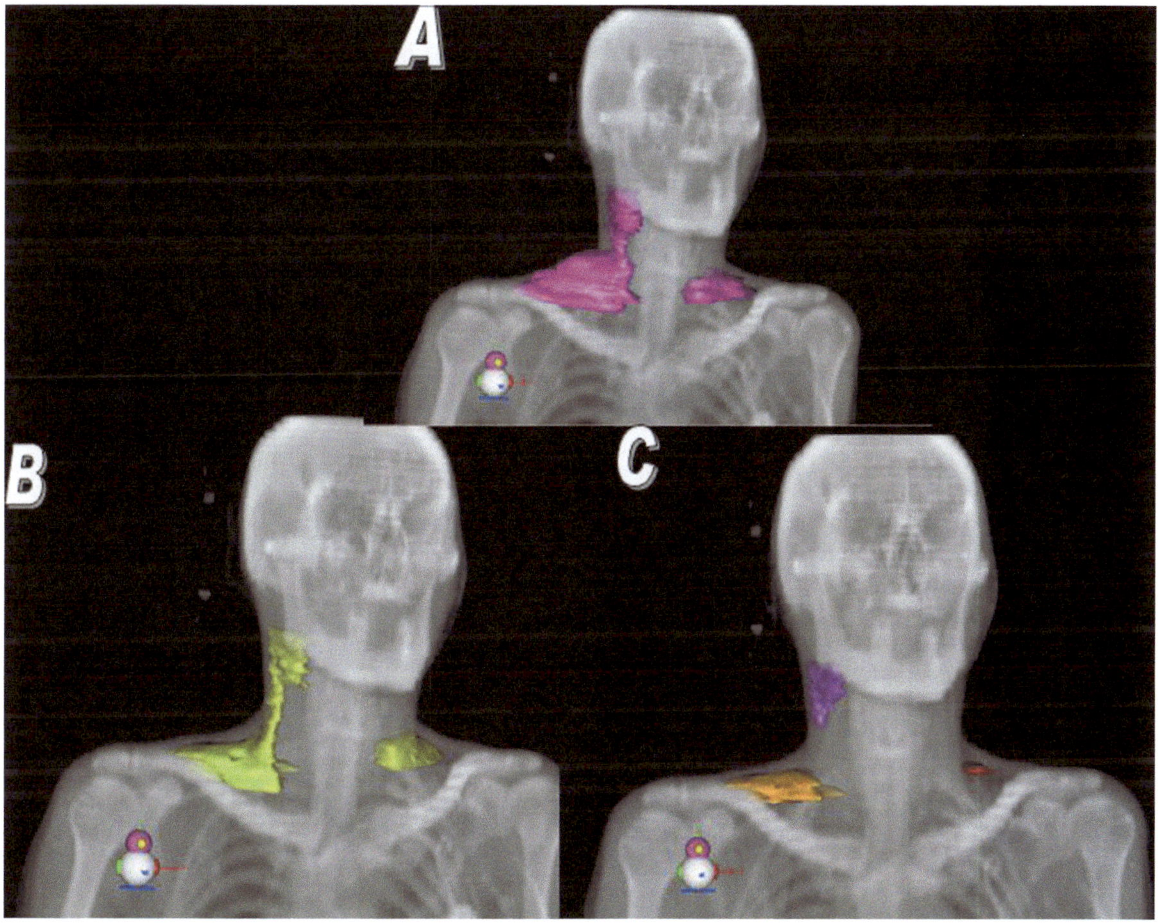

Fig. 9.31 (**a**) 3D representation of the initially involved nodes before chemotherapy. (**b**) 3D representation of the CTV. (**c**) 3D representation of the GTV

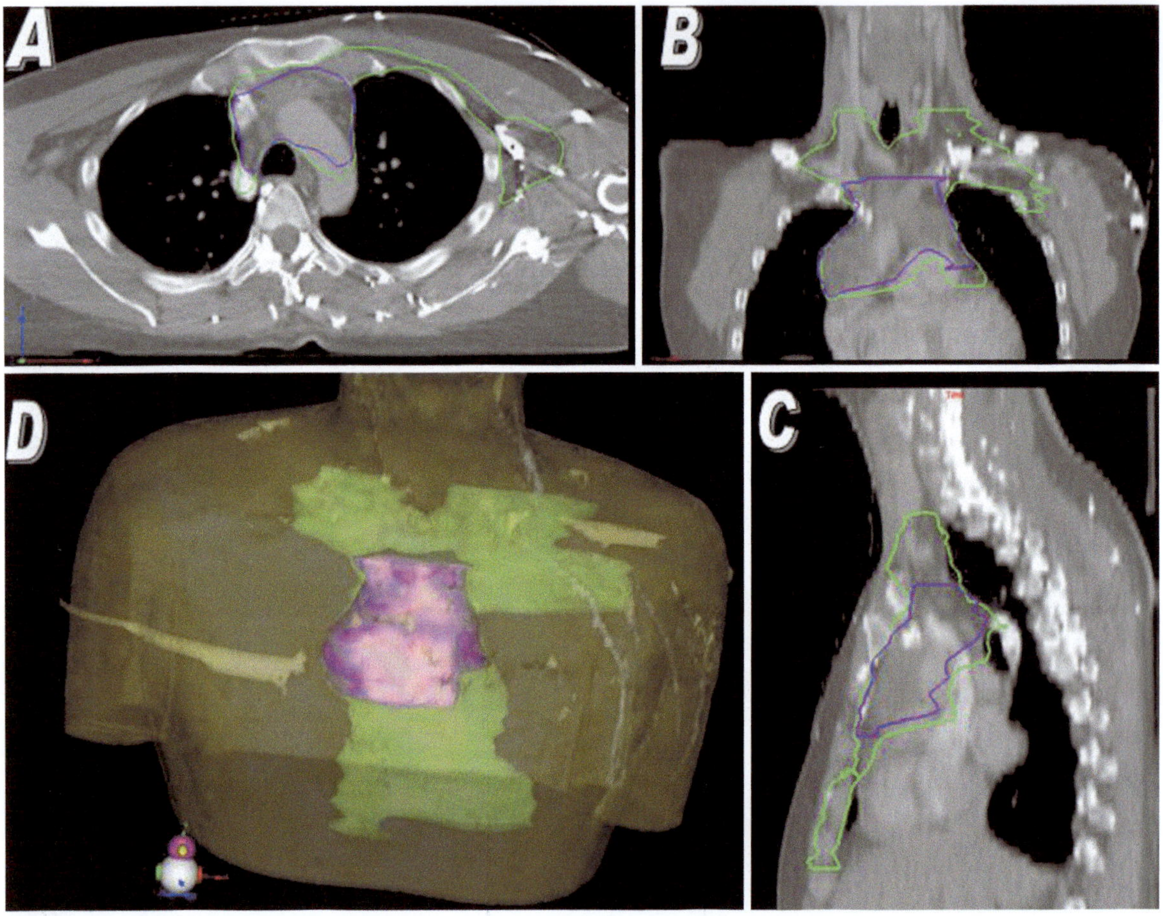

Fig. 9.32 (**a**) CTV (in *green color*) and GTV (*purple color*) are outlined on a post-chemotherapy CT scan. (**b**) Coronal view of the CTV and GTV. (**c**) Sagittal view of the CTV and GTV. (**d**) 3D representation of both volumes

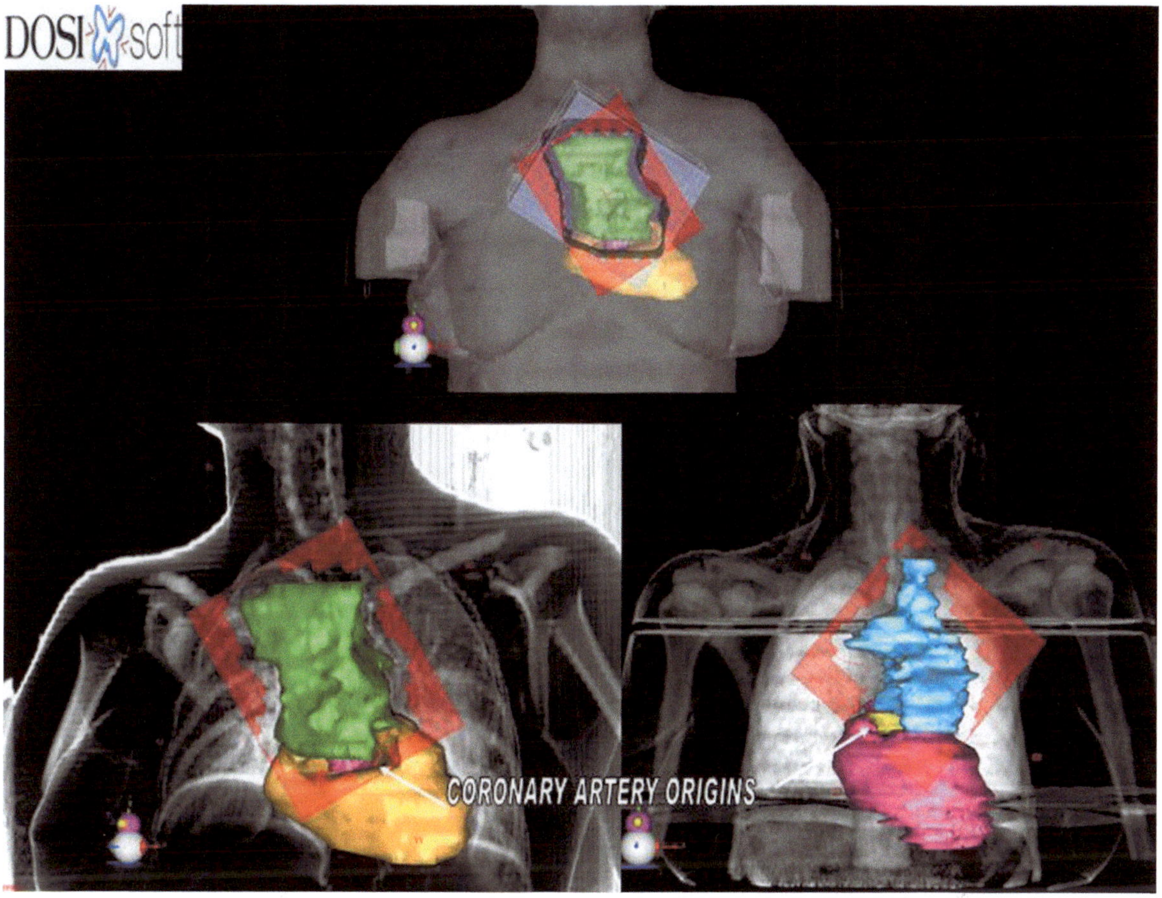

Fig. 9.33 3D-conformal radiotherapy for a mediastinal tumor mass allowing maximum sparing of the breasts, coronary artery origins and heart

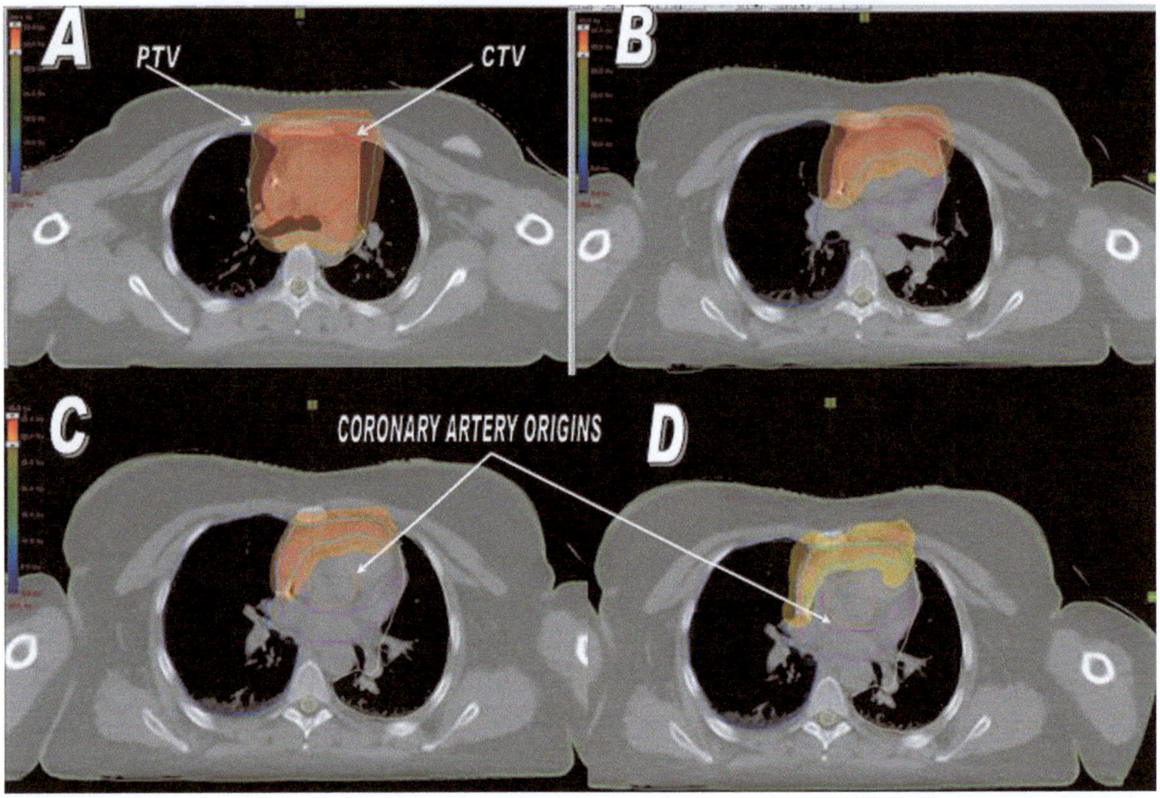

Fig. 9.34 Mediastinal tumor mass in CRu after chemotherapy treated with IMRT. The volume which will receive at least 95% of the prescribed dose is in *orange* (the 95% isodose line encompasses the PTV [*green color*]). Smaller radiation doses could be delivered to the origins of the coronary arteries with this technique

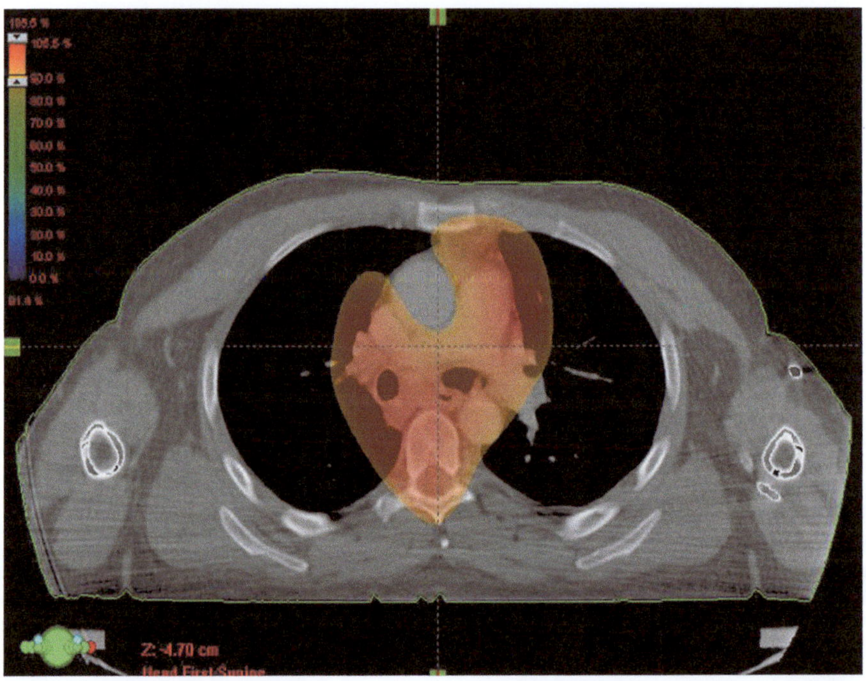

Fig. 9.35 Mediastinal tumor mass in CRu treated with IMRT allowing relative sparing of the aortic valve which required surgery

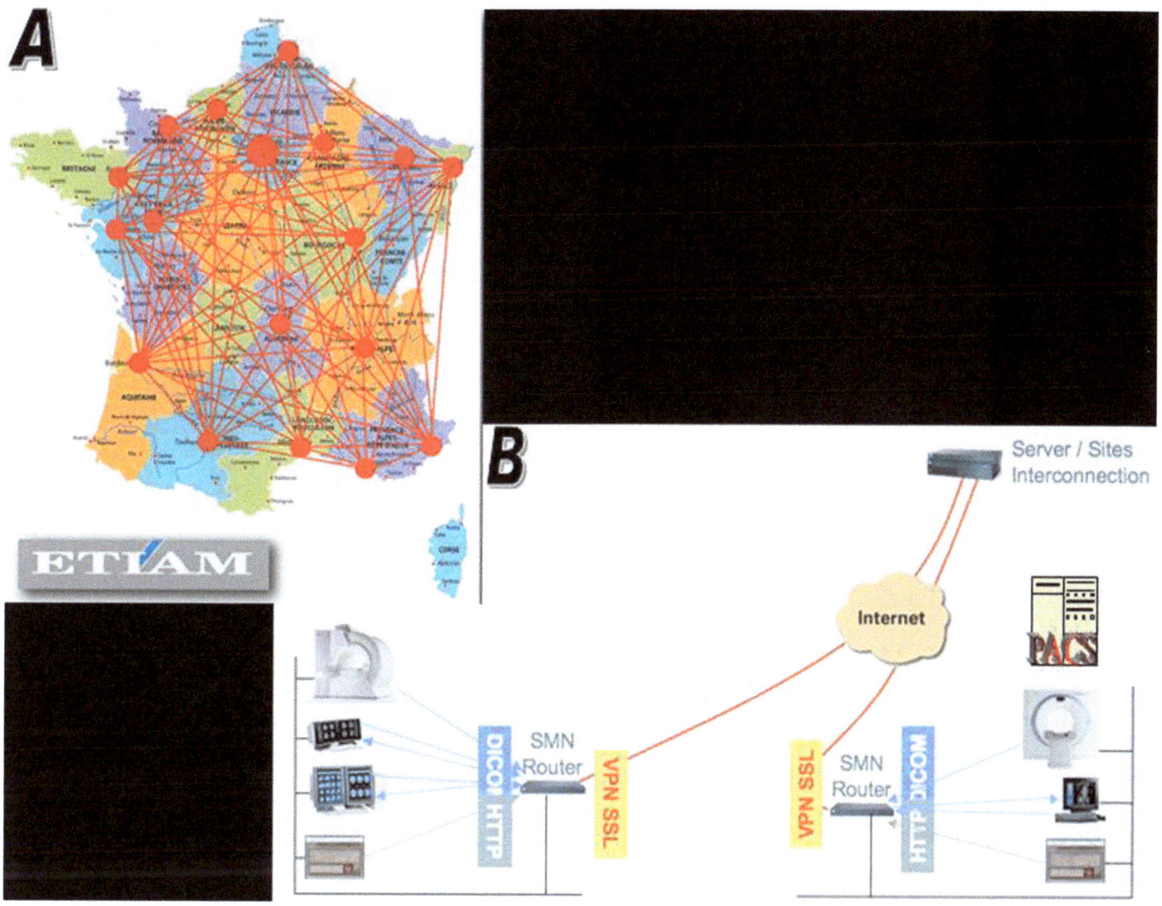

Fig. 9.36 (**a**) Overview of the internet network linking all French cancer centers. (**b**) The basic infrastructure of the internet communication system allowing the retrieval of DICOM and DICOM-RT data in various treatment planning systems and storage in hospital PACS servers

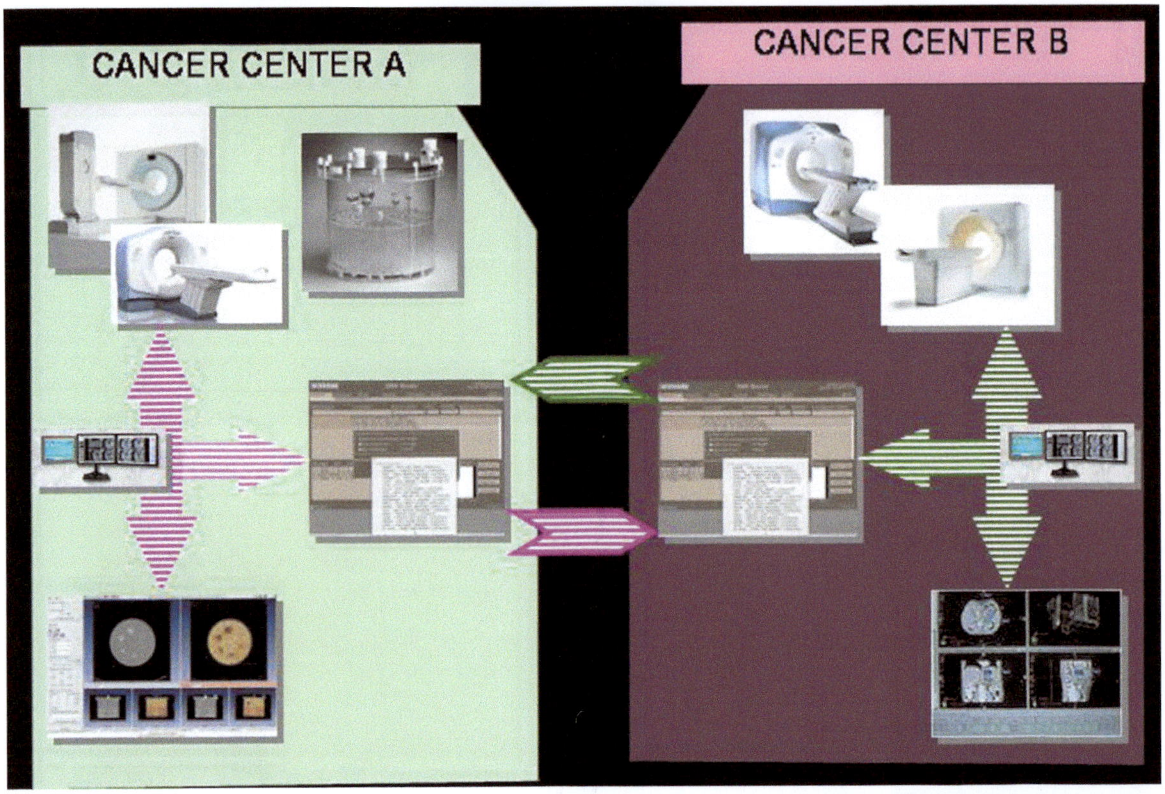

Fig. 9.37 A more detailed view of the information-sharing network system allowing the implementation of a prospective quality assurance program

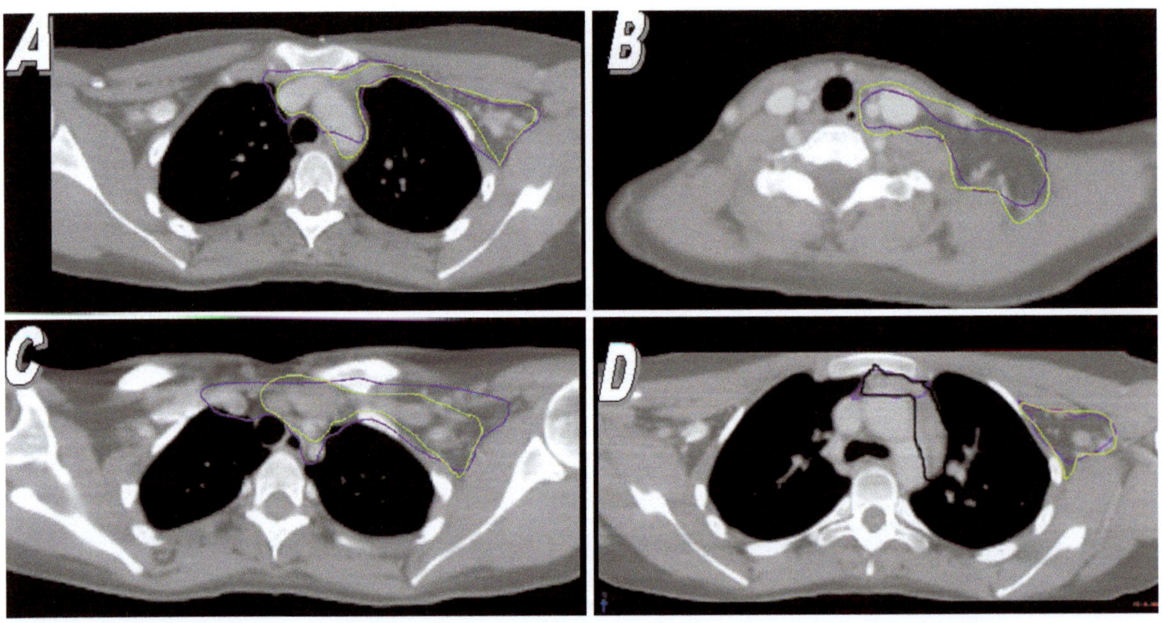

Fig. 9.38 (**a, b**) Full agreement between the local (*yellow outline*) and the reference center (*purple color*). (**c, d**) Slight disagreement between local and reference center. (**e, f**) Strong disagreement between centers as the areas outlined by the reference center were not included in the CTV by the local treating center

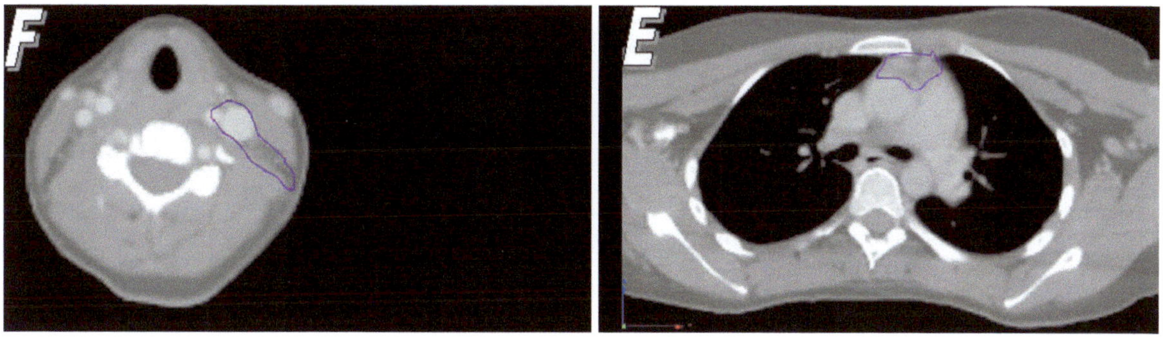

Fig. 9.38 (continued)

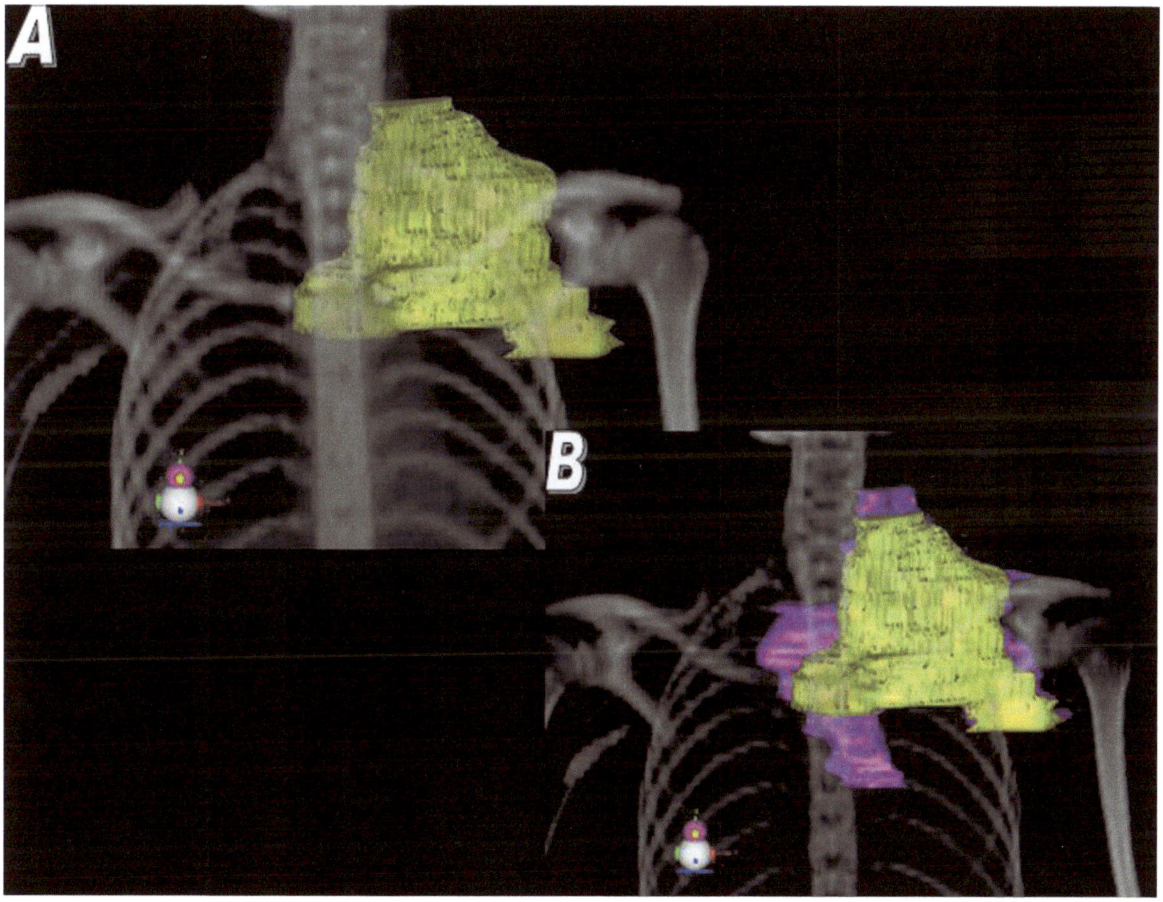

Fig. 9.39 (**a**) 3D CTV volume designed by the local center. (**b**) 3D CTV volume (in *purple*) proposed by the reference center

9.7 Conclusions

Hodgkin lymphoma remains a tremendous challenge for oncologists because of excellent overall survival rates but an unacceptable incidence of late complications. Better combined modality treatments substantially reducing late complications due to chemotherapy and radiotherapy could be achieved if the concept of involved node radiation is properly implemented.

Acknowledgements Lorna Saint Ange for editing the chapter, Claude Ruelle for help with the web-based quality assurance program, Dosisoft (Cachan 92000, France) for providing the software to analyze the imaging procedures and contourings from all major cancer centers, Etiam for providing the installation and maintenance of the web network and servers and finally the Clarence Westbury Foundation for financial assistance.

Laurence Gonzague M.D., Karine Peignaux M.D., Sawyna Provencher, M.D. Juliette Thariat M.D., Françoise Izar M.D., Bernard Dubray M.D., Christine Kerr M.D., Claire Brunaud M.D., Loic Feuvret M.D., Floriane Toudic M.D., Georges Noel M.D., Jean Leon Lagrange M.D. for providing patient data.

References

Aleman BM, van den Belt-Dusebout AW, Klokman WJ et al (2003) Long-term cause-specific mortality of patients treated for Hodgkin's disease. J Clin Oncol 21:3431–3439

Berthelsen AK, Holm S, Loft A et al (2005) PET/CT with intravenous contrast can be used for PET attenuation correction in cancer patients. Eur J Nucl Med Mol Imaging 32: 1167–1175

Bhatia S, Robison LL, Oberlin O et al (1996) Breast cancer and other second neoplasms after childhood Hodgkin's disease. N Engl J Med 334:745–751

Biti GP, Cimino G, Cartoni C et al (1992) Extended-field radiotherapy is superior to MOPP chemotherapy for the treatment of pathologic stage I–IIA Hodgkin's disease: eight-year update of an Italian prospective randomized study. J Clin Oncol 10:378–382

Bonadonna G, Bonfante V, Viviani S et al (2004) ABVD plus subtotal nodal versus involved-field radiotherapy in early-stage Hodgkin's disease: long-term results. J Clin Oncol 22:2835–2841

Castellino RA, Hoppe RT, Blank N et al (1984) Computed tomography, lymphography, and staging laparotomy: correlations in initial staging of Hodgkin disease. AJR Am J Roentgenol 143:37–41

Cheson BD, Horning SJ, Coiffier B et al (1999) Report of an international workshop to standardize response criteria for non-Hodgkin's lymphomas. NCI Sponsored International Working Group. J Clin Oncol 17:1244–1253

Cheson BD, Pfistner B, Juweid ME et al (2007) Revised response criteria for malignant lymphoma. J Clin Oncol 25:579–586

Donaldson SS, Link MP, Weinstein HJ et al (2007) Final results of a prospective clinical trial with VAMP and low-dose involved-field radiation for children with low-risk Hodgkin's disease. J Clin Oncol 25:332–337

Girinsky T, van der Maazen R, Specht L et al (2006) Involved-node radiotherapy (INRT) in patients with early Hodgkin lymphoma: concepts and guidelines. Radiother Oncol 79:270–277

Girinsky T, Ghalibafian M, Bonniaud G et al (2007) Is FDG-PET scan in patients with early stage Hodgkin lymphoma of any value in the implementation of the involved-node radiotherapy concept and dose painting? Radiother Oncol 85:178–186

Girinsky T, Specht L, Ghalibafian M et al (2008) The conundrum of Hodgkin lymphoma nodes: to be or not to be included in the involved node radiation fields. The EORTC-GELA lymphoma group guidelines. Radiother Oncol 88:202–210

Guermazi A (2001) Is it wise to eliminate lymphography from the staging of Hodgkin's disease? Leuk Lymphoma 42:655–660

Hancock SL, Tucker MA, Hoppe RT (1993) Factors affecting late mortality from heart disease after treatment of Hodgkin's disease. JAMA 270:1949–1955

Hanna SL, Fletcher BD, Boulden TF et al (1993) MR imaging of infradiaphragmatic lymphadenopathy in children and adolescents with Hodgkin disease: comparison with lymphography and CT. J Magn Reson Imaging 3:461–470

Hutchings M, Loft A, Hansen M et al (2007) Clinical impact of FDG-PET/CT in the planning of radiotherapy for early-stage Hodgkin lymphoma. Eur J Haematol 78:206–212

ICRU (1993) Prescribing, recording and reporting photon beam therapy. Report 50

ICRU (1999) Prescribing, recording and reporting photon beam therapy. Report 62

Kyzas PA, Evangelou E, Denaxa-Kyza D et al (2008) 18F-fluorodeoxyglucose positron emission tomography to evaluate cervical node metastases in patients with head and neck squamous cell carcinoma: a meta-analysis. J Natl Cancer Inst 100:712–720

Landman-Parker J, Pacquement H, Leblanc T et al (2000) Localized childhood Hodgkin's disease: response-adapted chemotherapy with etoposide, bleomycin, vinblastine, and prednisone before low-dose radiation therapy-results of the French Society of Pediatric Oncology Study MDH90. J Clin Oncol 18:1500–1507

Lister TA, Crowther D, Sutcliffe SB et al (1989) Report of a committee convened to discuss the evaluation and staging of patients with Hodgkin's disease: Cotswolds meeting. J Clin Oncol 7:1630–1636

Longo DL, Glatstein E, Duffey PL et al (1991) Radiation therapy versus combination chemotherapy in the treatment of early-stage Hodgkin's disease: seven-year results of a prospective randomized trial. J Clin Oncol 9:906–917

Mauch P (1995) Second malignancies after curative radiation therapy for good prognosis cancers. Int J Radiat Oncol Biol Phys 33:959–960

Ng AK, Bernardo MP, Weller E et al (2002) Long-term survival and competing causes of death in patients with early-stage Hodgkin's disease treated at age 50 or younger. J Clin Oncol 20:2101–2108

Pavlovsky S, Maschio M, Santarelli MT et al (1988) Randomized trial of chemotherapy versus chemotherapy plus radiotherapy for stage I–II Hodgkin's disease. J Natl Cancer Inst 80:1466–1473

Shahidi M, Kamangari N, Ashley S et al (2006) Site of relapse after chemotherapy alone for stage I and II Hodgkin's disease. Radiother Oncol 78:1–5

Specht L (2007) 2-[18F]fluoro-2-deoxyglucose positron-emission tomography in staging, response evaluation, and treatment planning of lymphomas. Semin Radiat Oncol 17:190–197

Valette F, Querellou S, Oudoux A et al (2007) Comparison of positron emission tomography and lymphangiography in the diagnosis of infradiaphragmatic Hodgkin's disease. Acta Radiol 48:59–63

van Leeuwen FE, Klokman WJ, Stovall M et al (2003) Roles of radiation dose, chemotherapy, and hormonal factors in breast cancer following Hodgkin's disease. J Natl Cancer Inst 95:971–980

Traditional and Modern Techniques for Radiation Treatment Planning

10

Stephanie A. Terezakis, Margie Hunt, Lena Specht, and Joachim Yahalom

Contents

10.1 Introduction

Radiation treatment-field design of Hodgkin lymphoma (HL) has markedly changed over the last decade. The addition of chemotherapy to HL treatment regimens has led to a reduction in radiation treatment-field size. Radiation therapy alone was delivered historically with an extended field. While extended-field treatment is still used under special circumstances, it is rarely used in the modern treatment of HL. Modern reduced-volume fields avoid normal tissue exposure and reduce the risk of long-term toxicity while avoiding in-field or marginal field failures. Several studies have suggested a decrease in second malignancy rate with the increasing use of involved-field lymph node irradiation, and smaller treatment fields may also reduce development of cardiovascular disease (Biti et al. 1994; Henry-Amar 1992; Swerdlow et al. 1992). Recent data suggest that patients treated with chemotherapy alone for early-stage HL most frequently relapse in the initially involved lymph node(s) (Shahidi et al. 2006). Thus, the European Organisation for Research and Treatment of Cancer–Groupe d'Etudes

S.A. Terezakis, M. Hunt, and J. Yahalom (✉)
Dept. of Radiation Oncology, Memorial Sloan-Kettering Cancer Center, 1275 York Ave., New York, NY 10021-6094, USA
e-mail: huntm@mskcc.org
e-mail: yahalomj@mskcc.org

L. Specht
Depts. of Oncology and Haematology, The Finsen Centre, Rigshospitalet, University of Copenhagen, 9 Blegdamsvej, 2100 Copenhagen, Denamark
e-mail: specht@dadlnet.dk

L. Specht and J. Yahalom (eds.), *Radiotherapy for Hodgkin Lymphoma*,
DOI: 10.1007/978-3-540-78944-4_10, © Springer-Verlag Berlin Heidelberg 2011

des Lymphomes de l'Adulte (EORTC-GELA) has introduced the concept of involved-node radiation that is delivered to the original pre-chemotherapy involved lymph node(s) (Girinsky et al. 2006b).

As fields have decreased in size, target volume definition has become an increasingly important dilemma for the radiation oncologist. Accurate treatment delivery is imperative for the adequate care of patients and for the protection of normal tissues. The advent of conformal techniques, including three-dimensional–conformal radiation treatment (3D-CRT) and intensity-modulated radiotherapy (IMRT) has also placed the onus on the treating physician to outline the treatment volume precisely. This chapter will focus on modern techniques, immobilization, imaging, and planning for involved-fields and emerging IMRT.

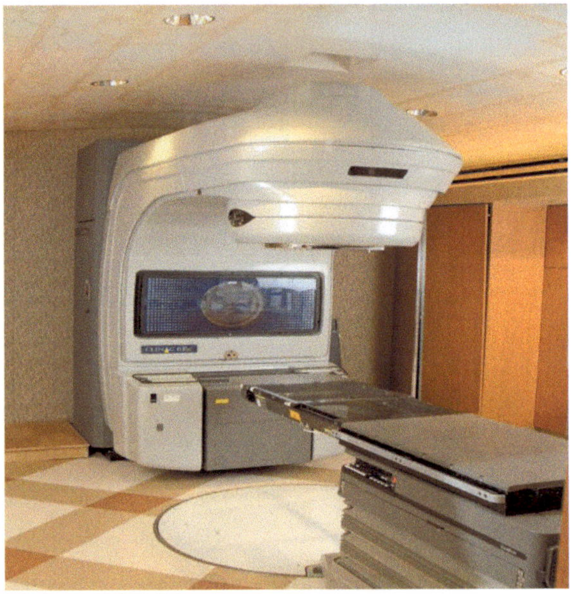

Fig. 10.1 Photograph of a linear accelerator

10.2 Historical Aspects

In the early 1920s, Rene Gilbert first demonstrated the use of radiation treatment to larger fields including both palpable and clinically uninvolved nodal areas. Radiation therapy as a curative modality for HL was first demonstrated by Vera Peters in 1950 (Peters 1950). Peters reported a 5- and 10-year survival rate of 88% and 72%, respectively, for 113 patients with stage I HL treated with fractionated radiation treatment at The Ontario Institute of Radiotherapy. In 1958, Peters and Middlemiss reported the results after longer follow-up of these patients and concluded that survival did not significantly change after 10 years (Peters and Middlemiss 1958).

Extended-field radiation for locally advanced disease became feasible with the introduction of the linear accelerator. Henry Kaplan collaborated with the Stanford Microwave Laboratory and developed the linear accelerator for radiation therapy use at Stanford in the 1950s. Linear accelerators allowed for the delivery of a large and accurate beam to target deeper tissues called high-dose extended-field radiation (Fig. 10.1). Kaplan reported significantly improved 2-year freedom from recurrence compared with low-dose involved-field radiation with palliative intent (Rosenberg and Kaplan 1985). The improvements in staging, and development of multimodality treatment using chemotherapy and radiation treatment, led to enhanced curability of HL. Extended-field radiation became standard treatment in the 1960s due to these promising outcomes.

Continued progress in the delivery of radiation from the extended field to the involved-field techniques used today enhanced conformality and dose homogeneity. The delivery of reduced fields requires detailed clinical information to delineate the target accurately. Pre-chemotherapy and post-chemotherapy imaging is required to define the tumor volume extent. The integration of computed tomography (CT) and positron emission tomography (PET)/CT treatment planning reduces the variability in treatment-field design. A margin of safety to address subclinical disease, and random and systematic error, is still necessary in field setup but techniques to minimize inaccuracies in treatment planning and delivery continue to improve.

10.3 Photon Energy

Linear accelerators with 6 MV photon-beam energy are commonly used in the treatment of patients with HL. A beam with 6 MV photon energy has a relatively flat beam profile and, therefore, allows for dose homogeneity throughout the treatment field. However, in large irregular treatment fields such as the mantle field, dose inhomogeneity in the range of 10–20% can occur

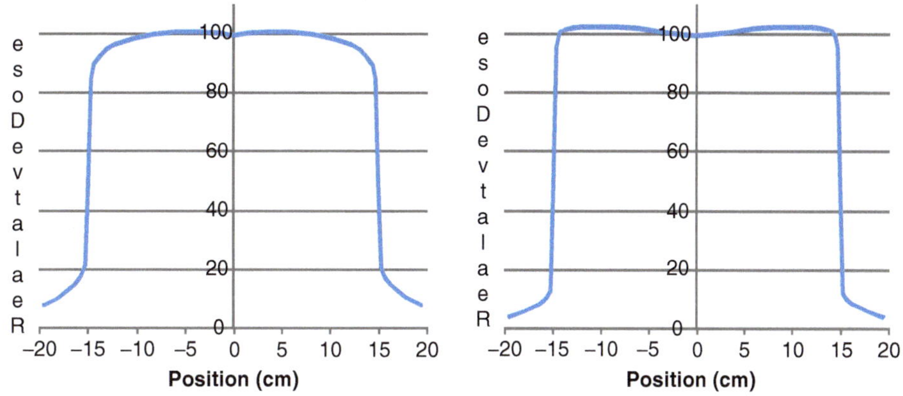

Fig. 10.2 Beam profile for a 6 MV beam for a 30 × 30 cm field (depth = 10 cm). *Left*, depth = 10 cm; *right*, depth = 1.4 cm

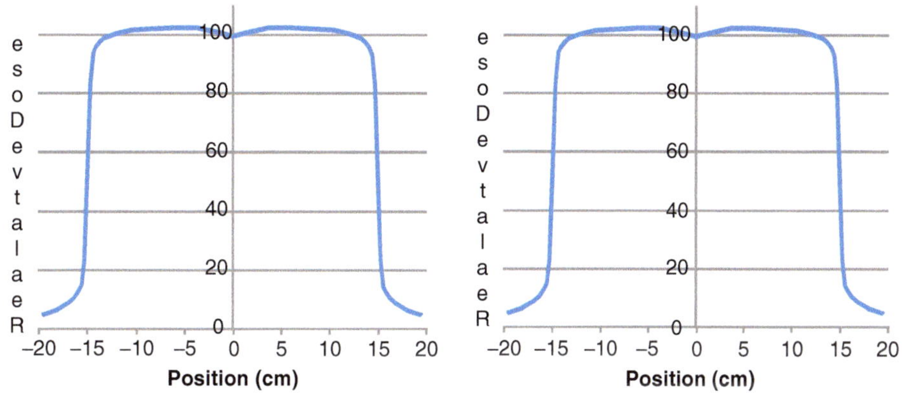

Fig. 10.3 Beam profile for a 15 MV beam for a 30 × 30cm field (depth = 1.4 cm). *Left*, depth = 10 cm; *right*, depth = 1.4 cm

due to differential separations in the superior and inferior regions of the field. Treatment at extended source-to-skin distances (SSD) of 120 cm or more not only leads to larger field sizes but can also help mitigate the irregularities in the dose distribution. The depth of maximum dose of a 6 MV beam is approximately 1.5 cm, close enough to the surface to avoid underdosing superficial lymph nodes while achieving penetration to treat deeper lymph node basins adequately (Fig. 10.2).

Higher beam energies can be used to treat patients with larger separations (>24 cm) and 10 or 15 MV beams are often used in the treatment of abdominal fields. In certain cases, the deeper penetration of a higher-energy beam is required, although superficial lymph nodes may be present that require treatment as well. For such cases, a "beam spoiler," a low-atomic-number absorber typically about 1 cm thick and placed approximately 20 cm from the surface of the patient, can be used to increase the superficial dose to an acceptable level while maintaining the depth-dose characteristics and dose homogeneity of a high-energy beam (Fig. 10.3).

10.4 Prescription Dose

Dose–response data reported by Kaplan suggested that a radiation dose of 40 Gy was necessary for the adequate treatment of Hodgkin and non-Hodgkin lymphomas (Kaplan 1966). However, multiple studies challenged this assumption and proposed a sigmoidal dose–response curve with a threshold dose of 30 Gy required to control disease, particularly subclinical disease (Fletcher and Shukovsky 1975; Hanks et al. 1982; Schewe et al. 1988; Thar et al. 1979).

Clinical factors likely to impact tumor control include tumor size, use of chemotherapy, disease extent, and technical considerations related to field design and accuracy of patient setup. The radiation dose is typically delivered in 1.8–2.0 Gy fractions. If significant portions of lung or heart are included, the dose per fraction can be reduced to 1.5 Gy. The available data indicate that the choice of fractionation is not critical for tumor control, and that a schedule with minimal risk of damage to normal structures should be selected (Brincker and Bentzen 1994).

The German Hodgkin Study Group clinically evaluated dose–response in patients with stage IA to IIB disease without risk factors in a randomized trial of 40 Gy extended-field radiation alone vs. 30 Gy extended-field radiation with a boost of 10 Gy to the involved site of disease (Duhmke et al. 1996, 2001). There was no significant difference in outcome between the two arms of the study indicating that 30 Gy is sufficient for clinically uninvolved areas. The optimum dose for clinically involved sites of disease with radiotherapy alone has not been tested in a randomized trial. Retrospective analyses of data from the literature have attempted to define a dose–response relationship depending on tumor burden (Vijayakumar and Myrianthopoulos 1992). However, a more stringent re-analysis of the available data concluded that there was no indication of a dose–response relationship at doses above 32.5 Gy and that there was not enough evidence to support the notion that various dose levels were required for different tumor burdens (Brincker and Bentzen 1994). Today, combined modality treatment is usually employed, and even lower doses may be sufficient in this setting (see Chap. 2, Sect. 2.3.1).

Radiation dose is an important determinant that influences the development of long-term complications. Both second solid tumors and cardiac complications are dose related (Hancock et al. 1993b; Travis et al. 2002, 2005).

10.5 Extended-Field Radiation Treatment

Extended-field radiation is loosely defined as the treatment of involved and adjacent uninvolved lymph node regions at risk of disease. This is determined primarily by literature elucidating the pattern of spread in patients with HL (Mauch et al. 1993; Rosenberg and Kaplan 1985). Treatment-field definitions vary in the literature and include the mantle and paraaortic fields, extended mantle, mini-mantle, subtotal lymphoid, and total lymphoid radiation.

Extended fields are rarely used today. Yet, in situation when RT is the primary treatment or in salvage programs (see Chap. 4), these fields are still employed and are therefore described with specific technical consideration below. Moreover, many long-term survivors were treated with these techniques in the past. In the evaluation of these patients the radiation oncologist needs to be familiar with these treatment techniques.

10.5.1 Radiation Field Terminology

Total lymphoid irradiation (TLI), also known as total nodal irradiation (TNI), involves treatment of the major nodal groups typically at risk for HL including the supradiaphragmatic lymph nodes in the so-called mantle field (cervical, supraclavicular, infraclavicular, axillary, mediastinal, and hilar lymph nodes) and the infradiaphragmatic lymph nodes in the so-called inverted Y field (paraaortic, pelvic and inguino-femoral lymph nodes). If a splenectomy has not been performed, the treatment field includes the spleen in the inverted Y field. The mantle and inverted Y fields are given sequentially in TLI to spare the patient significant acute toxicity (Fig. 10.4).

Subtotal lymphoid irradiation (STLI) of subtotal nodal irradiation (STNI) refers to the treatment of the mantle field and the paraaortic field (i.e., the upper part of the inverted Y field). The inferior border is placed at the aortic bifurcation and the spleen is included. Again, these fields are given sequentially so that they can be tolerated by the patient.

The extended mantle field, which includes the standard mantle field and the upper paraaortic lymph nodes with or without the spleen, can also be used to treat the upper abdominal lymph nodes. The use of the extended mantle field obviates the setup difficulties involved in the matching of the mantle and paraaortic fields for STLI; dose inhomogeneity and treatment time is reduced, although daily setup becomes more difficult due to the large field size and extended source-to-skin distance required for treatment delivery.

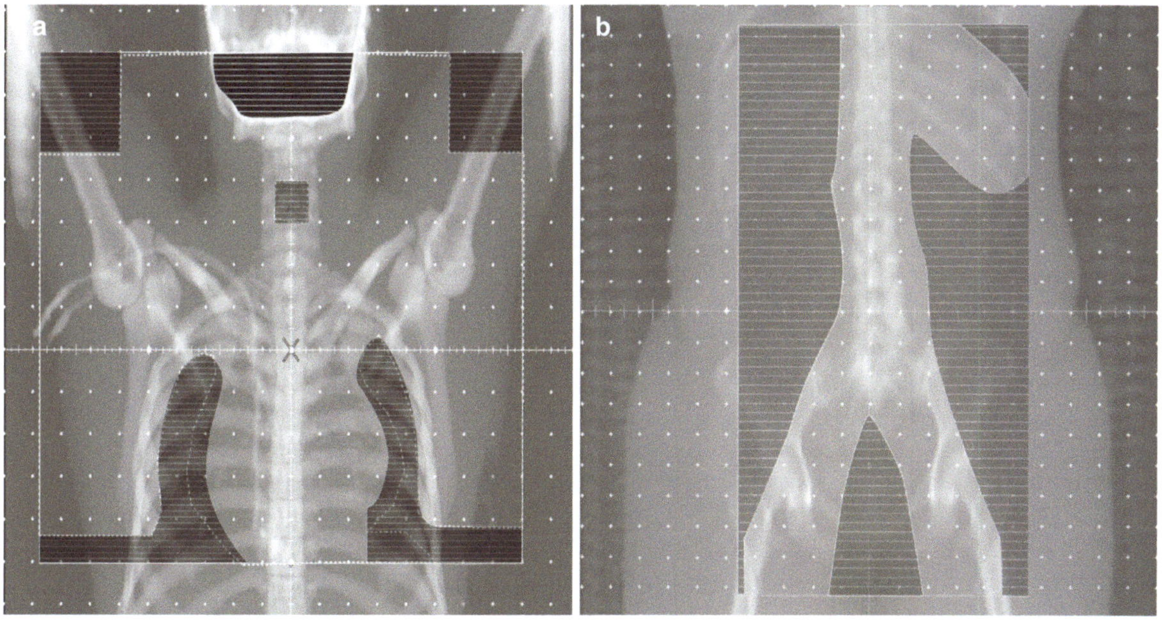

Fig. 10.4 Digitally reconstructed radiograph depicting TLI including treatment of the (**a**) mantle and (**b**) inverted Y fields, respectively

10.5.2 Mantle Field

The mantle field has traditionally been used to treat the supradiaphragmatic lymph node regions including the cervical, supraclavicular, infraclavicular, axillary, mediastinal, and hilar nodal basins (Fig. 10.5). The mini-mantle excludes the mediastinum but includes the cervical, supraclavicular, infraclavicular, and axillary lymph nodes. Design and accurate treatment delivery of this large field presents numerous challenges, particularly regarding the protection of the lungs and heart given their proximity to these lymph node regions.

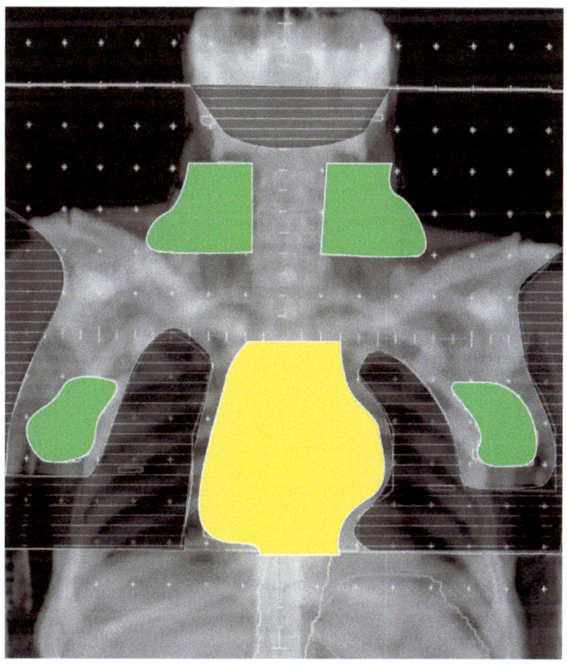

Fig. 10.5 Digitally reconstructed radiograph of the mantle field depicting CT-based contours of involved lymph nodes at the bilateral neck, bilateral axillae, and mediastinum

Significant dose inhomogeneities of 10% or more can be created by differences in patient thickness and depth of nodal basins across the neck and thorax (Gray and Prosnitz 1975; Jones and Hilko 1981; McCullough and Earle 1982; Vijayakumar et al. 1992). As a result, dose calculations at the neck, supraclavicular region, axilla, mediastinum, and spinal cord, or dose distributions through these regions, are often used to quantify the doses received by these regions. To improve dose homogeneity throughout the field, custom compensators or selective blocking have been used (Butts et al. 1997; Cantwell et al. 1989; Kessaris 1978). Such techniques achieve a uniform dose throughout the field by determining the treatment time needed to deliver the prescription dose to the mediastinum and then adding blocking or compensators to those sites where the prescribed dose is exceeded (such as the neck, supraclavicular, and axillary regions) due to variation in patient thickness. More recently, techniques using dynamic multileaf collimation, an intensity-modulated radiotherapy delivery method, have been proposed that simultaneously provide field shaping and missing tissue dose compensation throughout the mantle treatment field (Davis et al. 2006).

The dose to normal tissues protected by field blocking in a mantle field such as the breast and heart can also be quite variable. The shielded portions of the breast and heart can receive low, but still significant, doses during mantle irradiation due to internal scatter and transmission through the field blocks (Kowalski and Smith 1998; Wirth et al. 2008; Zellmer et al. 1991). Dose to the breast, in particular, is highly variable, since for many patients portions of the breast lie within both the open and blocked portions of the mantle field. As a result, dose to different regions of the breast for a typical course of mantle irradiation can range from several hundred cGy to doses close to the prescription dose.

The mantle field can be treated using a source-to-skin distance (SSD) or source-to-axis distance (SAD) technique (Fig. 10.6). Historically, SSD techniques have been used when field sizes larger than those possible with isocentric or SAD techniques were required. With early SSD techniques, the patient lies supine for delivery of the anterior field and prone for treatment with the posterior field. With the advent of "extended-range" treatment couches, however, it has become possible to treat the patient at an extended distance without repositioning. These so-called "extended SAD" techniques offer simplicity of patient setup compared with SSD techniques. With either SAD or extended-SAD techniques, rapid positioning can occur as the patient remains supine for the duration of treatment delivered using anterior and posterior fields. Unfortunately, it is difficult to visually verify gapping for adjacent posterior fields if the patient is supine for the entirety of treatment; instead, radiographic techniques must be the primary method of verification.

Although increased field size is the primary reason for using an extended-distance technique during mantle irradiation (120–140 cm), dose homogeneity can also be somewhat improved due to the improved depth-dose characteristics of the beam and decreased beam divergence between abutting fields in the match region. Ideally, 6 MV photons are used for treatment of the mantle field in conjunction with techniques to improve dose inhomogeneity. Although higher-energy photons may be considered, there is a risk of underdosing superficial nodal regions including the neck, and a method of increasing the dose within the first the first 1–2 cm of tissue (i.e., with the use of a beam spoiler or bolus) must be considered.

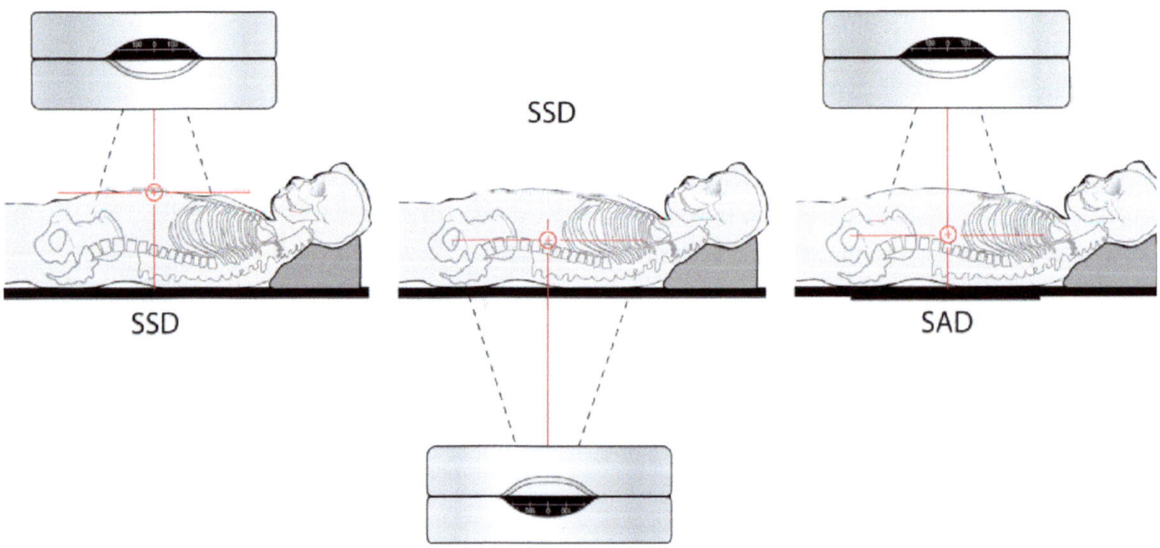

Fig. 10.6 Illustration of the SSD and SAD techniques

10.5.2.1 Technical Considerations of the Mantle Field

Patients receiving mantle irradiation can be positioned with the arms overhead or akimbo. Lymphangiography has been used in the past to estimate the position of axillary lymph nodes in lymphoma radiation planning (Pergolizzi et al. 2004; Weisenburger and Juillard 1974, 1977). The raising of the patient's arms alters the position of the axillary lymph nodes and lifts them superiorly and laterally (Fig. 10.7). As a result, humeral head blocking should be avoided so that the axillary lymph nodes are adequately covered within the treatment field (Fig. 10.8) (Mansur et al. 2005; Pergolizzi et al. 2000).

However, increased lung blocking can be readily performed when the axillary lymph nodes are pulled laterally from the chest wall. The humeral heads are adequately blocked in the akimbo position, although a strip of lung inside the rib may be treated to give adequate margin around the axillary lymph nodes. The akimbo technique is particularly preferred in prepubertal children so that the epiphyseal plate can be shielded. The akimbo position may also be more comfortable for patients and should be considered if the patients cannot tolerate their arms held above their heads. Increased skin reactions can occur when the arms are placed akimbo due to the skin folds at the level of the axilla.

To avoid blocking of the axillary lymph nodes, the location of the axillary structures can be precisely localized using CT simulation to allow for accurate target delineation (Mansur et al. 2005; Naida et al. 1996; Pergolizzi et al. 2004). Iodinated contrast should be used at the time of CT simulation to identify involved nodes and mediastinal structures to improve target delineation and normal organ identification.

An alpha cradle type mold should also be used for arm-positioning immobilization for enhanced reproducibility and the breasts should be taped most often in a lateral position to avoid inclusion within the mediastinal field (Fig. 10.9) especially when the axillae are not included in the field. The head should be placed in a neutral position as flexion may result in increased dose delivered to the oral cavity, while hyperextension may result in excessive radiation dose delivered to the infratentorial structures of the brain. The neck should be immobilized by use of a facemask, or a chinstrap if

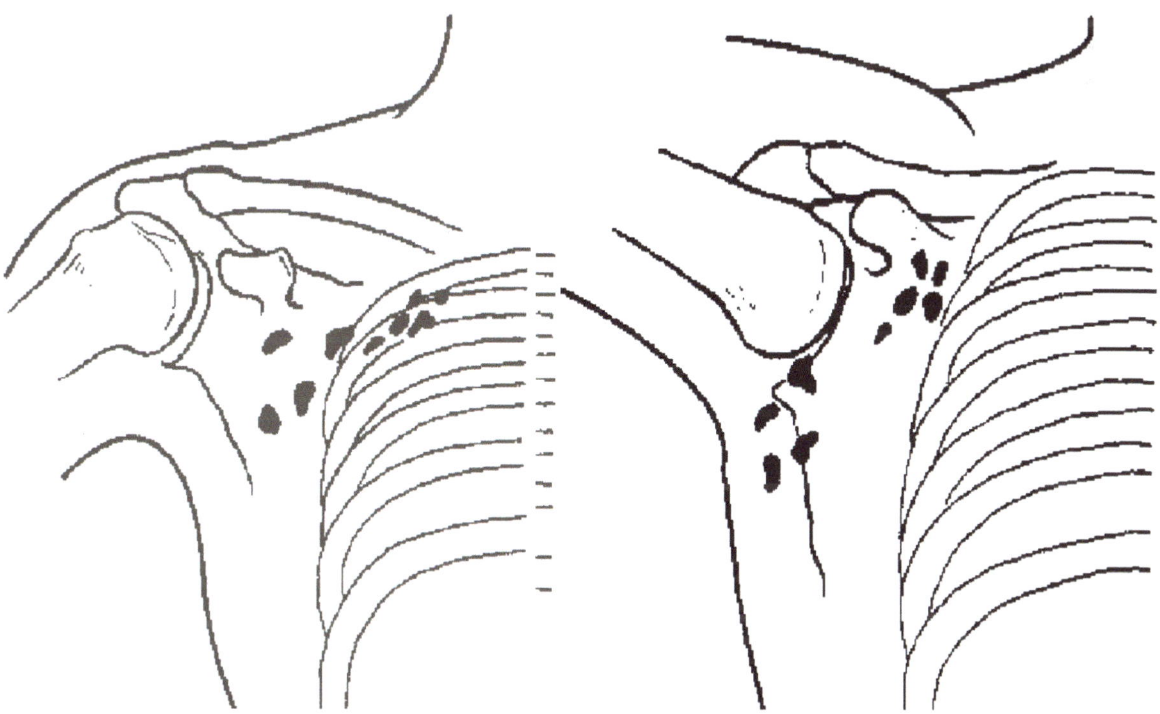

Fig. 10.7 Change in position of axillary lymph nodes in the arms-down (*left*) versus arms-up (*right*) positions

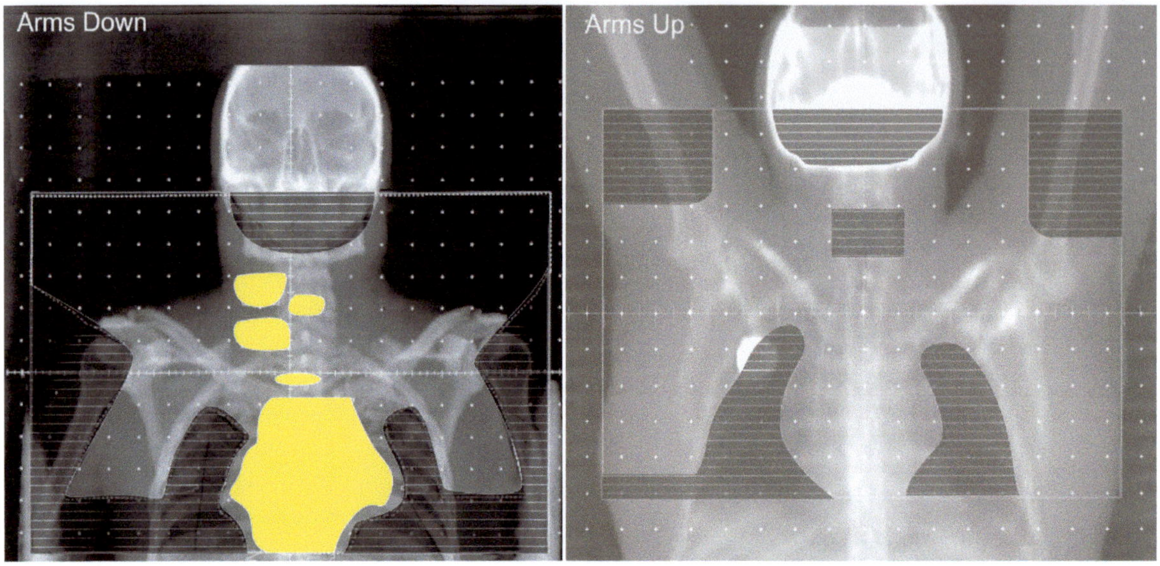

Fig. 10.8 Digitally reconstructed radiograph depicting a mantle field demonstrating humeral head blocking in the arms-down position (*left*). The humeral heads are not blocked when the arms are raised above the head to avoid blocking the axillary lymph nodes (*right*)

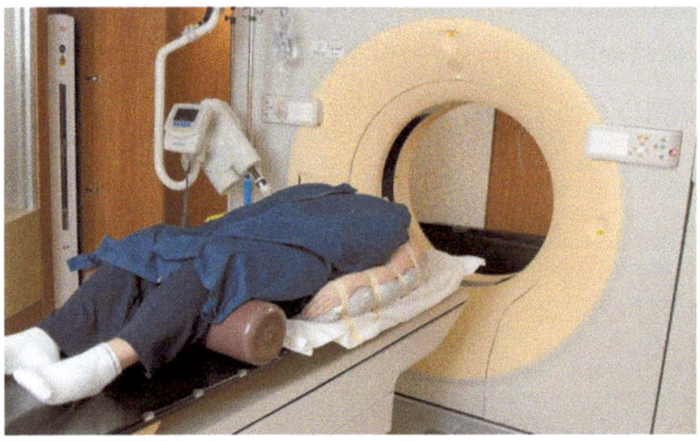

Fig. 10.9 Patient positioned for treatment of an involved field to the mediastinum while immobilized in an alpha cradle

the patient is unable to tolerate a mask. A cervical spine block, extending from the jaw to the bottom of the larynx, should be placed on the posterior neck field if the cord dose exceeds 40 Gy (Yahalom and Mauch 2002). The maximum cord dose should be calculated at mid-neck. Since the neck will normally receive a higher dose than the isocentric center (supra-sternal notch), in a patient with no midline neck disease, a laryngeal block extending from the notch of the thyroid cartilage to the inferior edge of the cricoid cartilage may be placed after 18–20 Gy or throughout the treatment as a half-value layer block. When bulky lymphadenopathy is present, the larynx block should be avoided so that cervical disease is adequately treated.

In patients who are undergoing extended-field radiation to supradiaphragmatic and infradiaphragmatic lymph nodes (i.e., mantle and paraaortic and/or pelvic fields), a 2 × 2 cm partial-transmission block may be placed on the posterior field at the match to protect against overdosing the spinal cord. Typically, a block of 2–2.5 cm thickness is sufficient to decrease the dose under the block to approximately 50%. Because the required thickness is energy and block-size dependent, measurements of the block transmission as a function of thickness should be made prior to implementing such a technique. Partial-transmission blocks can also be used to deliver a prophylactic dose of radiation to the lungs and heart while simultaneously delivering an adequate treatment dose to gross nodal disease. Carmel and Kaplan reported a decrease in acute radiation pneumonitis using this technique (Carmel and Kaplan 1976). Selective full-thickness field blocking can also be used to block the lungs or heart once the prescription dose has been achieved in these areas. A smaller nodal field can then be continued to a higher dose using the same fraction size after lung and heart blocks are inserted.

Patients with bulky mediastinal masses can be treated using a shrinking-field technique if a large volume of lung and heart are included within the treatment field. To preserve the tolerance of these normal structures, a low dose of approximately 1.5 Gy per fraction should be given initially until the patient can be rescanned for consideration of a cone-down field. Resimulation can be performed after a given period of time to allow for treatment response and modification of the treatment field to increase the size of the lung and heart blocks without significantly compromising the dose delivered to the tumor volume.

10.5.3 Paraaortic/Inverted Y Field

The inverted Y field has traditionally been used to treat the infradiaphragmatic lymph node regions including the paraaortic nodes, spleen, pelvic nodes and inguino-femoral nodes. A modification treating only the paraaortic nodes in patients with good prognostic characteristics was introduced to minimize toxicity. In the past, when the spleen was removed as part of the staging procedures, the splenic pedicle was included in the field.

10.5.3.1 Technical Considerations of the Paraaortic/Inverted Y Field

Equally weighted anterior and posterior fields are used to treat the paraaortic lymph nodes, spleen, pelvic, and/or inguino-femoral lymph nodes. Patients can be treated using the same setup as the mantle field. Treatment can be delivered supine using the SAD technique or supine and prone using the SSD technique. The superior border can be placed at the level of the T10/T11 junction when the infradiaphragmatic nodes are treated alone. If a supradiaphragmatic field is treated as well, the inferior border must be matched to the superior border of the infradiaphragmatic field accounting for divergence. An alpha cradle can be considered for immobilization of the abdomen and pelvis particularly if a conformal plan is designed for treatment.

CT and magnetic resonance imaging (MRI) can be used during simulation to ensure accurate localization of the kidneys and spleen when the patient is in the treatment position (Fig. 10.10). Iodinated contrast should be administered during CT simulation for localization of the paraaortic and pelvic lymph node chains. The positional changes of the spleen during respiration should be accounted for, particularly if volumes are transferred from a diagnostic CT that is normally taken in deep inspiration. The location of the kidneys must be identified to preserve function by limiting the total renal volume receiving dose. A pre-treatment renal scan can quantify kidney function and help avoid the radiation of a single functioning kidney so that adequate renal function is sustained.

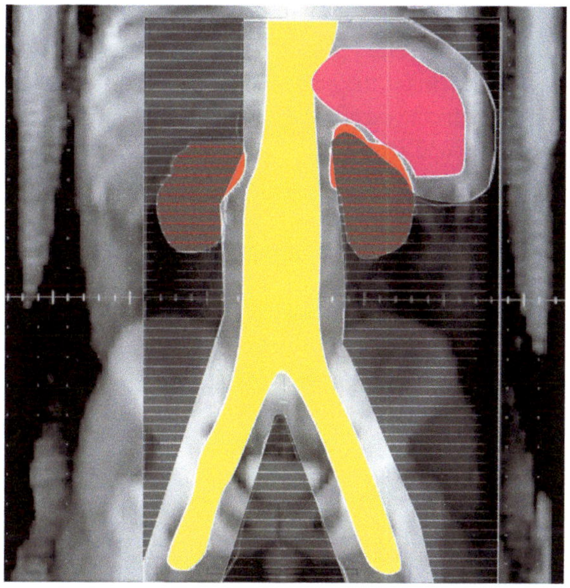

Fig. 10.10 Digitally reconstructed radiograph of the inverted Y field with contours depicting the position of the treated volume including the spleen, paraaortic, and pelvic lymph nodes with blocking of the bilateral kidneys

Because the spleen is difficult to identify on fluoroscopic films, CT or MRI simulation can ensure accurate target localization. The spleen abuts the diaphragm and, therefore, the diaphragm causes the spleen to move. To account for respiratory motion, the left diaphragm is included within the treatment field and a 1.5 cm margin should be added to the post-chemotherapy splenic volume (Yahalom and Mauch 2002). Since the spleen is also closely associated anatomically with the left kidney, the use of CT or MRI simulation can help accurately localize normal structures. Less than one-third of the kidney should be included within the treatment field. If the inclusion of more than one-third of kidney is necessary for adequate treatment of the infradiaphragmatic field, then the contralateral kidney dose should be constrained.

Gonadal dose is a special consideration in the treatment of the inverted Y field. The inferior border of a field that includes the pelvic nodes is generally placed inferiorly to the ischial tuberosities. With a standard treatment field including the pelvic lymph nodes, the testicles are not in the primary beam but receive internal scatter and head leakage radiation dose, which can cause permanent azoospermia (Centola et al. 1994; Lushbaugh and Casarett 1976). The testicular dose is generally 2–3% of the prescription dose, depending on the testicular shielding device used and the location of the treatment-field edge. Machine leakage may also result in increased scattered electrons at the skin surface (Fraass et al. 1985; Speiser et al. 1973). Unfortunately, it is not always possible to completely exclude the testes from the primary beam, particularly when the femoral nodes are included. As a result, the patient is at significantly higher risk for sterility and care must be taken to shield the testes as carefully as possible and ensure reproducibility of the shielding on a daily basis.

Testicular shielding using a "clamshell"-like device reduces dose primarily by reducing internal scatter and may help preserve fertility (Fig. 10.11). Clamshell shields can reduce the dose to the testes by approximately threefold to tenfold (Fraass et al. 1985). They are coated in 2 mm of a low-atomic number material such as plastic or rubber to absorb and minimize the dose from low-energy electrons created from within the shield itself. The testicles are placed within the clamshell behind the front wall with the lip of the shield overlapping the front wall. Patients at risk of receiving testicular doses are counseled and encouraged to undergo sperm banking prior to simulation or radiation treatment.

In the female patient, the ovaries are included within the standard pelvic treatment field, which results in the loss of fertility. Patients are counseled about the options for embryo or oocyte cryopreservation before initiation of radiotherapy. In an effort to preserve fertility, ovarian transposition can also be performed to move the ovaries outside the primary radiation treatment field or to relocate them to a site where blocking can be performed (Classe et al. 1998; Clough et al. 1996; Ray et al. 1970; Sola et al. 2008; Thibaud et al. 1992; Trueblood et al. 1970; Williams et al. 1999). Ovarian transposition at the time of staging laparotomy was common in the past. However, staging laparotomy is now rarely performed. The laparoscopic approach to oophoropexy has demonstrated effectiveness with a reduction in postoperative morbidity and is now increasingly used (Classe et al. 1998; Clough et al. 1996; Sola et al. 2008; Tinga et al. 1999; Williams et al. 1999; Williams and Mendenhall 1992). The surgeon must be informed of the intended radiation field to accurately relocate the ovaries. Radiopaque clips

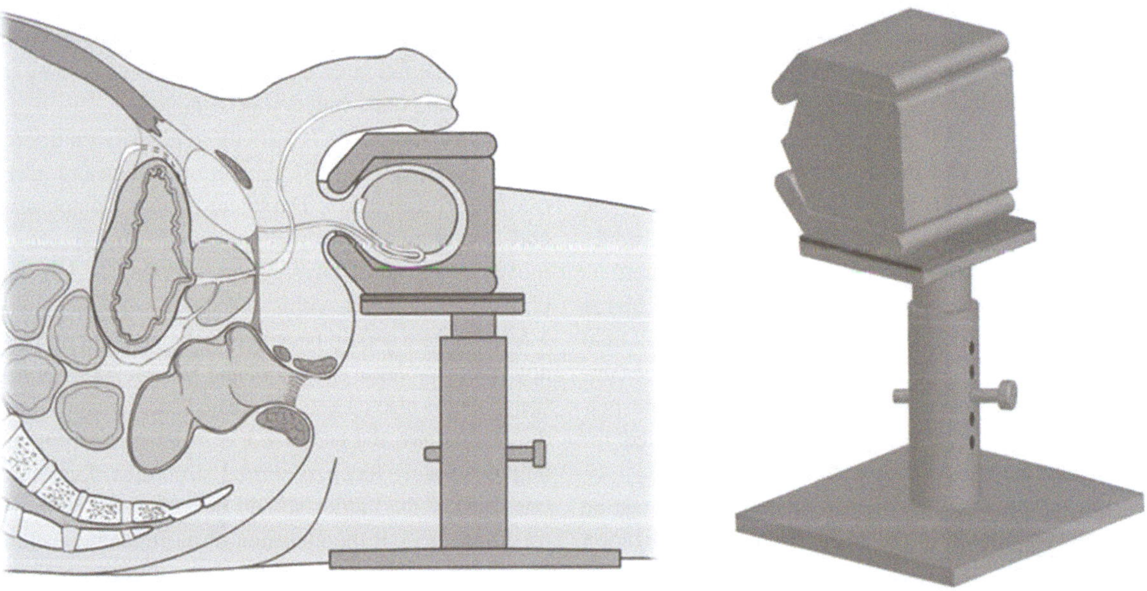

Fig. 10.11 Illustration of clamshell testicular shielding

should be placed at the proximal and distal end of the ovaries. This helps ensure that the treatment field can be designed to avoid them. Movement of the ovaries from their oophoropexy location can be identified during simulation and ovarian position should be confirmed before treatment is delivered.

Ovarian dose is affected by scattered radiation generated within the treatment field as well as primary transmission through the block. A number of technical factors can affect the total dose delivered to the ovaries including the field size, distance of the ovaries from the edge of the field, and suboptimal location of the ovaries relative to the field edge. Combined modality therapy can be used to reduce the treatment-field size so that involved-field radiation may be considered. Ovarian function is more likely to be preserved with a reduced treatment-field size and increased distance from the primary beam.

10.6 Involved-Field Radiation

Several trials have demonstrated that in the combined modality setting with modern chemotherapy regimens much smaller radiation fields are needed (Bonadonna et al. 2004; Engert et al. 2003; Ferme et al. 2007). The involved field (IF) is generally perceived as encompassing the site of the initial clinically involved lymph node group. The "grouping" of lymph nodes has not been clearly defined, and there has been a tendency to use the regions defined for the Ann Arbor staging classification (Kaplan and Rosenberg 1966), although they were never meant to be used for radiotherapy planning. In the following are given definitions of types of radiation fields used in the treatment of Hodgkin lymphoma.

10.6.1 Technical Considerations for Involved-Field Radiation

Radiation treatment of the involved lymph node region after chemotherapy requires accurate treatment-field design. The cervical (including supraclavicular lymph nodes), axillary, mediastinal, paraaortic/spleen, or pelvic lymph nodes are commonly designated as sites for involved-field treatments based on patterns of disease spread. Both pre-chemotherapy and post-chemotherapy clinical information and imaging must be available for definition of the involved site. Pre-chemotherapy identification of initially involved lymph node groups is required to define the treatment field. Post-chemotherapy imaging is also necessary to assess response and reduce treatment-field size appropriately. Technical guidelines for treatment-field setup, positioning, and immobilization exist for each involved-field site. Unless contraindicated, iodinated contrast should be administered at the time of CT simulation to highlight the vasculature, normal organs at risk, and potential sites of disease. In general, 6 MV photons are optimal for treating sites above the diaphragm while higher energies (10 MV or 15 MV) can be used below the diaphragm.

10.6.1.1 Cervical (Including Supraclavicular Lymph Nodes) Field

Treatment of the cervical region includes the unilateral or bilateral neck and supraclavicular lymph nodes extending from the base of the skull to the clavicles. The patient is positioned supine and the neck is immobilized using a thermoplastic mask extending over the head, neck, and shoulder region (Figs. 10.12 and 10.13). A chin strap can be used for reproducibility if the patient is unable to tolerate a mask but consideration must then be given during field design to the increased risk and magnitude of positioning errors

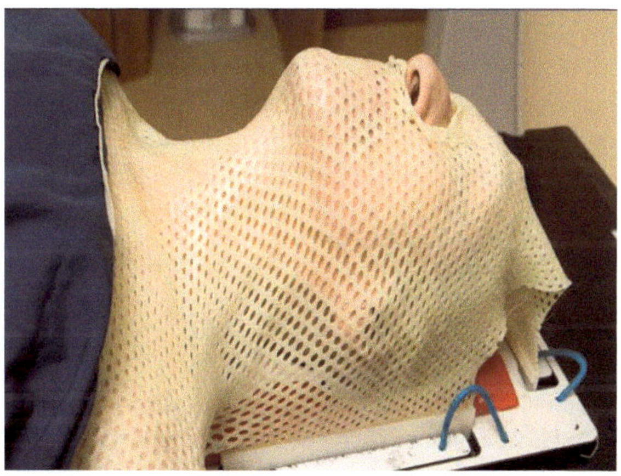

Fig. 10.12 Immobilization of a patient undergoing simulation for treatment to the unilateral neck using an Aquaplast mask

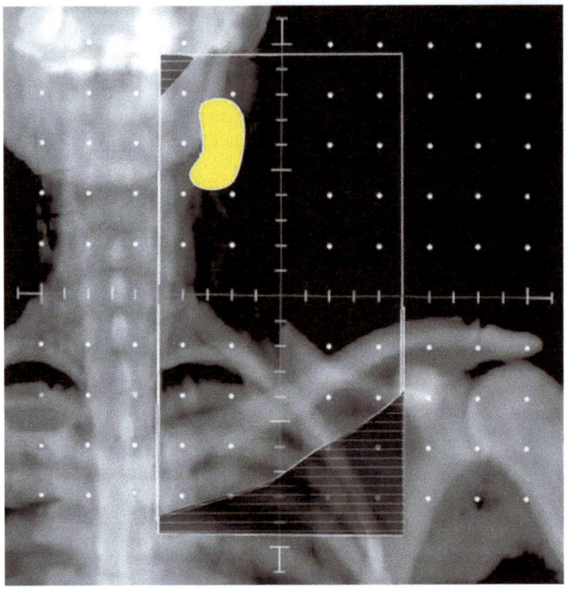

Fig. 10.13 Digitally reconstructed radiograph of the unilateral neck involved field with CT-based contours outlining the involved node

during treatment. When the supraclavicular lymph nodes are not involved, the lateral border is placed at the ipsilateral transverse processes unless an adequate margin is necessary for coverage of medially placed lymph nodes. If the supraclavicular lymph nodes are involved, the lateral border should be extended to the contralateral border of the transverse processes.

The maximum cord dose should be calculated at the mid-neck with a cervical cord block placed posteriorly if it exceeds 36 Gy. A larynx block should be used unless an adequate margin cannot be achieved due to medial cervical lymph nodes or bulky disease involvement. The larynx block should be implemented at 1,800 cGy or a 50% partial-transmission larynx block can be used for the full duration of treatment (Yahalom and Mauch 2002). A posterior mouth block should be used if the patient is treated supine to block divergence through the mouth.

10.6.1.2 Axillary Field

Treatment of the axilla includes the ipsilateral axillary, infraclavicular, and supraclavicular lymph nodes. The superior border is set at the C5–C6 interspace and the inferior border is placed at the tip of the scapula or at least 2 cm below the lowest initially involved axillary lymph node. The medial border is placed at the ipsilateral transverse process but should include the vertebral bodies if the supraclavicular lymph nodes are clinically involved. The lateral border should flash the axilla. The arms should be preferably placed above the head and immobilized using a custom mold to enhance reproducibility.

Based on information derived from lymphangiograms, axillary lymph node position changes with arm abduction to overlap with the humeral head (Weisenburger and Juillard 1974, 1977). In a study by Mansur et al., CT simulation performed on 61 patients determined that the degree of overlap of axillary lymph nodes and the humeral head significantly increased as the degree of arm abduction increased (Mansur et al. 2005). Humeral head blocking when the arm is abducted greater than 55° blocks axillary lymph nodes. Therefore, humeral head blocking should be avoided in adult patients who are positioned with their arms above their heads. For pre-pubertal children, the arms should be placed akimbo to allow humeral head shielding to protect the epiphyseal plate for bone growth. CT simulation enables accurate delineation of the axillary lymph node region and appropriate blocking depending on the clinical scenario (Fig. 10.14).

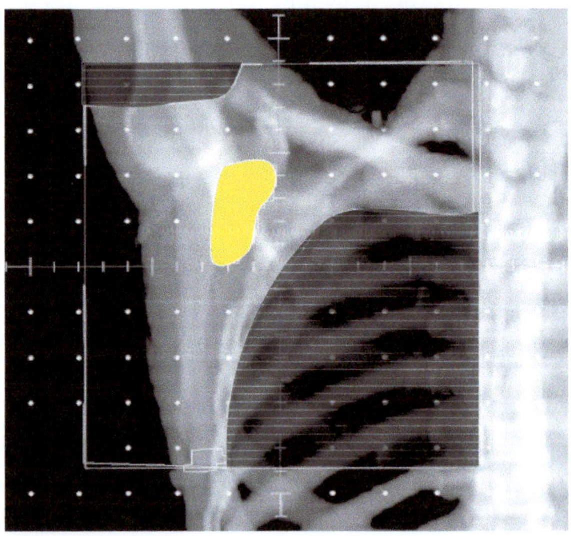

Fig. 10.14 Digitally reconstructed radiograph depicting an axillary involved field with CT-based contours of the involved axillary lymph nodes

10.6.1.3 Mediastinal Field

The mediastinal treatment field should include the hilar, pretracheal, paratracheal, paraesophageal, internal mammary, subcarinal, anterior superior mediastinal lymph nodes, and bilateral medial supraclavicular lymph nodes. These lymph nodes are difficult to identify using radiographic simulation films but can be precisely localized using CT simulation. The upper border should be placed at the C5–C6 interspace and at the top of the larynx if the supraclavicular lymph nodes are involved. A half-value layer (HVL) block can be placed over the larynx. The lower border should be placed 2 cm below the pre-chemotherapy inferior border or 5 cm below the carina, while the lateral border should be placed 1.5 cm from the post-chemotherapy volume (Fig. 10.15) (Yahalom and Mauch 2002).

For treatment, the patient is placed supine with the arms akimbo or at the side. If the axillary lymph nodes are involved, the arms may be raised above the head. Due to the known association of secondary breast cancer and HL radiation treatment, the breasts should be moved away from the field and taped for immobilization. The breasts can be outlined with a wire during simulation for better visualization during treatment planning so that normal breast tissue can be avoided within the treatment field (Bhatia et al. 1996; Boivin et al. 1995; Boivin and O'Brien 1988; Colvett 1995; Cook et al. 1990; Dershaw et al. 1992; Goss and Sierra 1998; Hancock et al. 1993a; Hancock and Hoppe 1996; Henry-Amar 1988; Janjan et al. 1988; Kaldor et al. 1987; Lavey et al. 1990; Prior and Pope 1988; Sankila et al. 1996; Swerdlow et al. 1992; Tester et al. 1984; Tinger et al. 1997; Tucker et al. 1988; Tucker 1993; van Leeuwen et al. 1994; Wolden et al. 1998; Yahalom et al. 1992).

10.6.1.4 Paraaortic/Pelvic Lymph Nodes Field(s)

The standard paraaortic field includes a volume extending from the top of T11 to the bottom of L4 including 2 cm above and below the pre-chemotherapy volume (Yahalom and Mauch 2002). The lateral borders of the field include the edge of the transverse processes or 2 cm around the post-chemotherapy volume. The position of the paraaortic lymph nodes and bilateral kidneys can be confirmed using CT simulation (Fig. 10.16). The spleen should be included within the paraaortic treatment field if imaging suggests disease involvement. If the patient has undergone splenectomy, the field can be extended laterally to include the splenic hilar region. The splenic hilum may be marked by

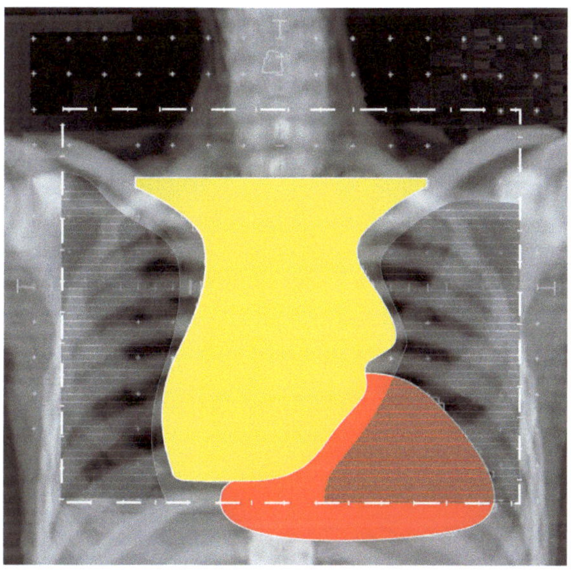

Fig. 10.15 Digitally reconstructed radiograph of a mediastinal involved field with CT-based contours of the involved mediastinum and normal heart

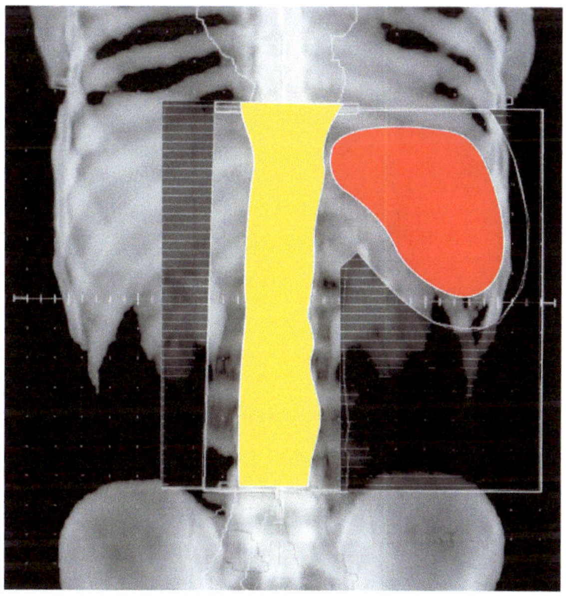

Fig. 10.16 Digitally reconstructed radiograph of the paraaortic treatment field with CT-based contours of the involved paraaortic lymph nodes and spleen

radiopaque clips during surgical resection. If clips were not placed at the time of surgery, the field can be extended laterally at T12–L1, where the splenic hilar lymph nodes are located along the splenic vasculature. The post-chemotherapy splenic volume should be treated with 1.5 cm margins. Patients may be immobilized with a custom mold, particularly if a three-dimensional conformal treatment is planned.

The external iliac, femoral, and inguinal lymph nodes are included within an involved field when one of these lymph node groups requires treatment. The upper border is placed at the middle of the sacro-iliac joint while the lower border is placed 5 cm below the lesser trochanter (Yahalom and Mauch 2002). The lateral border is set at the greater trochanter at least 2 cm lateral to the initially involved lymph nodes. The medial border is placed at the obturator foramen or at least 2 cm medial to the pre-chemotherapy lymph nodes. When there is evidence of common iliac nodal involvement, the treatment field is extended to L4–L5 at least 2 cm beyond the pre-chemotherapy volume. The patient can be placed in a "frog-leg" position to separate the leg from the external genitalia as well as flatten any inguinal skin folds to minimize a potential skin reaction (Fig. 10.17).

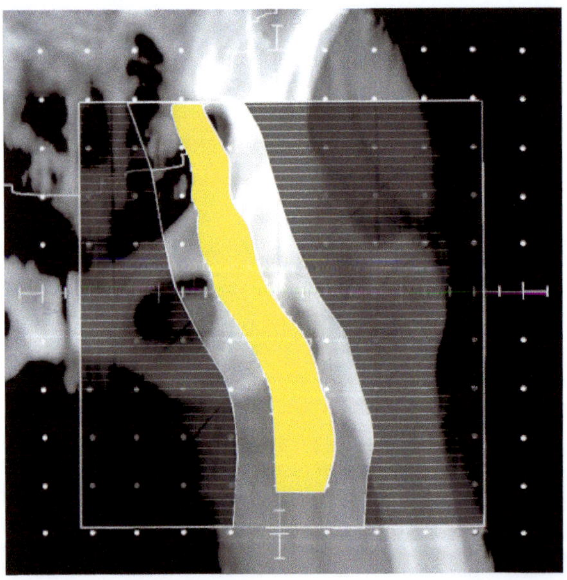

Fig. 10.17 Digitally reconstructed radiograph of a unilateral pelvic treatment field depicting CT-based contours of the involved pelvic and inguinal lymph nodes

10.7 Involved-Node Radiation

The lymphatic system is a continuous system throughout the body, and the division into lymph node regions and lymph node groups is really artificial, created with the aim of systematically staging patients (Kaplan and Rosenberg 1966). The goal of radiotherapy in the combined modality setting is to irradiate the macroscopically involved lymphoma volume, but no more than that, in order to avoid unnecessary radiation to normal tissues. With the introduction of much more accurate imaging and treatment delivery techniques the trend is now to disregard the old definitions of regions and lymph node groups and to focus radiotherapy on the initial macroscopically involved lymph nodes (and the relatively rare extranodal involved structures) with tight margins. This concept is called involved-node radiotherapy (INRT), and it is described in detail in Chap. 9.

10.8 Field Matching

A patient frequently requires treatment to multiple sites, contiguous and non-contiguous, and field matching is required to abut adjacent treatment fields. Extended-field radiation requires matching techniques when patients are treated to mantle and paraaortic and/or pelvic lymph node fields. These fields are often treated sequentially to reduce toxicity. Depending on the extent of treatment, involved sites can often be treated simultaneously (i.e., cervical and axillary). Perfect geometric matching of abutting treatment fields is often not possible, particularly when large field sizes are needed. As a result, diverging field edges in the match region must be aligned so as to minimize dose inhomogeneity. Several techniques for geometrically matching adjoining fields have evolved to prevent overlap at these sites and improve dose distributions.

10.8.1 Skin-Gap Technique

The most commonly used technique is the skin-gap technique, whereby pairs of diverging fields are aligned by calculating the gap needed at the surface of the patient to match the fields at depth. Abutting fields can be matched at midplane, at the depth of a tumor, or at the depth of a critical structure such as the spinal cord. The match plane should be selected after consideration of the relative locations of the tumor volume and normal tissues. Although the fields geometrically align in the match plane, in most situations, high- and low-dose regions are created in other planes due to the unequal divergence of the fields. This technique is most appropriate when the tumor volume lies relatively deep in the body and the superficial tissues are not at high risk for disease. It is also the most commonly used technique when the required field sizes are too large for the half beam technique.

Proper field matching can be verified by directly measuring the skin gap on the anterior patient surface where small tattoos are placed at the inferior border of the upper field and at the superior border of the lower field. Verification films should then be obtained to confirm the inferior upper field edge and the superior lower field edge of the opposing fields. The divergent field edges must be identified in relation to the spine to protect against overlap at the cord. When two sets of treatment fields are matched through a critical structure, a small HVL block can be added at each field border in the match region. For example, a 2 × 2 cm HVL block is placed over the spinal cord when matching mantle and paraaortic fields. Oh et al. evaluated different techniques for HVL block placement and found that placement of HVL blocks on both posterior fields ensured a maximum spinal cord dose less than the prescription without a significant loss in target coverage (Fig. 10.18) (Oh et al. 2000).

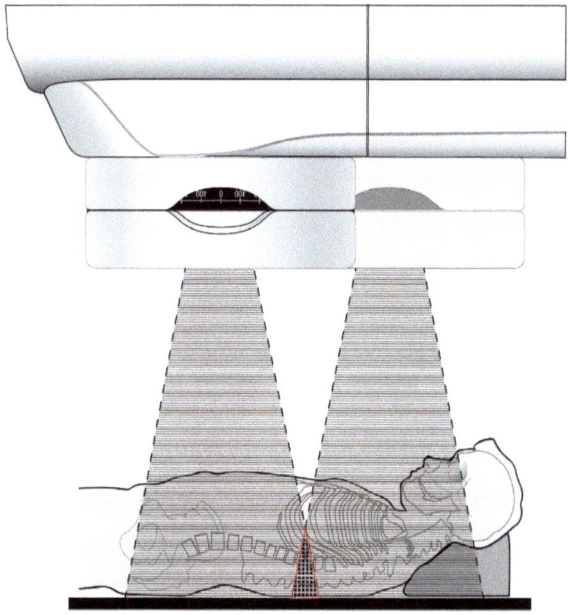

Fig. 10.18 Matching treatment fields with the skin-gap technique

10.8.2 Half-Beam Technique

Using the half-beam technique, the geometric divergence between two sets of opposing fields can be reduced or eliminated. Half of each beam is blocked using either Cerrobend® blocks or asymmetric collimator jaws so that the field edge passes through the central axis of the beam, eliminating divergence at the field border. If the half-beam technique is applied to both sets of opposing fields, a perfect geometric match is created. Just as often, the half-beam technique is applied to one set of beams, reducing the field divergence and associated dose heterogeneity in the match region by roughly half. HVL blocks can still be applied to the field edges in the match region, but if they are omitted, it is essential that treatment machine mechanical tolerances and patient setup be accurate and reproducible to reduce the potential for unanticipated hot spots in the region of the spinal cord. Limitations to the half-beam technique include the reduced field size and the fact that it can be used to create a perfect geometric match between no more than two sets of fields (Fig. 10.19).

10.8.3 Matching-Divergence Technique

The matching-divergence technique can also result in a perfect match but it is less commonly used because it is cumbersome. In this technique, the divergence from the inferior anterior field is matched with the divergence of the superior posterior field while the divergence of the superior anterior field is matched with the divergence of the inferior posterior field. The angles of divergence of the inferior field must be coincident with the divergence of the superior field. The gap is calculated at midplane. Tattoos should be placed

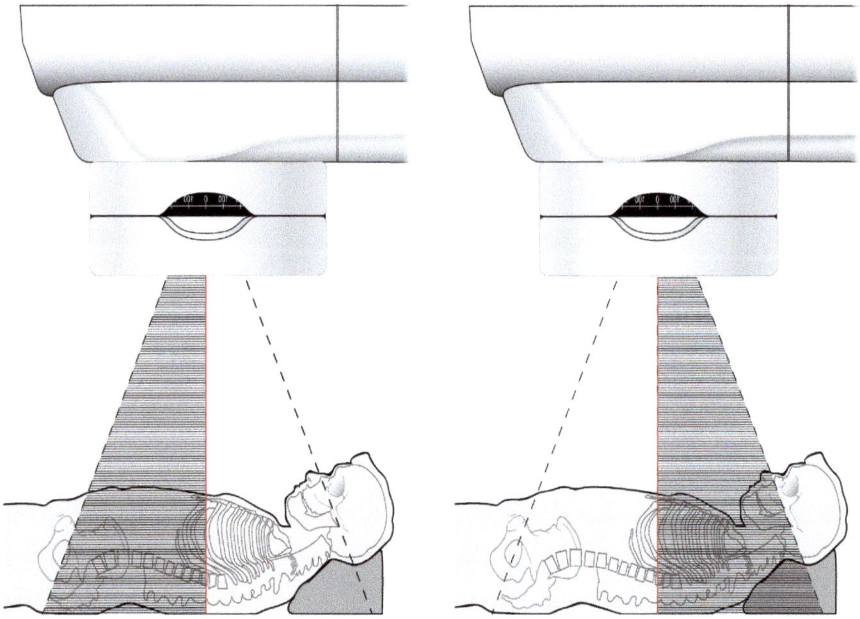

Fig. 10.19 Matching treatment fields with the half-beam technique

at the inferior edge of the superior field and at the superior edge of the inferior field. Again, film verification of the field edges must be obtained to assess for overlap. A small 2 × 2 cm HVL or full-thickness block can be placed at the site of field abutment to reduce the risk of exceeding the tolerance dose of the spinal cord (Fig. 10.20).

10.9 Blocking

Custom blocks for the delivery of radiation can be fabricated using a bismuth-lead-tin-cadmium alloy with a low melting point known as Lipowitz's alloy or commercially as Cerrobend® (Fig. 10.21). Full-thickness Cerrobend® blocks typically reduce the

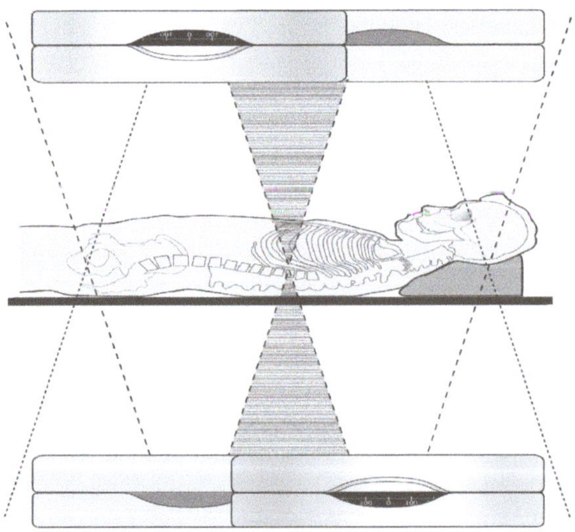

Fig. 10.20 Matching treatment fields by matching divergence of opposing beams

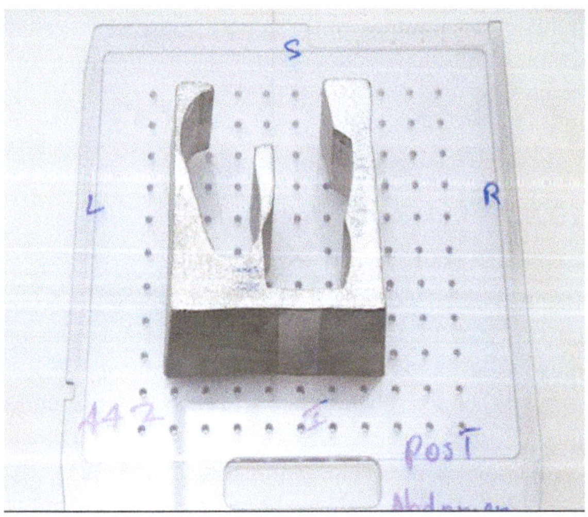

Fig. 10.21 Cerrobend® blocks used for blocking of normal structures

primary beam by five HVLs to a transmission of approximately 3%. Dose underneath the block is invariably higher than 3%, however, because of dose contribution from scattered radiation originating within the irradiated field. The magnitude of this scatter and the dose to a point under a block is dependent on the size of the irradiated field, the proximity of the point of interest from the block or field edge, and the energy of the radiation. Large fields, small blocks, close proximity to the field or block edge and lower beam energy all serve to increase scatter dose, resulting in low, but measurable, doses to normal tissues under blocks.

Historically, partial-transmission blocks have found several uses in the treatment of lymphomas. Partial-transmission blocks reduce transmission of the primary radiation beam so that only a percentage of the prescribed dose will be delivered. The transmission reduction achieved is a function of the block thickness, usually specified in terms of the number of HVLs, which is the block thickness needed to reduce the primary beam intensity in half. HVL blocks, which reduce the primary beam transmission to 50% of the dose in the open field, are used at the junction of adjacent treatment fields to reduce the potential of overdose in the junction area. In the design of the mantle field, HVL blocks are also used to reduce dose to the cervical spine and the larynx. When the clinical indication arises, partial-transmission blocks can also be used to deliver low-dose irradiation to the whole lungs or liver when a higher dose is prescribed to the mediastinum or paraaortic lymph node regions, respectively. Because the contribution of scattered radiation to the total dose under a block depends on block size, field size and beam energy, the block thickness required to reduce the radiation to a specified level must usually be measured to ensure accuracy.

A multileaf collimator (MLC) is composed of "shielding leaves" that are built into the head of the treatment machine and can move independently into and out of the radiation beam (Fig. 10.22). MLCs provide a flexible method of conformal field shaping that can be used in place of Cerrobend® blocks. However, certain types of field shaping such as blocking in the center of a treatment field (i.e., "island" shielding) and the creation of certain concave apertures cannot be accomplished using MLC; in these cases, a block must still be fabricated. These limitations have hindered MLC use in field shaping for large mantle and pelvic fields. Benefits of MLC include the fact that the field apertures can be designed quickly and changes can be readily accommodated. Whereas field edges defined with blocks are smooth, MLC leaf widths are typically 0.5 or 1.0 cm, and, therefore, the MLC-defined field edge has some irregularity. Most clinics have deemed MLCs to be sufficiently smooth for most applications and their flexibility and increased accuracy compared with custom blocking have led to their widespread use for most disease sites.

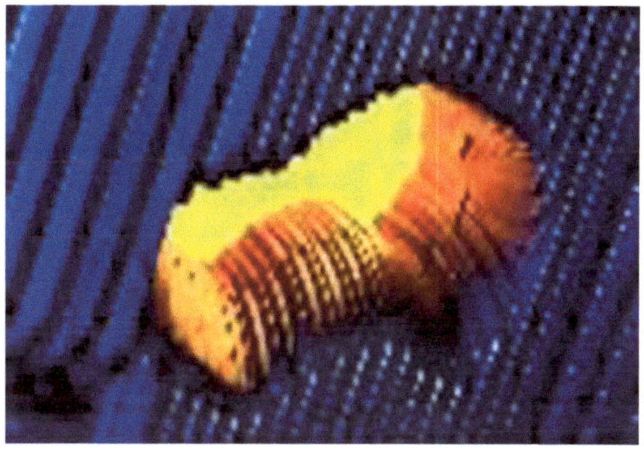

Fig. 10.22 Multileaf collimator (MLC) leaves used for treatment-field design with projection

10.10 CT-Based Treatment Planning

The definition of treatment fields using conventional radiographic simulation is limited by the visualization of bony landmarks and the two-dimensional nature of the images. CT simulation, on the other hand, provides three-dimensional imaging of the patient in the treatment position and, consequently, more precise anatomic localization of tumor and normal structures (Fig. 10.23). Several studies performed have demonstrated improved localization rates using CT simulation compared with fluoroscopic simulation (Brown et al. 1991; Dinges et al. 1998; Naida et al. 1996).

CT simulators provide the user with a variety of computer-based "virtual simulation" tools including sophisticated contour drawing or segmentation tools as well as tools for creating a variety of images from the CT data such as 3D surface views and projection images. Digitally reconstructed radiographs, or DRRs, are probably the most useful type of two-dimensional projection images reconstructed from the CT data. DRRs can be used in place of conventional radiographic images for field definition and verification. In the planning of lymphomas, the tools of CT simulation are particularly useful since they allow the physician to combine CT image-based segmentation of the gross disease with DRR-based field design for subclinical disease, an efficient and accurate method to design many lymphoma fields (Fig. 10.24).

CT simulation does not easily allow the evaluation of respiratory motion, however, and the availability of fluoroscopy on conventional simulators is still useful for this important assessment. Recent advances in time-dependent or “four-dimensional (4D)” CT imaging technology are leading to methods for evaluating respiratory motion using CT alone that will be applicable to a variety of radiation-treatment sites. These

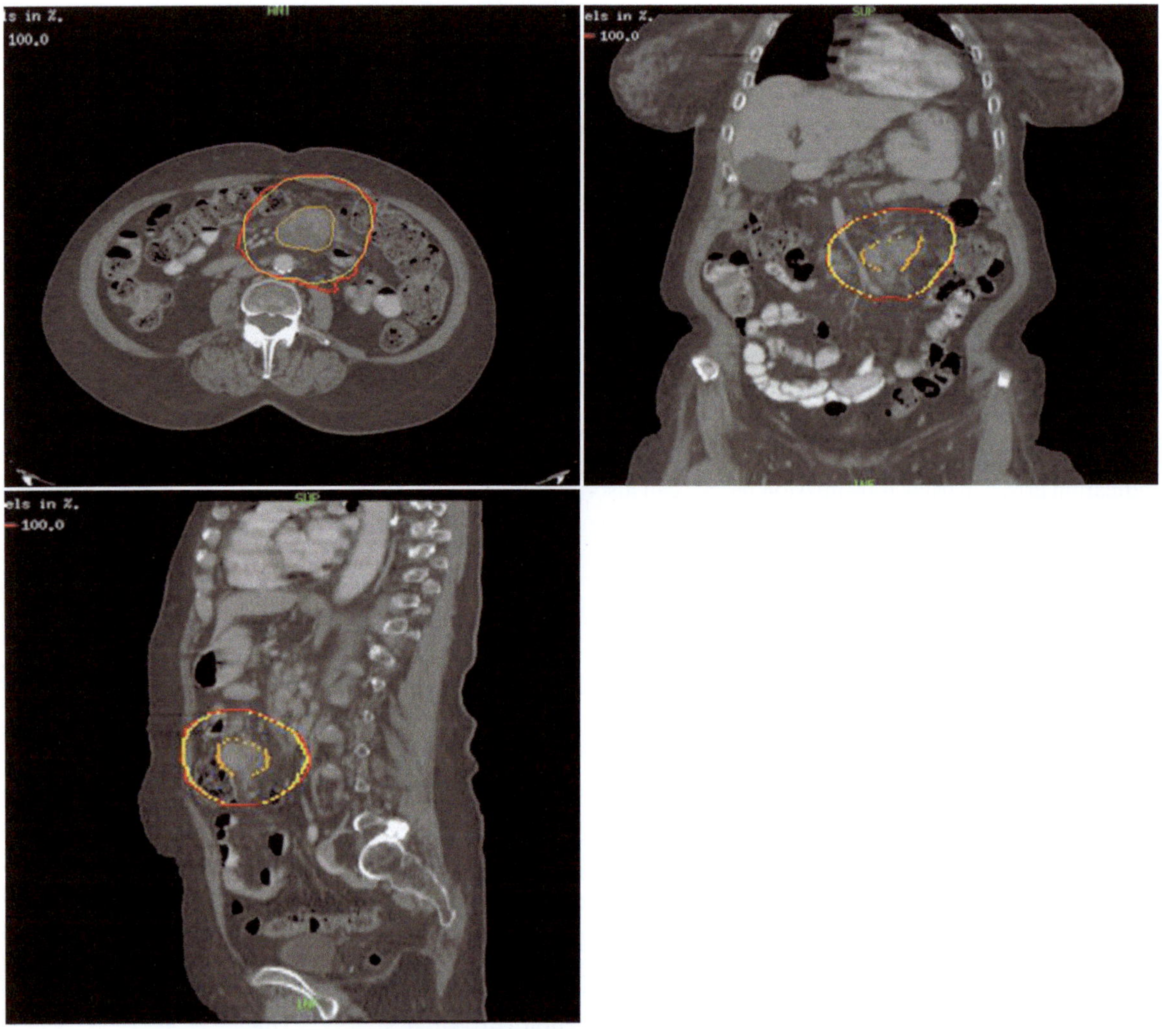

Fig. 10.23 Tumor-volume contours (gross tumor volume in *orange* and planning tumor volume in *red*) using CT-based planning depicted in coronal, axial, and sagittal planes

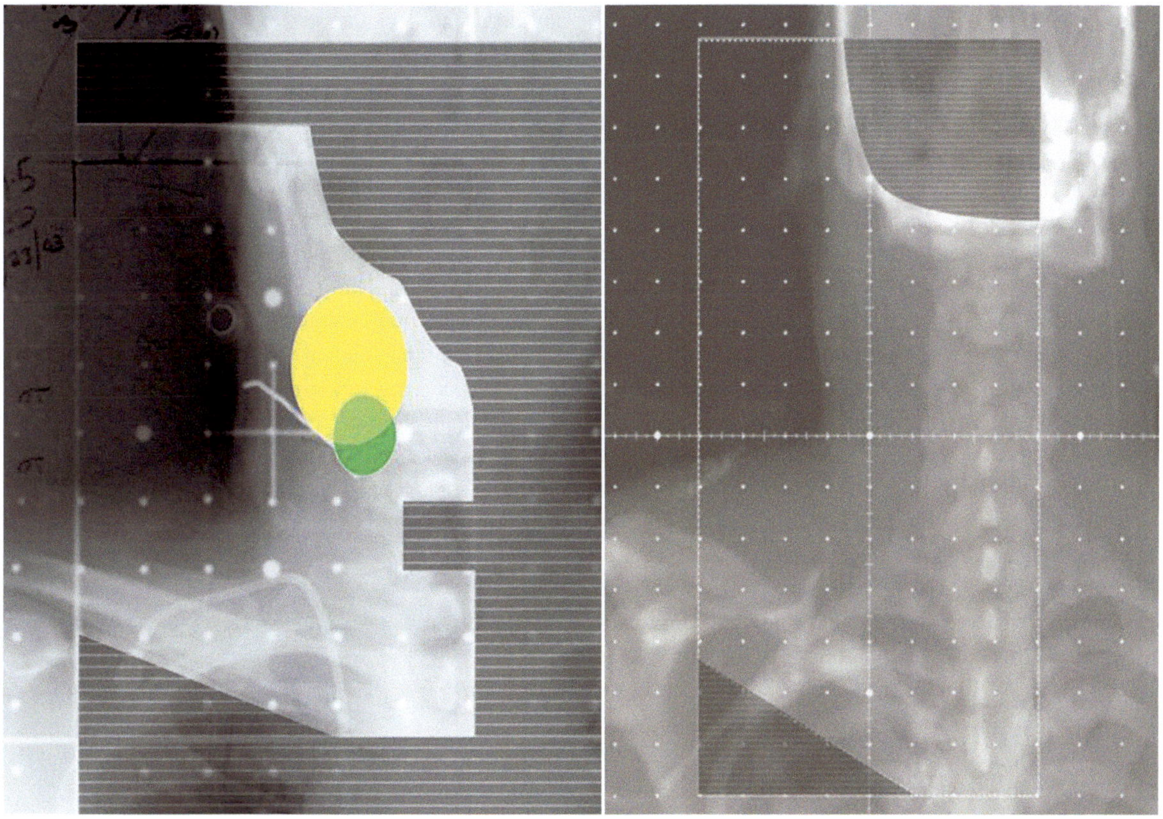

Fig. 10.24 Treatment-planning images derived from conventional simulation (*left*) compared with digitally reconstructed radiographs (*right*) derived from CT-based treatment planning in the treatment of the unilateral neck

methods may prove useful in the treatment of lymphoma.

10.11 Conformal Radiation Planning and Delivery Techniques

The development of three-dimensional conformal radiotherapy (3D-CRT) technology in the 1980s and 1990s led to improvements in our ability to deliver conformal radiation to a highly complex target while sparing surrounding normal tissues. A natural extension of the use of CT imaging for simulation and target localization, 3D planning uses CT images as the basis for field design and dose calculation. 3D-CRT relies on so-called "forward planning" to create radiation dose distributions. The radiation-treatment intent is specified by the physician, and a physicist or dosimetrist then defines the number, direction, weight, and shape of the radiation beams. Evaluation of the plan is accomplished using 3D tools, including the review of isodose distributions created in a variety of planes as well as dose-volume histograms, which are graphical representations of the dose delivered throughout the target and normal tissues of interest.

Intensity-modulated radiotherapy (IMRT) is an incremental improvement on 3D planning that utilizes radiation beams with varying intensities across the field. The intensity map of each beam is determined by sophisticated optimization algorithms in a method known as "inverse planning" (Chui and Spirou 2001; Spirou and Chui 1998; Ten Haken and

Lawrence 2006; Verhey 2002). To start the IMRT planning process, the planner specifies the number and direction of treatment fields much as he or she would for conventional "forward planning." Rather than specifying the weight and shape of each beam, however, the planner provides the desired doses to the physician-defined target and normal tissues as input to specialized optimization software. This software determines the intensity patterns for each field that will yield a dose distribution as close as possible to the physician's intent. The resulting IMRT dose distribution is typically highly conformal and, unlike conventional 3D distributions, can contain multiple concavities that improve normal tissue sparing. IMRT plans are characterized by a fair number of treatment fields (typically five to nine), which improves conformality and also spreads the radiation dose over a larger volume of tissue (Fig. 10.25). Delivery of the irregular intensity patterns needed for IMRT is usually accomplished by dynamically moving MLC leaves during treatment (dynamic multileaf collimation) or by delivering a series of irregular, static MLC shapes (segmental IMRT or step-and-shoot) (Galvin et al. 1993; Spirou and Chui 1998). Dynamic delivery can produce higher resolution intensity patterns but requires more intensive and complex treatment machine quality assurance than step-and-shoot methods. Both techniques are widely in use.

Although IMRT has gained widespread acceptance in the treatment of many malignancies including prostate and head and neck cancers, its use for lymphomas has been limited due to the relatively large treatment volumes that a typical extended field encompassed, and the low doses routinely used for this disease. Nonetheless, IMRT may provide significant advantage in select cases and is better suited for the involved-field or involved-node approach. Patients who present with bulky mediastinal lymphadenopathy may benefit from IMRT for sparing of heart and lung tissue (Fig. 10.26). The sparing of lung tissue may also have particular importance for patients who are at higher risk for radiation pneumonitis after stem-cell transplant or bleomycin administration. Many patients who are referred for involved-field radiation therapy before or after stem-cell transplants have had prior radiation. These patients may not be candidates for further radiotherapy if conventional techniques

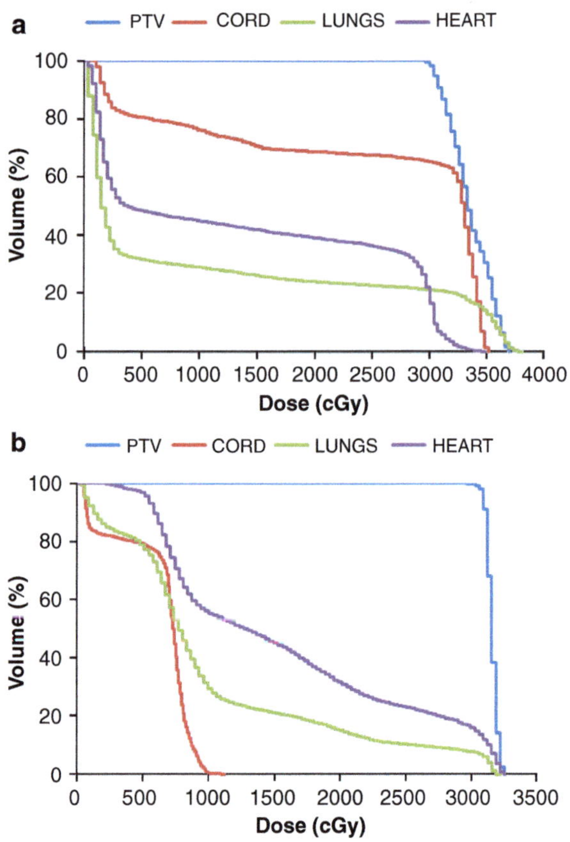

Fig. 10.26 Dose-volume histograms (DVHs) of conventional and IMRT plans, respectively, for a patient who presented with bulky mediastinal (**a**) and anterior abdominal (**b**) disease. The DVHs demonstrate reduced dose to normal structures and decreased hot spots using an IMRT plan compared with conventional AP/PA fields. PTV = planned tumor volume

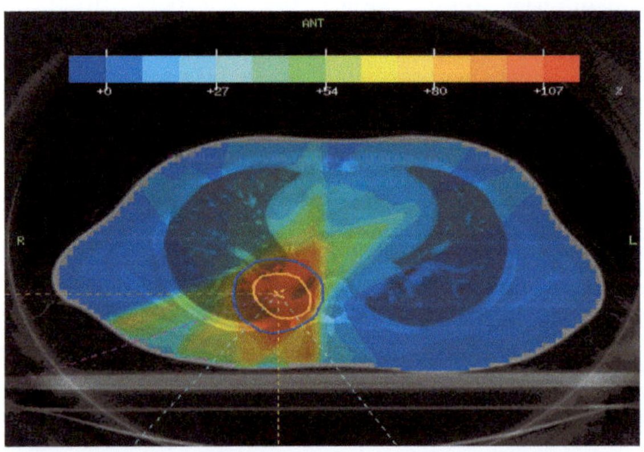

Fig. 10.25 Patient who underwent prior radiation now with recurrent lymphoma in the mediastinum. The patient's retreatment was planned using IMRT; the color-wash image depicts adequate tumor volume coverage while minimizing dose to the surrounding normal lung and heart

are used; however, re-irradiation may become feasible as a result of the improved normal tissue sparing afforded by IMRT.

Multiple studies have compared normal tissue doses for lymphoma patients using conventional 2D radiation, 3D-CRT, and IMRT. Goodman et al. analyzed 16 patients with Hodgkin's lymphoma or non-Hodgkin's lymphoma mediastinal disease who had either received prior mediastinal radiation or had extremely large mediastinal masses (Goodman et al. 2005). The planning target volume dose was improved using IMRT and 3D-CRT compared with conventional anterior-posterior/posterior-anterior fields. Both mean lung dose and the probability of pneumonitis as assessed with a biological model that evaluates damage to organ sub-units known as the fractional damage were less with IMRT compared with 2D and 3D plans (Jackson et al. 1993). However, the volume of lung receiving at least 20 Gy (V_{20}) increased with IMRT (Goodman et al. 2005). The parameter most predictive for the development of lung toxicity, including radiation pneumonitis, is still uncertain. Yorke et al. demonstrated that both mean dose and fractional damage correlated significantly with the development of radiation pneumonitis for non-small-cell lung-cancer patients treated to higher doses (range, 57.6–81 Gy) but it is not known whether these observations apply to the lymphoma population (Yorke et al. 2002).

Girinsky et al. also compared IMRT, 3D-CRT, and anterior-posterior/posterior-anterior plans for HL patients with mediastinal masses. IMRT improved the dose distribution to the heart, coronary arteries, esophagus, and spinal cord. However, conventional treatment resulted in a lung mean dose that was slightly lower than 3D-CRT and IMRT, and a lung V_{20} that was similar to IMRT but significantly lower than that of 3D-CRT. The median dose to the breasts was lower with conventional planning and 3D-CRT compared to IMRT plans but there were no differences in the breast V_{20} (the volume of the breast receiving 20 Gy) comparing the three plans (Girinsky et al. 2006a). Nieder et al. studied eight females with mediastinal targets and identified reduced median heart and breast doses with IMRT. However, an increased volume of breast received low doses (15% or less) using IMRT (Nieder et al. 2007).

IMRT delivery, particularly when delivered using dynamic multileaf collimation, requires more monitor units then conventional or 3D treatment, resulting in increased leakage radiation and, consequently, increased dose to regions of the patient that lie beyond the treatment volume. As a result, patients can be exposed to higher total body doses with IMRT even though IMRT's increased dose conformality results in lower doses within the treatment volume. It has been hypothesized that an increase in total body dose may lead to an elevation in rates of radiation-induced second malignancies, which could be doubled in long-term survivors (Hall 2006). Whether a low dose to a larger volume is preferred over a higher dose to a smaller volume still remains controversial.

Another feature of IMRT is that the variable intensity patterns can be used to selectively escalate the dose to subvolumes within the patient, "dose painting" or "simultaneous integrated boost." Dose painting can deliver higher doses to areas at risk for macroscopic disease while delivering a substantial but lower dose to surrounding subclinical disease. The use of IMRT dose painting can integrate a boost treatment that would normally be delivered after conventional treatment (albeit at a higher dose per fraction) so that the overall treatment course can be shortened (Fig. 10.27).

IMRT results in a relatively steeper dose fall-off beyond the planning target volume compared to

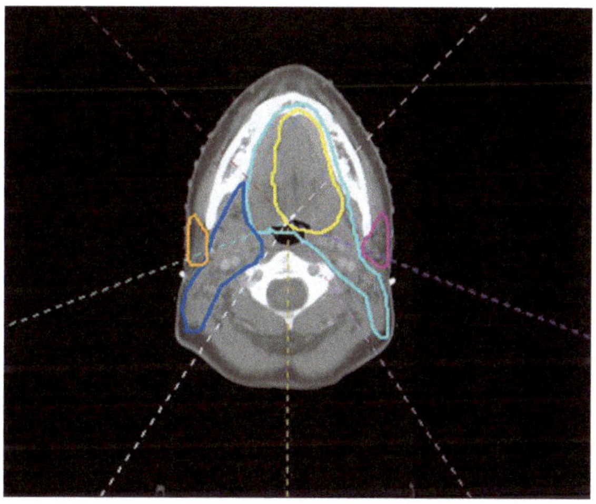

Fig. 10.27 Dose-painting to the head and neck region; yellow contour, gross tumor volume; turquoise contour, planned tumor volume of a high-risk subclinical region at the ipsilateral neck; dark blue contour, planned tumor volume of a low-risk subclinical region including contralateral lymph nodes

conventional and 3D-CRT techniques. This increased conformality leads to an increased risk of geographic misses and highlights the crucial need for accurate target delineation. Advances in imaging have enhanced our ability to accurately identify tumor volumes, and multiple diagnostic modalities can now be incorporated directly into the treatment planning process using sophisticated image fusion and registration software to aid in target delineation. Long-term clinical outcomes are eagerly awaited to determine if such techniques can improve the therapeutic ratio.

10.12 PET/CT Radiation Treatment Planning

PET using 2-[^{18}F]fluoro-2-deoxyglucose (FDG) has been increasingly utilized as a diagnostic tool in lymphoma management. Multiple studies have demonstrated increased sensitivity and specificity of FDG-PET compared with CT scan alone (Jerusalem et al. 2001; Sasaki et al. 2002; Schiepers et al. 2003; Schoder et al. 2001; Stumpe et al. 1998; Weihrauch et al. 2002; Wirth et al. 2002). A specificity of 41% for CT scan in staging HL was determined in a study by Stumpe et al. while a specificity of 96% was identified for FDG-PET (Stumpe et al. 1998). FDG-PET frequently results in the upstaging of lymphoma patients and, therefore, management decisions may be altered once PET information is acquired (Hutchings et al. 2006).

CT simulation remains standard for radiation planning both because of its tremendous usefulness in defining the anatomic extent of tumors and normal structures, and because the Hounsfield units acquired from CT images are proportional to electron density, a parameter essential for dose calculations in heterogeneous media. PET contributes functional information about the tumor and, as such, complements the anatomical detail of a CT scan. FDG-PET and CT scan have been increasingly used in conjunction for radiation-treatment planning. An FDG-PET scan obtained in a nuclear medicine department can be co-registered to a CT treatment-planning scan obtained in a department of radiation oncology. The patient can be placed in the treatment-planning position using an appropriate immobilization device for both scans for reproducibility.

The FDG-PET scan can be fused with the CT treatment-planning scan. However, co-registration may be difficult if the patient's position varies between the two scans. With the introduction of dedicated PET/CT scanners for simulation, PET and CT images can be acquired simultaneously, and information derived from the FDG-PET portion of the scan can be immediately co-registered for use in tumor-volume delineation.

PET/CT simulation can be used to plan radiation-treatment fields. Multiple studies have now demonstrated that PET/CT treatment planning can affect management and tumor-volume definition in lymphoma patients (Figs. 10.28 and 10.29) (Girinsky et al. 2007; Hutchings et al. 2007; Lee et al. 2004; Terezakis et al. 2007). In the treatment of early-stage HL, patients often receive chemotherapy prior to radiation treatment. Hutchings et al. recently studied 30 patients with early-stage HL who received a staging FDG-PET/CT. A short course of adriamycin, bleomycin, vinblastine, and dacarbazine was delivered prior to radiation treatment. Involved-field radiation therapy planning was initially performed using a CT treatment-planning scan alone but patients were then planned using contours delineated on PET/CT. The integration of FDG-PET information would have resulted in an increase in the treated volume in seven patients. In these patients the volume receiving 90% of the prescription dose was increased by 8–87%. A decrease in the treated volume would have occurred in two patients (Hutchings et al. 2007). It was concluded that the use of PET/CT should be further investigated, particularly as the treatment volume may increase for some patients.

Girinsky et al. also specifically studied patients with early-stage HL and addressed the challenge of contouring a pre-chemotherapy volume on a post-chemotherapy CT planning scan. Pretreatment CT and FDG-PET scans were performed in the treatment position and were co-registered with a post-chemotherapy CT simulation planning scan. FDG-PET helped to delineate lymph nodes that were otherwise undetectable on CT scan in 36% of patients. Hence, pre-chemotherapy FDG-PET scans can identify lymph node sites that require consolidative radiation (Girinsky et al. 2007).

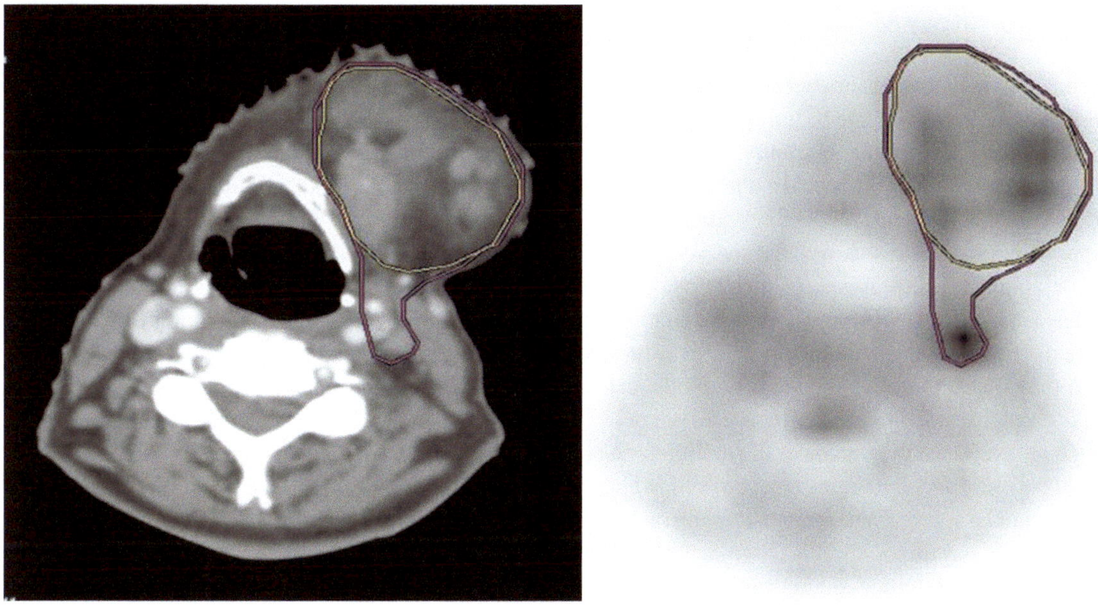

Fig. 10.28 The target volume was altered in this patient presenting with diffuse large B-cell lymphoma after PET/CT simulation (CT shown to the left, PET to the right). Yellow contour, gross tumor volume based on CT information alone. Pink contour, gross tumor volume based on PET/CT simulation incorporating an ipsilateral cervical lymph node that was FDG-avid but not enlarged by radiographic criteria

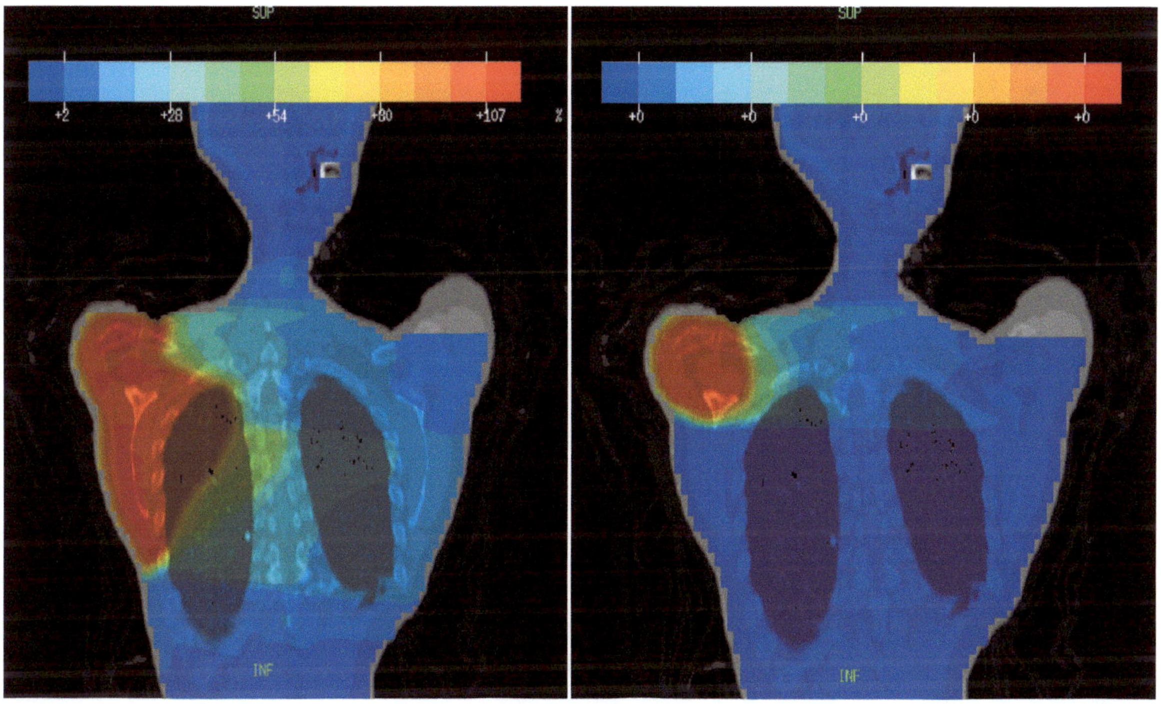

Fig. 10.29 Color-wash images of IMRT plans of a patient with multiple myeloma of the shoulder comparing CT (*left*) versus PET/CT (*right*) volumes. The PET/CT volume was significantly smaller, enabling reduction of dose to the lungs and heart

10.13 Respiratory Motion Management

The accuracy of radiation treatment-field design, target, and normal tissue definition can be limited by intrafractional movement due to organ motion. Respiratory motion can affect tumor position in the thorax and abdomen significantly and can lead to unnecessary treatment of normal tissues as well as underdosing of the tumor volume. The presence of significant organ motion also limits the development of tightly conformal dose distributions since additional margin must be added to the clinical target volume to ensure adequate coverage during treatment. In the absence of accurate imaging that reveals the magnitude of the motion for an individual patient, generic margins must be used, which may or may not be appropriate, given that organ motion is highly patient and tumor specific. Significant variation in extent of lung-tumor motion ranging from >3 cm to several millimeters has been identified leading to both targeting errors and systematic errors in treatment planning (Erridge et al. 2003; Keall et al. 2006; Liu et al. 2007; Seppenwoolde et al. 2002).

Respiration movements may also lead to spatial separation between the target volume and critical normal structures which can be exploited to the advantage of the patient. It was pointed out many years ago that by irradiating mediastinal lymphomas in inspiration significant sparing of lung tissue could be achieved compared to treatment in ordinary free breathing (Willett et al. 1987). This finding has been confirmed in a couple of later studies, indicating a relative reduction in the irradiated lung volume of almost 25% (Claude et al. 2007; Stromberg et al. 2000) (Fig. 10.30).

Several techniques to account for tumor motion have been developed. Respiratory gating is one method used to ensure the delivery of radiation only during a favorable segment of the respiratory cycle identified during the treatment-planning process (Kubo and Hill 1996; Ohara et al. 1989; Tada et al. 1998). During CT simulation, infrared markers, placed on the patient skin surface, are imaged to provide a trace of the thoracic motion resulting from respiration. Simultaneously, the patient is CT scanned. In prospective gating the scanner is programmed to acquire images only in the prespecified part of the respiratory cycle. This CT-scanning is then used for treatment planning. In retrospective gating the patient is imaged using a multislice helical scanner and a very low pitch so that multiple images are obtained at each couch position. The images are tagged with the time of acquisition and then correlated with the breathing trace obtained from the infrared markers. The images are later separated or "binned"

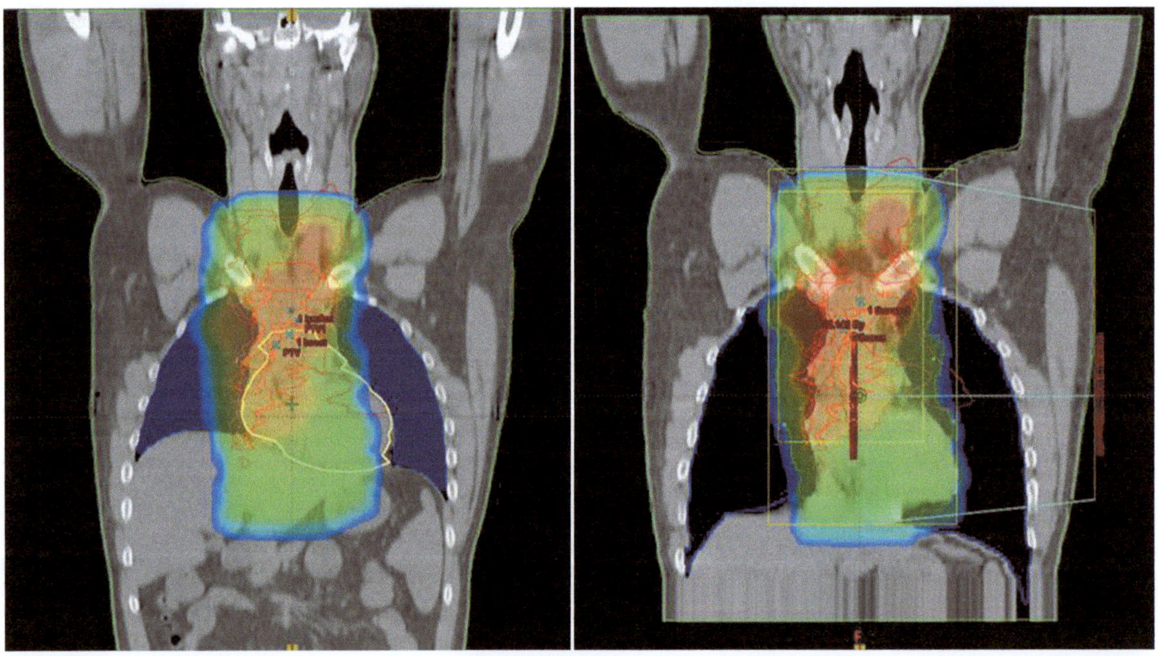

Fig. 10.30 Dose distribution for a patient treated for extensive mediastinal HL with radiotherapy in free breathing (*left*) or in inspiration (*right*) demonstrating significant sparing of the lungs with treatment in inspiration.

typically into 10 segments spread out over the respiratory cycle. For each bin, a full 3D rendering of the patient's anatomy is obtained that can then be viewed as a 4D "movie," demonstrating the effects of organ motion during respiration. This technique is known as 4D CT or respiration-correlated CT. Each of the image segments can also be separately reviewed to evaluate the magnitude of tumor motion and determine the best portion of the respiratory cycle and corresponding breathing trace for radiation treatment. The selected CT images are then used for treatment planning. At the time of treatment, the infrared markers are repositioned on the patient skin surface and a new breathing trace is obtained. As long as the patient's breathing is regular and similar to that obtained during simulation, the trace is used to automatically trigger the radiation beam, thereby "gating" the treatment during the appropriate segments of the respiratory cycle. Given the magnitude of intra- and inter-fraction motion identified during respiration, image-guided radiation delivery is recommended for the verification of gated treatment (Bissonnette et al. 2009; Guckenberger et al. 2007; Juhler Nottrup et al. 2007, 2008; Korreman et al. 2006, 2008; Sonke et al. 2005, 2008).

4D CT scans can also be used to create an internal target volume to account for respiratory motion. In this approach, the physician must define the target volume on each of the 10 4D CT image bins. The envelope of the 10 target volumes defines the internal target volume (Fig. 10.31). Radiation can then be delivered using a plan based on the internal target volume. This approach provides a more accurate delineation of the target volume since it provides the physician with direct visualization of the effects of respiration. This visualization facilitates both target definition and further minimization of normal tissue within the treated volume (Harsolia et al. 2008; Wang et al. 2009).

Modern radiotherapy for HL is usually part of combined modality treatment, and the radiotherapy planning process usually involves co-registration of pre-chemotherapy CT-scans or more often PET/CT-scans. When planning gated radiotherapy for HL it is therefore necessary to obtain gated imaging already before chemotherapy is started. As mentioned above, for patients receiving mediastinal irradiation treatment in inspiration enables significant sparing of lung tissue. For these patients a pre-chemotherapy PET/CT-scan gated in inspiration is needed to enable the full advantage of the respiratory gated radiotherapy (Fig. 10.32).

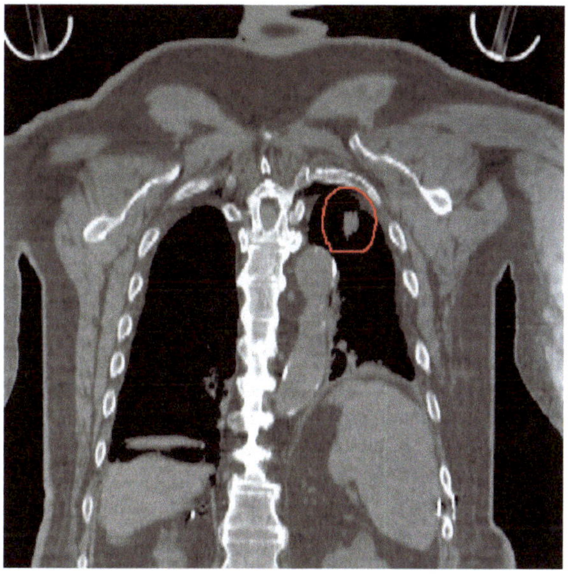

Fig. 10.31 Delineation of the internal target volume (*red*) from the gross tumor volume after accounting for respiratory motion identified using a 4D-CT scan.

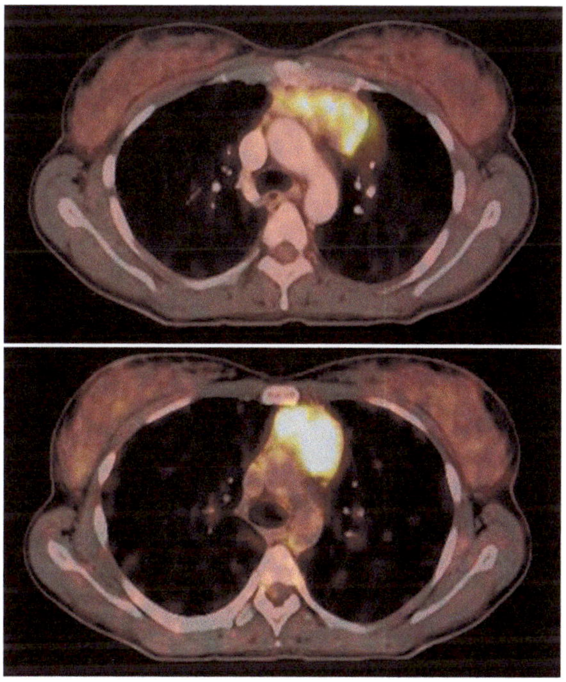

Fig. 10.32 Pre-chemotherapy PET/CT-scan in a patient with HL with mediastinal involvement. Upper panel shows scan in free breathing with smeared out PET + volume. Lower panel shows scan in inspiration, demonstrating a much more homogenously PET + (and much narrower) lymphoma volume

10.14 Conclusion

Radiotherapy is an important part of the treatment of HL. In the past very extensive radiotherapy with total or subtotal nodal irradiation was used, techniques which are not often used today. In the modern combined modality setting prophylactic irradiation of clinically uninvolved areas has been abandoned. Much smaller radiation fields, involved-field radiotherapy or the even more conformal involved-node radiotherapy, are used. Modern advanced imaging and treatment delivery techniques enable drastic reductions in the irradiation of normal tissue, thus reducing very significantly the risk of long-term complications from radiotherapy. Hence, with further refinements and with widespread use of these techniques radiotherapy may be used to even greater advantage for HL patients in the future.

References

Bhatia S, Robison LL, Oberlin O et al (1996) Breast cancer and other second neoplasms after childhood Hodgkin's disease. N Engl J Med 334:745–751

Bissonnette JP, Purdie TG, Higgins JA et al (2009) Cone-beam computed tomographic image guidance for lung cancer radiation therapy. Int J Radiat Oncol Biol Phys 73:927–934

Biti G, Cellai E, Magrini SM et al (1994) Second solid tumors and leukemia after treatment for Hodgkin's disease: an analysis of 1121 patients from a single institution. Int J Radiat Oncol Biol Phys 29:25–31

Boivin JF, O'Brien K (1988) Solid cancer risk after treatment of Hodgkin's disease. Cancer 61:2541–2546

Boivin JF, Hutchison GB, Zauber AG et al (1995) Incidence of second cancers in patients treated for Hodgkin's disease. J Natl Cancer Inst 87:732–741

Bonadonna G, Bonfante V, Viviani S et al (2004) ABVD plus subtotal nodal versus involved-field radiotherapy in early-stage Hodgkin's disease: long-term results. J Clin Oncol 22:2835–2841

Brincker H, Bentzen SM (1994) A re-analysis of available dose–response and time–dose data in Hodgkin's disease. Radiother Oncol 30:227–230

Brown AP, Urie MM, Barest G et al (1991) Three-dimensional photon treatment planning for Hodgkin's disease. Int J Radiat Oncol Biol Phys 21:205–215

Butts JR, Abell GA, Morrison JC et al (1997) Dose uniformity from a computerized three-dimensional tissue compensating system. Med Dosim 22:113–116

Cantwell JP, Renner WD, O'Connor TP et al (1989) A dosimetric comparison of three compensator design methods for the mantle field. Med Dosim 14:257–263

Carmel RJ, Kaplan HS (1976) Mantle irradiation in Hodgkin's disease. An analysis of technique, tumor eradication, and complications. Cancer 37:2813–2825

Centola GM, Keller JW, Henzler M et al (1994) Effect of low-dose testicular irradiation on sperm count and fertility in patients with testicular seminoma. J Androl 15:608–613

Chui CS, Spirou SV (2001) Inverse planning algorithms for external beam radiation therapy. Med Dosim 26:189–197

Classe JM, Mahe M, Moreau P et al (1998) Ovarian transposition by laparoscopy before radiotherapy in the treatment of Hodgkin's disease. Cancer 83:1420–1424

Claude L, Malet C, Pommier P et al (2007) Active breathing control for Hodgkin's disease in childhood and adolescence: feasibility, advantages, and limits. Int J Radiat Oncol Biol Phys 67:1470–1475

Clough KB, Goffinet F, Labib A et al (1996) Laparoscopic unilateral ovarian transposition prior to irradiation: prospective study of 20 cases. Cancer 77:2638–2645

Colvett KT (1995) Bilateral breast carcinoma after radiation therapy for Hodgkin's disease. South Med J 88:239–242

Cook KL, Adler DD, Lichter AS et al (1990) Breast carcinoma in young women previously treated for Hodgkin disease. AJR Am J Roentgenol 155:39–42

Davis QG, Paulino AC, Miller R et al (2006) Mantle fields in the era of dynamic multileaf collimation: field shaping and electronic tissue compensation. Med Dosim 31:179–183

Dershaw DD, Yahalom J, Petrek JA (1992) Breast carcinoma in women previously treated for Hodgkin disease: mammographic evaluation. Radiology 184:421–423

Dinges S, Koswig S, Buchali A et al (1998) Comparison of conventional and virtual simulation for radiation treatment planning of malignant lymphoma. Strahlenther Onkol 174(Suppl 2):28–30

Duhmke E, Diehl V, Loeffler M et al (1996) Randomized trial with early-stage Hodgkin's disease testing 30 Gy vs. 40 Gy extended field radiotherapy alone. Int J Radiat Oncol Biol Phys 36:305–310

Duhmke E, Franklin J, Pfreundschuh M et al (2001) Low-dose radiation is sufficient for the noninvolved extended-field treatment in favorable early-stage Hodgkin's disease: long-term results of a randomized trial of radiotherapy alone. J Clin Oncol 19:2905–2914

Engert A, Schiller P, Josting A et al (2003) Involved-field radiotherapy is equally effective and less toxic compared with extended-field radiotherapy after four cycles of chemotherapy in patients with early-stage unfavorable Hodgkin's lymphoma: results of the HD8 trial of the German Hodgkin's Lymphoma Study Group. J Clin Oncol 21:3601–3608

Erridge SC, Seppenwoolde Y, Muller SH et al (2003) Portal imaging to assess set-up errors, tumor motion and tumor shrinkage during conformal radiotherapy of non-small cell lung cancer. Radiother Oncol 66:75–85

Ferme C, Eghbali H, Meerwaldt JH et al (2007) Chemotherapy plus involved-field radiation in early-stage Hodgkin's disease. N Engl J Med 357:1916–1927

Fletcher GH, Shukovsky LJ (1975) The interplay of radiocurability and tolerance in the irradiation of human cancers. J Radiol Électrol Méd Nucl 56:383–400

Fraass BA, Kinsella TJ, Harrington FS et al (1985) Peripheral dose to the testes: the design and clinical use of a practical and effective gonadal shield. Int J Radiat Oncol Biol Phys 11:609–615

Galvin JM, Chen XG, Smith RM (1993) Combining multileaf fields to modulate fluence distributions. Int J Radiat Oncol Biol Phys 27:697–705

Girinsky T, Pichenot C, Beaudre A et al (2006a) Is intensity-modulated radiotherapy better than conventional radiation treatment and three-dimensional conformal radiotherapy for mediastinal masses in patients with Hodgkin's disease, and is there a role for beam orientation optimization and dose constraints assigned to virtual volumes? Int J Radiat Oncol Biol Phys 64:218–226

Girinsky T, van der Maazen R, Specht L et al (2006b) Involved-node radiotherapy (INRT) in patients with early Hodgkin lymphoma: concepts and guidelines. Radiother Oncol 79:270–277

Girinsky T, Ghalibafian M, Bonniaud G et al (2007) Is FDG-PET scan in patients with early stage Hodgkin lymphoma of any value in the implementation of the involved-node radiotherapy concept and dose painting? Radiother Oncol 85:178–186

Goodman KA, Toner S, Hunt M et al (2005) Intensity-modulated radiotherapy for lymphoma involving the mediastinum. Int J Radiat Oncol Biol Phys 62:198–206

Goss PE, Sierra S (1998) Current perspectives on radiation-induced breast cancer. J Clin Oncol 16:338–347

Gray L, Prosnitz LR (1975) Dosimetry of Hodgkin's disease therapy using a 4 MV linear accelerator. Radiology 116:423–428

Guckenberger M, Meyer J, Wilbert J et al (2007) Intra-fractional uncertainties in cone-beam CT based image-guided radiotherapy (IGRT) of pulmonary tumors. Radiother Oncol 83:57–64

Hall EJ (2006) Intensity-modulated radiation therapy, protons, and the risk of second cancers. Int J Radiat Oncol Biol Phys 65:1–7

Hancock SL, Hoppe RT (1996) Long-term complications of treatment and causes of mortality after Hodgkin's disease. Semin Radiat Oncol 6:225–242

Hancock SL, Tucker MA, Hoppe RT (1993a) Breast cancer after treatment of Hodgkin's disease. J Natl Cancer Inst 85:25–31

Hancock SL, Tucker MA, Hoppe RT (1993b) Factors affecting late mortality from heart disease after treatment of Hodgkin's disease. JAMA 270:1949–1955

Hanks GE, Kinzie JJ, Herring DF et al (1982) Patterns of care outcome studies in Hodgkin's disease: results of the national practice and implications for management. Cancer Treat Rep 66:805–808

Harsolia A, Hugo GD, Kestin LL et al (2008) Dosimetric advantages of four-dimensional adaptive image-guided radiotherapy for lung tumors using online cone-beam computed tomography. Int J Radiat Oncol Biol Phys 70:582–589

Henry-Amar M (1988) Quantitative risk of second cancer in patients in first complete remission from early stages of Hodgkin's disease. NCI Monogr 65–72

Henry-Amar M (1992) Second cancer after the treatment for Hodgkin's disease: a report from the International Database on Hodgkin's Disease. Ann Oncol 3(Suppl 4):117–128

Hutchings M, Loft A, Hansen M et al (2006) Positron emission tomography with or without computed tomography in the primary staging of Hodgkin's lymphoma. Haematologica 91:482–489

Hutchings M, Loft A, Hansen M et al (2007) Clinical impact of FDG-PET/CT in the planning of radiotherapy for early-stage Hodgkin lymphoma. Eur J Haematol 78:206–212

Jackson A, Kutcher GJ, Yorke ED (1993) Probability of radiation-induced complications for normal tissues with parallel architecture subject to non-uniform irradiation. Med Phys 20:613–625

Janjan NA, Wilson JF, Gillin M et al (1988) Mammary carcinoma developing after radiotherapy and chemotherapy for Hodgkin's disease. Cancer 61:252–254

Jerusalem G, Beguin Y, Fassotte MF et al (2001) Whole-body positron emission tomography using 18F-fluorodeoxyglucose compared to standard procedures for staging patients with Hodgkin's disease. Haematologica 86:266–273

Jones D, Hilko R (1981) Measurements of the dose distribution in mantle fields. Int J Radiat Oncol Biol Phys 7:1733–1735

Juhler Nottrup T, Korreman SS, Pedersen AN et al (2007) Intra- and interfraction breathing variations during curative radiotherapy for lung cancer. Radiother Oncol 84:40–48

Juhler-Nottrup T, Korreman SS, Pedersen AN et al (2008) Interfractional changes in tumour volume and position during entire radiotherapy courses for lung cancer with respiratory gating and image guidance. Acta Oncol 47:1406–1413

Kaldor JM, Day NE, Band P et al (1987) Second malignancies following testicular cancer, ovarian cancer and Hodgkin's disease: an international collaborative study among cancer registries. Int J Cancer 39:571–585

Kaplan HS (1966) Evidence for a tumoricidal dose level in the radiotherapy of Hodgkin's disease. Cancer Res 26:1221–1224

Kaplan HS, Rosenberg SA (1966) The treatment of Hodgkin's disease. Med Clin N Am 50:1591–1610

Keall PJ, Mageras GS, Balter JM et al (2006) The management of respiratory motion in radiation oncology report of AAPM Task Group 76. Med Phys 33:3874–3900

Kessaris ND (1978) A dose compensator for mantle fields. Int J Radiat Oncol Biol Phys 4:889–894

Korreman S, Mostafavi H, Le QT et al (2006) Comparison of respiratory surrogates for gated lung radiotherapy without internal fiducials. Acta Oncol 45:935–942

Korreman SS, Juhler-Nottrup T, Boyer AL (2008) Respiratory gated beam delivery cannot facilitate margin reduction, unless combined with respiratory correlated image guidance. Radiother Oncol 86:61–68

Kowalski A, Smith S (1998) Measurement of radiation dose delivered to breast tissue during mantle field irradiation for Hodgkin's disease. Med Dosim 23:31–36

Kubo HD, Hill BC (1996) Respiration gated radiotherapy treatment: a technical study. Phys Med Biol 41:83–91

Lavey RS, Eby NL, Prosnitz LR (1990) Impact on second malignancy risk of the combined use of radiation and chemotherapy for lymphomas. Cancer 66:80–88

Lee YK, Cook G, Flower MA et al (2004) Addition of 18F-FDG-PET scans to radiotherapy planning of thoracic lymphoma. Radiother Oncol 73:277–283

Liu HH, Balter P, Tutt T et al (2007) Assessing respiration-induced tumor motion and internal target volume using four-dimensional computed tomography for radiotherapy of lung cancer. Int J Radiat Oncol Biol Phys 68:531–540

Lushbaugh CC, Casarett GW (1976) The effects of gonadal irradiation in clinical radiation therapy: a review. Cancer 37:1111–1125

Mansur DB, Kong FM, El N, I et al (2005) CT localization of axillary lymph nodes in relation to the humeral head: significance of arm position for radiation therapy planning. Radiother Oncol 77:191–193

Mauch PM, Kalish LA, Kadin M et al (1993) Patterns of presentation of Hodgkin disease. Implications for etiology and pathogenesis. Cancer 71:2062–2071

McCullough EC, Earle JD (1982) A measurement of doses to the neck for mantle field treatment of lymphomas with cobalt-60, 4-, and 10-MV photon beams. Radiology 144:432–434

Naida JD, Eisbruch A, Schoeppel SL et al (1996) Analysis of localization errors in the definition of the mantle field using a beam's eye view treatment-planning system. Int J Radiat Oncol Biol Phys 35:377–382

Nieder C, Schill S, Kneschaurek P et al (2007) Comparison of three different mediastinal radiotherapy techniques in female patients: Impact on heart sparing and dose to the breasts. Radiother Oncol 82:301–307

Oh CE, Hunt M, Silva JJ et al (2000) Optimal matchline blocking and matchline dosimetry for lymphoma patients. Med Dosim 25:231–236

Ohara K, Okumura T, Akisada M et al (1989) Irradiation synchronized with respiration gate. Int J Radiat Oncol Biol Phys 17:853–857

Pergolizzi S, Settineri N, Gaeta M et al (2000) What is the best position of the arms in mantle field for Hodgkin's disease? Int J Radiat Oncol Biol Phys 46:119–122

Pergolizzi S, Settineri N, Ascenti G et al (2004) Enlarged axillary nodes and position of the arms in axillary irradiation – a computed tomography and magnetic resonance imaging evaluation. Acta Oncol 43:182–185

Peters MV (1950) A study of survivals in Hodgkin's disease treated radiologically. Am J Roentgenol 63:299–311

Peters MV, Middlemiss KCH (1958) A study of Hodgkin's disease treated by irradiation. Am J Roentgenol 79:114–121

Prior P, Pope DJ (1988) Hodgkin's disease: subsequent primary cancers in relation to treatment. Br J Cancer 58:512–517

Ray GR, Trueblood HW, Enright LP et al (1970) Oophoropexy: a means of preserving ovarian function following pelvic megavoltage radiotherapy for Hodgkin's disease. Radiology 96:175–180

Rosenberg SA, Kaplan HS (1985) The evolution and summary results of the Stanford randomized clinical trials of the management of Hodgkin's disease: 1962–1984. Int J Radiat Oncol Biol Phys 11:5–22

Sankila R, Garwicz S, Olsen JH et al (1996) Risk of subsequent malignant neoplasms among 1, 641 Hodgkin's disease patients diagnosed in childhood and adolescence: a population-based cohort study in the five Nordic countries. Association of the Nordic Cancer Registries and the Nordic Society of Pediatric Hematology and Oncology. J Clin Oncol 14:1442–1446

Sasaki M, Kuwabara Y, Koga H et al (2002) Clinical impact of whole body FDG-PET on the staging and therapeutic decision making for malignant lymphoma. Ann Nucl Med 16:337–345

Schewe KL, Reavis J, Kun LE et al (1988) Total dose, fraction size, and tumor volume in the local control of Hodgkin's disease. Int J Radiat Oncol Biol Phys 15:25–28

Schiepers C, Filmont JE, Czernin J (2003) PET for staging of Hodgkin's disease and non-Hodgkin's lymphoma. Eur J Nucl Med Mol Imaging 30(Suppl 1):S82–S88

Schoder H, Meta J, Yap C et al (2001) Effect of whole-body (18) F-FDG PET imaging on clinical staging and management of patients with malignant lymphoma. J Nucl Med 42:1139–1143

Seppenwoolde Y, Shirato H, Kitamura K et al (2002) Precise and real-time measurement of 3D tumor motion in lung due to breathing and heartbeat, measured during radiotherapy. Int J Radiat Oncol Biol Phys 53:822–834

Shahidi M, Kamangari N, Ashley S et al (2006) Site of relapse after chemotherapy alone for stage I and II Hodgkin's disease. Radiother Oncol 78:1–5

Sola V, Ricci P, Baeza MR et al (2008) Preservation of ovarian function in young woman with hodgkin disease by laparoscopic medial transposition before abdominal irradiation. Surg Laparosc Endosc Percutan Tech 18:423–425

Sonke JJ, Zijp L, Remeijer P et al (2005) Respiratory correlated cone beam CT. Med Phys 32:1176–1186

Sonke JJ, Lebesque J, van HM (2008) Variability of four-dimensional computed tomography patient models. Int J Radiat Oncol Biol Phys 70:590–598

Speiser B, Rubin P, Casarett G (1973) Aspermia following lower truncal irradiation in Hodgkin's disease. Cancer 32:692–698

Spirou SV, Chui CS (1998) A gradient inverse planning algorithm with dose-volume constraints. Med Phys 25:321–333

Stromberg JS, Sharpe MB, Kim LH et al (2000) Active breathing control (ABC) for Hodgkin's disease: reduction in normal tissue irradiation with deep inspiration and implications for treatment. Int J Radiat Oncol Biol Phys 48:797–806

Stumpe KD, Urbinelli M, Steinert HC et al (1998) Whole-body positron emission tomography using fluorodeoxyglucose for staging of lymphoma: effectiveness and comparison with computed tomography. Eur J Nucl Med 25:721–728

Swerdlow AJ, Douglas AJ, Hudson GV et al (1992) Risk of second primary cancers after Hodgkin's disease by type of treatment: analysis of 2846 patients in the British National Lymphoma Investigation. BMJ 304:1137–1143

Tada T, Minakuchi K, Fujioka T et al (1998) Lung cancer: intermittent irradiation synchronized with respiratory motion–results of a pilot study. Radiology 207:779–783

Ten Haken RK, Lawrence TS (2006) The clinical application of intensity-modulated radiation therapy. Semin Radiat Oncol 16:224–231

Terezakis TA, Hunt MA, chmidtlein CR et al (2007) 18FDG-PET with CT scan co-registration for radiation treatment planning of lymphoma patients. Int J Radiat Oncol Biol Phys 69:S535–S536

Tester WJ, Kinsella TJ, Waller B et al (1984) Second malignant neoplasms complicating Hodgkin's disease: the National Cancer Institute experience. J Clin Oncol 2:762–769

Thar TL, Million RR, Hausner RJ et al (1979) Hodgkin's disease, stages I and II: relationship of recurrence to size of disease, radiation dose, and number of sites involved. Cancer 43:1101–1105

Thibaud E, Ramirez M, Brauner R et al (1992) Preservation of ovarian function by ovarian transposition performed before pelvic irradiation during childhood. J Pediatr 121:880–884
Tinga DJ, Dolsma WV, Tamminga RY et al (1999) Preservation of ovarian function in 2 young women with Hodgkin disease by laparoscopic transposition of the ovaries prior to abdominal irradiation. Ned Tijdschr Geneeskd 143:308–312
Tinger A, Wasserman TH, Klein EE et al (1997) The incidence of breast cancer following mantle field radiation therapy as a function of dose and technique. Int J Radiat Oncol Biol Phys 37:865–870
Travis LB, Gospodarowicz M, Curtis RE et al (2002) Lung cancer following chemotherapy and radiotherapy for Hodgkin's disease. J Natl Cancer Inst 94:182–192
Travis LB, Hill D, Dores GM et al (2005) Cumulative absolute breast cancer risk for young women treated for Hodgkin lymphoma. J Natl Cancer Inst 97:1428–1437
Trueblood HW, Enright LP, Ray GR et al (1970) Preservation of ovarian function in pelvic radiation for Hodgkin's disease. Arch Surg 100:236–237
Tucker MA (1993) Solid second cancers following Hodgkin's disease. Hematol Oncol Clin N Am 7:389–400
Tucker MA, Coleman CN, Cox RS et al (1988) Risk of second cancers after treatment for Hodgkin's disease. N Engl J Med 318:76–81
van Leeuwen FE, Klokman WJ, Hagenbeek A et al (1994) Second cancer risk following Hodgkin's disease: a 20-year follow-up study. J Clin Oncol 12:312–325
Verhey LJ (2002) Issues in optimization for planning of intensity-modulated radiation therapy. Semin Radiat Oncol 12:210–218
Vijayakumar S, Myrianthopoulos LC (1992) An updated dose–response analysis in Hodgkin's disease. Radiother Oncol 24:1–13
Vijayakumar S, Rosenberg I, Brandt T et al (1992) Quantification of doses to mediastinal lymph nodes in Hodgkin's disease. Med Dosim 17:87–94
Wang L, Hayes S, Paskalev K et al (2009) Dosimetric comparison of stereotactic body radiotherapy using 4D CT and multiphase CT images for treatment planning of lung cancer: evaluation of the impact on daily dose coverage. Radiother Oncol 91:314–324
Weihrauch MR, Re D, Bischoff S et al (2002) Whole-body positron emission tomography using 18F-fluorodeoxyglucose for initial staging of patients with Hodgkin's disease. Ann Hematol 81:20–25
Weisenburger TH, Juillard G (1974) Axillary lymphangiograms in radiation therapy of lymphomas. Preliminary report. Radiology 113:463–465
Weisenburger TH, Juillard GJ (1977) Upper extremity lymphangiography in the radiation therapy of lymphomas and carcinoma of the breast. Radiology 122:227–230
Willett CG, Linggood RM, Stracher MA et al (1987) The effect of the respiratory cycle on mediastinal and lung dimensions in Hodgkin's disease. Implications for radiotherapy gated to respiration. Cancer 60:1232–1237
Williams RS, Mendenhall N (1992) Laparoscopic oophoropexy for preservation of ovarian function before pelvic node irradiation. Obstet Gynecol 80:541–543
Williams RS, Littell RD, Mendenhall NP (1999) Laparoscopic oophoropexy and ovarian function in the treatment of Hodgkin disease. Cancer 86:2138–2142
Wirth A, Seymour JF, Hicks RJ et al (2002) Fluorine-18 fluorodeoxyglucose positron emission tomography, gallium-67 scintigraphy, and conventional staging for Hodgkin's disease and non-Hodgkin's lymphoma. Am J Med 112:262–268
Wirth A, Kron T, Wittwer H et al (2008) Phantom measurements and computed estimates of breast dose with radiotherapy for Hodgkin's lymphoma: dose reduction with the use of the involved field. J Med Imaging Radiat Oncol 52:394–402
Wolden SL, Lamborn KR, Cleary SF et al (1998) Second cancers following pediatric Hodgkin's disease. J Clin Oncol 16:536–544
Yahalom J, Mauch P (2002) The involved field is back: issues in delineating the radiation field in Hodgkin's disease. Ann Oncol 13(Suppl 1):79–83
Yahalom J, Petrek JA, Biddinger PW et al (1992) Breast cancer in patients irradiated for Hodgkin's disease: a clinical and pathologic analysis of 45 events in 37 patients. J Clin Oncol 10:1674–1681
Yorke ED, Jackson A, Rosenzweig KE et al (2002) Dose-volume factors contributing to the incidence of radiation pneumonitis in non-small-cell lung cancer patients treated with three-dimensional conformal radiation therapy. Int J Radiat Oncol Biol Phys 54:329–339
Zellmer DL, Wilson JF, Janjan NA (1991) Dosimetry of the breast for determining carcinogenic risk in mantle irradiation. Int J Radiat Oncol Biol Phys 21:1343–1351

Quality Assurance of Radiotherapy for Hodgkin Lymphoma

11

Rolf-Peter Müller and Hans Theodor Eich

Contents

R.-P. Müller (✉) and H.T. Eich
Department of Radiation Oncology, University of Cologne, Kerpener Straße 62, 50937, Cologne, Germany
e-mail: rolf-peter.mueller@uk-koeln.de; hans.eich@uk-koeln.de

11.1 Introduction

The quality of radiotherapy in Hodgkin lymphoma (HL) depends on the successful completion of each of the following steps: (1) Correct identification of sites of involvement and sites at significant risk for microscopic disease. This requires true information of an accurate and complete physical examination, correct interpretation of the diagnostic images used for staging, and knowledge about the regions at risk and patterns of spread of HL. (2) Selection and design of treatment field that will adequately cover the volume at risk and optimal spare of normal tissues. (3) Prescription of the optimal dose for disease control. (4) Meticulous delivery of the treatment plan. Failure to execute any of these steps properly will affect the quality and success of the overall treatment. Despite the excellent overall success rate by radiation therapy within combined-modality treatment, a need for quality assurance programs to assure the success of each of these steps has been documented in the literature. Large cooperative groups, e.g., the German Hodgkin Study Group (GHSG) or the European Organization for Research and Treatment of Cancer (EORTC), established extensive quality assurance programs within their multicenter trials. The objective of this article is to show recent achievements and developments in quality control of radiotherapy for HL exemplified by the GHSG trials. Their programs will be discussed in the context of the strategy of other cooperative group trials.

Since its beginning, more than 14,000 patients with HL have been enrolled into the multicenter randomized trials of the GHSG. Within four completed study generations the treatment of HL has developed in a stepwise manner by using the results of the completed protocols. With respect to radiotherapy, the

L. Specht and J. Yahalom (eds.), *Radiotherapy for Hodgkin Lymphoma*,
DOI: 10.1007/978-3-540-78944-4_11, © Springer-Verlag Berlin Heidelberg 2011

study group successfully evaluated different dose–effect relationships and could also prove the radiation efficacy of involved-field (IF) radiotherapy in early stages in combination with effective chemotherapy (Engert et al. 2003, 2007). The GHSG with 460 participating study institutions set up a radiotherapy reference center within the Department of Radiation Oncology at the University of Cologne to undertake quality assurance of the group's clinical studies (Muller and Eich 2005b). The HD4 study (early-favorable-stages) (randomization 1988–1993) had demonstrated that major protocol violations, especially the design of the extended-field (EF) radiotherapy fields, were associated with a statistically significant reduction in freedom from treatment failure (FFTF) (Duhmke et al. 1996, 2001). In this trial, an expert panel reviewed after finishing of treatment the radiation therapy treatment plan, simulation and verification films, technique, and dosimetry of 393 patients and classified each case as compliant with the protocol or as a violation. About 30% of cases were classified as having a major protocol violation; two-thirds of violations were related to inadequate treatment volume, while most of the remainder of violations were related to excessively protracted treatment time, technical inadequacies, and excessive radiation dose. Twenty-two patients (19%) with protocol violations subsequently had recurrence of HL, compared with 26 patients (11%) whose treatment was consistent with the protocol. FFTF at 5 years was 82% in patients treated without a protocol violation compared with 70% in patients with a protocol violation ($p < 0.04$). The quality control program in this trial was retrospective post treatment and highlighted two key factors : (1) the need for a real-time quality control program which could influence the actual delivery of treatment and (2) a close cooperation between diagnostic radiology and radiotherapy to use all imaging information for an optimal design of the individual radiotherapy treatment plan as required by the protocol prescriptions. As a consequence, new radiotherapy quality assurance programs were initiated, based on the design of the new trials and former programs were enhanced:

1. Central prospective radiation oncological review of cross-sectional imaging in early-stage HL
2. Retrospective quality control of the IF-radiotherapy

11.2 Central Prospective Radiation Oncological Review of Cross-Sectional Imaging in Early-Stage Hodgkin Lymphoma

Treatment strategies in HL have changed dramatically during recent years. For many decades the optimal and standard treatment for early-stage favorable HL was EF-radiotherapy. Today major study groups have changed from EF-radiotherapy to IF-radiotherapy preceded by short-term chemotherapy to reduce the extent of late toxicities without the risk of lowering the overall survival rates (Muller and Eich 2005a). For the first time, the IF-treatment technique was applied to all study patients in the HD10 (early-favorable stages) and HD11 (early-unfavorable stages) trials (30 versus 20 Gy) within a combined-modality approach (randomization 1998–2002) (Figs. 11.1 and 11.2) (Diehl et al. 2005; Eich et al. 2005). To guarantee the treatment quality of IF-radiotherapy a central prospective radiation oncological review of all patients' entire diagnostic imaging and clinical findings was performed (Eich et al. 2004b; Muller and Eich 2005b). An individual radiotherapy prescription was provided for every study patient.

All participating study centers (both, the responsible radiation oncologist and the medical oncologist) were requested to score disease involvement at a total of 34 possible anatomical sites on case report forms (CRF) (Fig. 11.3) and to determine the stage of disease according to the Ann Arbor classification before starting chemotherapy. The metric size of involved

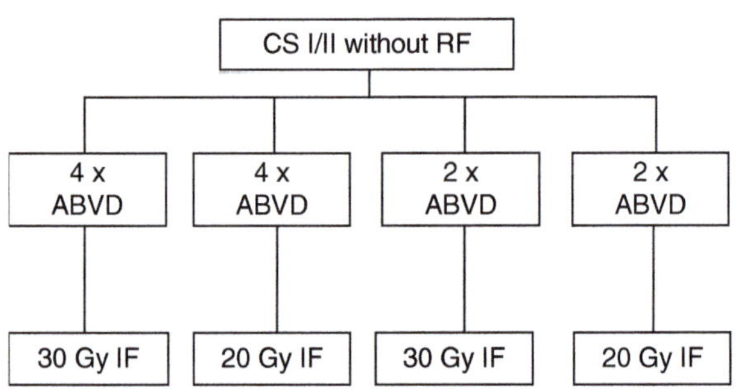

Fig. 11.1 Design of the HD10 trial. RF: risk factor; Large mediastinal mass; extranodal disease; high ERS; three or more areas involved; ABVD: adriamycin 25 mg/m^2; bleomycin 10 mg/m^2; vinblastine 6 mg/m^2; dacarbazine 375 mg/m^2

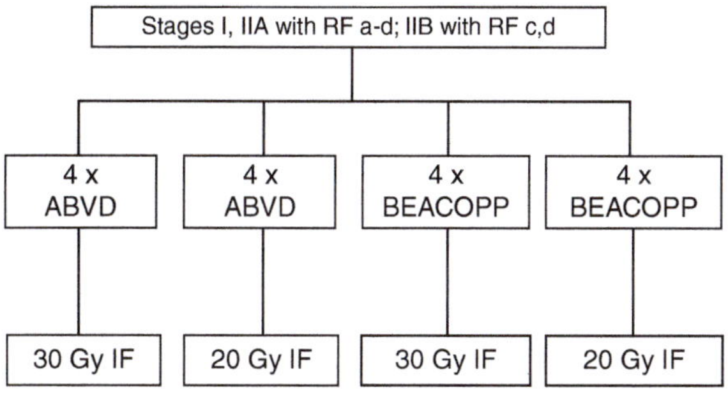

Fig. 11.2 Design of the HD11 trial. RF: risk factor: (a) large mediastinal mass; (b) extranodal disease; (c) high ERS; (d) three or more areas; ABVD: adriamycin 25 mg/m²; bleomycin 10 mg/m²; vinblastine 6 mg/m²; dacarbazine 375 mg/m²; BEACCOPP: bleomycin 10 mg/m²; etoposide 100 mg/m²; adriamycin 25 mg/m²; cyclophosphamide 650 mg/m²; vincristine 1.4 mg/m²; procarbazine 100 mg/m²; prednisone 40 mg/m²

nodes should also be reported. Lymph nodes of more than 5 cm in diameter were classified as bulky disease. In the GHSG trials, the tracheal bifurcation reflected the anatomical border between the upper and lower mediastinum. Lymph node involvement limited up to the tracheal bifurcation was differentiated from involvement below the bifurcation. In case of a superior mediastinal involvement only, the lower field border was one vertebral body below the tracheal bifurcation.

The CRF as well as all diagnostic images (CT, MRI, and X-rays) were sent to the radiotherapy reference center in Cologne, Germany. Besides conventional mailing, the delivery and processing of digital imaging on CD-ROM or via the internet was possible since January 2001.

At the reference center the diagnostic images were reviewed by a panel of expert radiation oncologists and radiologists and compared with the documentation on the CRF. Criteria for reevaluation were any abnormalities on chest radiographs and CT/MRT scans suspicious of disease, in particular taking into account the size and form of lymph nodes (>1.5 cm) and any extra-lymphatic disease based on widely accepted standards in radiology. Differences between the disease involvement documented by the participating study center and the reference center were recorded. In cases of significant discrepancy the physician in charge of the participating center was contacted and the individual disease extension and stage were discussed. Usually, a consensus between the reference center and the participating study center could be achieved. Subsequently an individualized treatment proposal

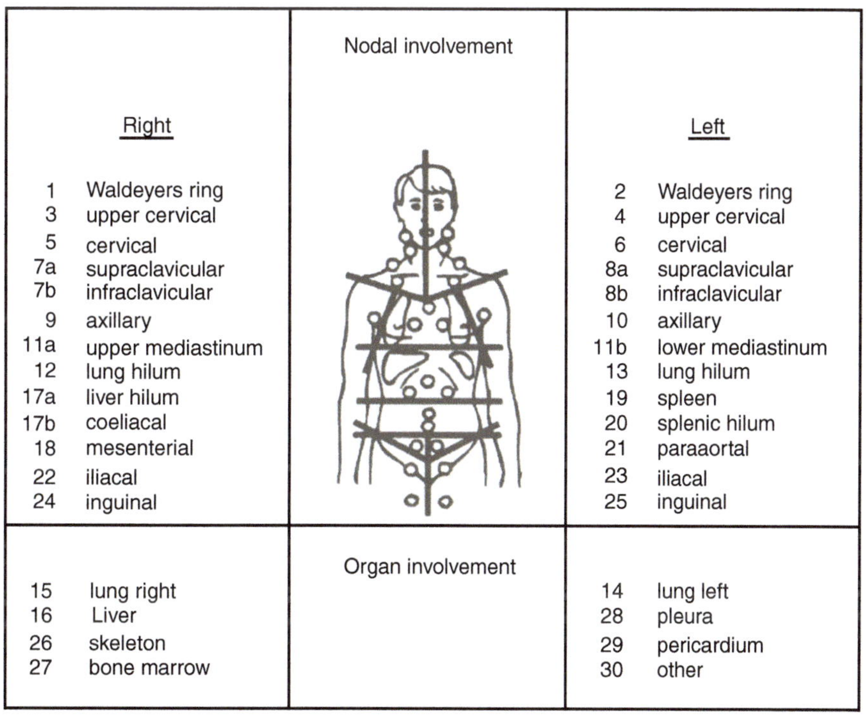

Fig. 11.3 Scoring system of anatomical sites according to the German Hodgkin Study Group (GHSG) protocol guidelines

was compiled. Site, extent, and spread of disease were marked in a schematic figure, as was the resulting individual treatment field for the IF-radiotherapy.

Complete sets of documentation (CRF as well as CT, MRI, and X-ray images) of 1,214/1,371 patients (89%) in HD10 and 1,397/1,570 patients (89%) in HD11 were submitted to the reference center. The introduction of electronic image transfer optimized and simplified the workflow of this quality assurance programs. Rapid online consultation and real-time teleconferences regarding disease involvement, patient management, and communication of the radiotherapy treatment prescription with connected hospitals were helpful (Eich et al. 2004a).

The evaluation of the quality assurance program showed that a considerable proportion of involved sites were not or incorrectly recorded on the corresponding CRF by the participating center. For patients with early-stage HL (HD10) there was a correction of disease involvement in 49%, for patients with intermediate stages (HD11) in 67%. Most discrepancies were seen in the lower mediastinum (23%), infraclavicular- (17%), upper cervical- (16%), supraclavicular- (13%), and pulmonary hilar region (13%) (Fig. 11.4).

The comparison of the documented disease by the participating study centers and the expert's statement resulted in a change of disease stage in 41 patients. Considering disease stage as revised and the guidelines of the protocol, 93 patients had to be treated in a different protocol. Due to the incorrect lymph node documentation of the participating study centers the radiotherapy treatment volume had to be enlarged in 891/2,611 (34%) patients and reduced in 82/2,611 (3%) patients. According to the most frequently corrected lymph node sites, the changes of the involved-field treatment volume particularly affected the lower mediastinum, pulmonary hilar, and neck lymph nodes.

The most common site of disagreement was the mediastinum, created by the study protocol definition of the tracheal bifurcation being the anatomical border between the upper and lower mediastinum. Inconsistent CT interpretation of hilar lymphadenopathy has been recognized previously and was apparent here. The relatively frequent disagreement associated with infraclavicular sites may reflect difficulties in defining the precise anatomic border relative to the clavicles, supraclavicular fossae, and axillae. Since radiation oncologists in Germany have to spend at least 1 year of training in diagnostic radiology during their education, they should be familiar with the interpretation of cross-sectional imaging. In the routine use of IF-radiotherapy in combined-modality treatment protocols for HL, it is mandatory that the treating radiation oncologist looks at the CT scans personally in order to plan the radiation fields. The responsibility of the treatment still rests with the treating radiation oncologist. Apparently, the external medical and radiation oncologists sometimes documented the disease involvement on the basis of the radiological report but the primary radiologists were not always familiar with the scoring systems in HL or might have had no sufficient information. This underlines the need for standardized reporting in oncological imaging as well as continuing medical education. This would provide clinicians with the radiological

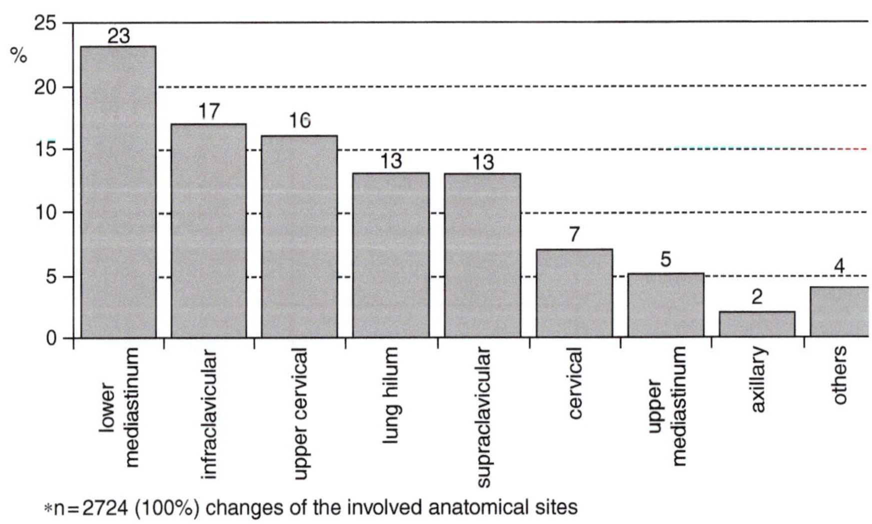

Fig. 11.4 Proportion of disagreements of involved anatomical regions between the expert's statement and the documentation form. This is shown anatomic site-based*

information they require before making treatment decisions.

Recently the German-Austrian pediatric HD study group described their experiences of a centralized data review of 578 patients from 71 participating hospitals. Similar to the procedure of the GHSG, the study participants had to send clinical patient data as well as radiographs and CT to the study coordination center where a centralized review had been conducted (Dieckmann et al. 2002). Dieckmann et al. reported that the reference center received chest CT scans from 84.6% of the patients and CT scans of the abdomen of 76.8%. The pediatric study group observed a revision of stage in 20% of all reviewed patients and 13.3% of these patients had to be shifted into a different treatment group.

11.3 Retrospective Quality Control of the Involved-Field Radiotherapy

Based on the simulation films, verification films and radiation treatment protocols of the patients in the HD10 and HD11 trials, an expert radiotherapy panel evaluated retrospectively the adequacy of irradiated IF-treatment portals, applied radiation doses, treatment time, and technical parameters. Between 1999 and 2006 a total of 825/1,370 randomized patients of the HD10 (60%) and 954/1,422 patients of the HD11 trial (67%) were evaluated by the panel (Eich et al. 2008). RT was rated as suboptimal in 47% of all reviewed cases. Although the participating radiotherapy centers got a precise radiotherapy prescription, most difficulties occurred in the adequate coverage of the IF as defined in the study protocol (40%) followed by technical faults (12%). Deviations from the prescribed single daily dose (1.8–2 Gy), weekly dose as well as total reference dose were rare (1%).

Since there is no international consensus on the definition of IF-radiotherapy in HL available (Yahalom and Mauch 2002), the GHSG described their definition, all technical parameters as well as dosage extensively in the written study protocol, so that there was consistency in the criteria between the panel and the local radiotherapy center. Most difficulties occurred in the adequate coverage of the IF, especially in the neck region, upper mediastinum, and infraclavicular region. A significant number of participating radiation oncologists reluctantly irradiated the spinal cord in the case of cervical involvement. According to the protocol the medial field border had to include the whole cervical spine to secure that all regional lymph nodes were adequate covered (Fig. 11.5). Since the total dose was only 20 or 30 Gy, a risk for toxicity of the spinal cord was unlikely. Also the implementation of 3D treatment planning, which could be used, seemed to be a problem. The delineation of only the involved lymph nodes with a safety margin was not according to protocol in a reasonable number of patients. To follow the protocol guidelines the whole lymph node region according to anatomical landmarks had to be treated. The GHSG definition of an upper and lower mediastinum to spare the heart was widely accepted by the participating centers. Fortunately the compliance to apply the total dose of 30 Gy as well as 20 Gy was good, so that the study question can be answered as planned. At the start of the trials HD10 and HD11 a lot of radiation oncologists were reluctant to apply only 20 Gy, especially when a significant residual tumor after chemotherapy was left.

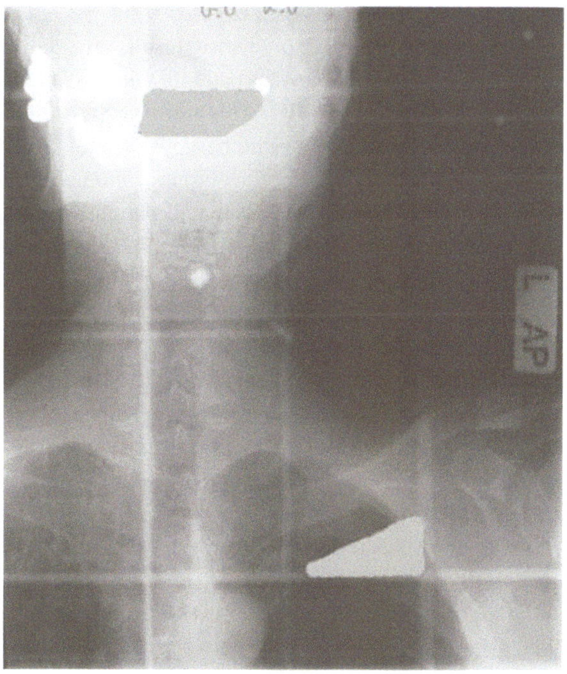

Fig. 11.5 Involved-field irradiation for a patient with stage I Hodgkin lymphoma involving the left neck. Upper Border: mastoid process. Lower Border: 1.5–2 cm below the bottom of the clavicle. Lateral Border: To include the medial two-thirds of the clavicle. Medial Border: entire vertebral body (spinal cord) is included

But they were told that very consequent stopping rules would prevent a higher risk of recurrence. According to the technical faults the usage of more than 10 MeV photons was a protocol violation according to the panel if there was no adequate documentation of a bolus on the radiotherapy CRF or a CT plan available. Whether these objections detected by the panel are relevant for relapses in the era of combined-modality treatment needs to be established.

Since the implementation of combined-modality treatment, no study group could ever prove that the quality of radiotherapy is still a prognostic factor as demonstrated in the HD4 trial (Duhmke et al. 1996, 2001). The GHSG recently reported on the final results of the HD7 trial (1994–1998) for early-favorable stages (Engert et al. 2007). This trial investigated whether combined-modality treatment with two cycles ABVD followed by EF-radiotherapy is superior to EF-radiotherapy alone. A retrospective radiotherapy quality control of 529 patients demonstrated that most protocol violations were classified as volume too small (44%), protracted in time of radiotherapy (24%), or dose too low (12%). FFTF did not differ significantly, between patients with and without protocol violations (Engert et al. 2007).

Recently the EORTC published results of quality control for IF-radiotherapy in patients with advanced stages (Aleman et al. 2005). This retrospective study demonstrated that a major radiotherapy protocol violation, predominantly concerning target volumes, was observed in 47% of all 135 evaluated patients. There was no relationship between the pattern of relapse and major violations of the protocol.

The Patterns of Care studies in the United States on HL demonstrated that patients with adequate portal margins had significantly fewer in-field or marginal recurrences, or relapses of any type (Kinzie et al. 1983). However, the expertise of the radiation oncologist, use of a dedicated simulator, performance of routine port films to ensure set-up accuracies, and use of individually shaped blocks, linear accelerators, and EF-treatment were all associated with an improved treatment outcome. In the Patterns of Care study published in 1995, discrepancies between the consensus guidelines developed in 1993 and the surveyed United States practice were noted in a number of areas (Hoppe et al. 1994; Hughes et al. 1995). The authors suggested that specific changes in treatment techniques and utilization of appropriate equipment, may improve the quality of treatment planning and delivery.

As the follow-up of the trials HD10 and HD11 (randomization 1998–2002) is still not mature, we are not able to do a relapse analysis at this time, but potential correlations between radiotherapy quality and relapse rate will be investigated as soon as possible. However, a detailed analysis of possible faults and pitfalls in IF-radiotherapy is now available (Eich et al. 2008). As a consequence, radiation oncologists were trained on the definition of IF-radiotherapy at the GHSG meetings and at the annual meetings of the German Society for Therapeutic Radiation Oncology (DEGRO). This quality control program is again being implemented in the ongoing trials HD13 (early-favorable stages) and HD14 (early-unfavorable stages) (active since 2002) where all patients receive 30 Gy IF-radiotherapy within a combined-modality approach. Thus we intend to compare the results of the quality control of HD10 and HD11 with that of HD13 and HD14 to see whether any improvement of the quality based on the initiated training programs for radiation oncologists is to be seen comparable to the results of the Patterns of Care studies in the United States.

11.4 Conclusion

Central review of the diagnostic imaging and clinical findings of HL patients show a considerable number of discrepancies compared with the local evaluation. Meticulous evaluation of all imaging information in a collaboration between radiation oncologist and diagnostic radiologist is mandatory. Stringent quality assurance programs must be implemented.

References

Aleman BM, Girinsky T, van der Maazen RW et al (2005) Quality control of involved-field radiotherapy in patients with advanced Hodgkin's lymphoma (EORTC 20884). Int J Radiat Oncol Biol Phys 63:1184–1190

Dieckmann K, Potter R, Wagner W et al (2002) Up-front centralized data review and individualized treatment proposals in a multicenter pediatric Hodgkin's disease trial with 71 participating hospitals: the experience of the German-Austrian pediatric multicenter trial DAL-HD-90. Radiother Oncol 62:191–200

Diehl V, Brillant C, Engert A et al (2005) Recent interim analysis of the HD11 trial of the GHSG: intensification of chemotherapy and reduction of radiation dose in early unfavourable stage Hodgkin's lymphoma. Blood 106:240a–241a

Duhmke E, Diehl V, Loeffler M et al (1996) Randomized trial with early-stage Hodgkin's disease testing 30 Gy vs. 40 Gy extended field radiotherapy alone. Int J Radiat Oncol Biol Phys 36:305–310

Duhmke E, Franklin J, Pfreundschuh M et al (2001) Low-dose radiation is sufficient for the noninvolved extended-field treatment in favorable early-stage Hodgkin's disease: long-term results of a randomized trial of radiotherapy alone. J Clin Oncol 19:2905–2914

Eich HT, Muller RP, Schneeweiss A et al (2004a) Initiation of a teleradiotherapeutic network for patients in German lymphoma studies. Int J Radiat Oncol Biol Phys 58:805–808

Eich HT, Staar S, Gossmann A et al (2004b) Centralized radiation oncologic review of cross-sectional imaging of Hodgkin's disease leads to significant changes in required involved field-results of a quality assurance program of the German Hodgkin Study Group. Int J Radiat Oncol Biol Phys 58:1121–1127

Eich H, Mueller R, Engert A et al (2005) Comparison of 30 Gy versus 20 Gy involved field radiotherapy after two versus four cycles ABVD in early stage Hodgkin's lymphoma: interim analysis of the German Hodgkin Study Group trial HD10. Int J Radiat Oncol Biol Phys 63:1–2

Eich HT, Engenhart-Cabillic R, Hansemann K et al (2008) Quality control of involved field radiotherapy in patients with early-favorable (HD10) and early-unfavorable (HD11) Hodgkin's lymphoma: an analysis of the German Hodgkin Study Group. Int J Radiat Oncol Biol Phys 71:1419–1424

Engert A, Schiller P, Josting A et al (2003) Involved-field radiotherapy is equally effective and less toxic compared with extended-field radiotherapy after four cycles of chemotherapy in patients with early-stage unfavorable Hodgkin's lymphoma: results of the HD8 trial of the German Hodgkin's Lymphoma Study Group. J Clin Oncol 21:3601–3608

Engert A, Franklin J, Eich HT et al (2007) Two cycles of doxorubicin, bleomycin, vinblastine, and dacarbazine plus extended-field radiotherapy is superior to radiotherapy alone in early favorable Hodgkin's lymphoma: final results of the GHSG HD7 trial. J Clin Oncol 25:3495–3502

Hoppe RT, Hanlon AL, Hanks GE et al (1994) Progress in the treatment of Hodgkin's disease in the United States, 1973 versus 1983. The patterns of care study. Cancer 74:3198–3203

Hughes DB, Smith AR, Hoppe R et al (1995) Treatment planning for Hodgkin's disease: a patterns of care study. Int J Radiat Oncol Biol Phys 33:519–524

Kinzie JJ, Hanks GE, MacLean CJ et al (1983) Patterns of care study: Hodgkin's disease relapse rates and adequacy of portals. Cancer 52:2223–2226

Muller RP, Eich HT (2005a) Current role of radiotherapy in the treatment of Hodgkin's disease. In: Perez CA, Brady LW, Halperin EC et al (eds) Update principles and practice of radiation oncology. Lippincott Williams & Wilkins, Philadelphia, PA

Muller RP, Eich HT (2005b) The development of quality assurance programs for radiotherapy within the German Hodgkin Study Group (GHSG). Introduction, continuing work, and results of the radiotherapy reference panel. Strahlenther Onkol 181:557–566

Yahalom J, Mauch P (2002) The involved field is back: issues in delineating the radiation field in Hodgkin's disease. Ann Oncol 13(Suppl 1):79–83

Evaluation of Response After Radiotherapy for Hodgkin Lymphoma

12

Lena Specht and Martin Hutchings

Contents

L. Specht (✉) and M. Hutchings
Departments of Oncology and Haematology, The Finsen Centre, Rigshospitalet, University of Copenhagen, 9 Blegdamsvej, 2100, Copenhagen, Denmark
e-mail: specht@dadlnet.dk
e-mail: hutchings@dadlnet.dk

12.1 Introduction

The evaluation of response after treatment is important for treating physicians and patients alike. Response is an important surrogate for other measures of clinical benefit, notably progression-free survival (PFS) and overall survival (OS). It is also an important guide for determining the need for further therapy or for change in treatment strategy. It is therefore extremely important to use widely accepted and readily applied standard criteria based on the anatomical tumor burden.

Response criteria were developed by the World Health Organization (WHO) in 1981 (Miller et al. 1981), introducing the concept of an overall assessment of the tumor burden by summing the products of bidimensional measurements and evaluation of change from baseline measurements. However, these criteria were often modified to accommodate new technologies and special situations in specific tumor types.

An international collaboration was established to standardize and simplify response criteria for solid tumors, and the so-called Response Evaluation Criteria in Solid Tumors (RECIST) criteria were published in 2000 (Therasse et al. 2000). Important features of these response criteria were the definition of minimum size of measurable lesions and the introduction of unidimensional, rather than bidimensional, measures for evaluation. However, the evaluation of lymph nodes was not specifically dealt with.

An update of the RECIST criteria was published in 2009 (Eisenhauer et al. 2009), dealing with a number of issues left unanswered by the original RECIST publication, including how to handle assessment of lymph nodes and how to use newer imaging technologies. With regard to the evaluation of lymph nodes it was recognized that they, unlike other malignant deposits, have a normal size when nonmalignant, and that the measured size of a

L. Specht and J. Yahalom (eds.), *Radiotherapy for Hodgkin Lymphoma*,
DOI: 10.1007/978-3-540-78944-4_12, © Springer-Verlag Berlin Heidelberg 2011

lymph node is highly dependent on the manner in which it is measured and the spatial orientation of the lymph node relative to the CT scan (Schwartz et al. 2009).

The RECIST criteria were developed for solid tumors, and it is recognized that the assessment of lymph nodes in lymphomas is more complex. Still, the large systematic effort in clarification of assessment of response in the RECIST publications may be used as guidance in the evaluation of lymphomas.

12.2 Evaluation of Response Using Size Criteria

The fundamental approach to assessment of response has been primarily based on measurements of the anatomical extent of disease. In Hodgkin lymphoma (HL), the vast majority of involved sites are lymph nodes. The finding by CT or physical examination most suggestive of malignant involvement is nodal size. Since lymph nodes occur normally in the body they will have a normal size. Hence, the crucial point is to define criteria to differentiate normal lymph nodes from lymph nodes involved with HL.

In a report from an international meeting on the evaluation of patients with HL, the so-called Cotswolds meeting, it was decided that lymph nodes of more than 1.5 cm cross-sectional diameter should be regarded as unequivocally abnormal and representing HL (Lister et al. 1989). Moreover, it was decided that partial remission (PR) should be defined as a decrease by at least 50% in the sum of the products of the largest perpendicular diameters (SPD) of all measurable lesions.

However, others used different size criteria. The German Hodgkin Study Group (GHSG) used 1.0 cm cross-sectional diameter as the upper threshold of normal lymph node size (Vorwerk et al. 2008). Whatever cutoff value is used, there will be false-negatives (e.g., microscopic involvement of lymph nodes of normal size) and false-positives (e.g., reactive hyperplasia in enlarged nodes). The choice of cutoff value does, however, have a significant impact on the evaluation of the disease status of the individual patients (Vorwerk et al. 2008).

The measurement of the transverse diameter of lymph nodes on CT scans is dependent on the orientation of the axis of the lymph node relative to the CT slices. Moreover, the size of normal lymph nodes varies between different anatomic locations. It has been shown that the measurement of the short axis of lymph nodes is the most reliable parameter, and an upper limit of normal lymph node size in the short axis of 1 cm has been suggested (Glazer et al. 1985). These criteria have been implemented in the most recent update of the RECIST criteria (Eisenhauer et al. 2009; Schwartz et al. 2009).

However, the assessment of lymph nodes in lymphomas may be more complex. Lymph nodes involved with lymphoma may decrease in size after treatment but develop fibrosis, necrosis or inflammation resulting in persistent enlargement of the node even if no longer histologically involved by lymphoma. This led to the definition in the report from the Cotswolds meeting of the response category complete remission unconfirmed/uncertain (CRu), denoting patients in whom remission status is unclear (Lister et al. 1989). Patients in this category have no clinical evidence of HL but some radiological abnormality persists at a site of previous disease, the significance of which is uncertain.

The response category CRu was included in the response criteria for non-Hodgkin lymphomas developed and published by an International Working Group (IWG) (Cheson et al. 1999). In these criteria, lymph nodes greater than 1.5 cm in greatest transverse diameter are considered abnormal, and should decrease to less than 1.5 cm to be considered normal in size. Lymph nodes between 1.1 and 1.5 cm in greatest diameter may be considered abnormal from the outset, and they must decrease to 1.0 cm or less or by more than 75% in the SPD to be considered normal after treatment. However, if a lymph node mass greater than 1.5 cm in greatest transverse diameter persists after treatment, the patient can be considered in CRu if the residual lymph node has regressed by more than 75% in SPD compared with the size of the original mass.

The IWG response criteria were widely used also for the evaluation of HL patients. However, the CRu concept in the response assessment of both HL and non-Hodgkin lymphomas was always problematic.

12.3 Evaluation of Response Using Anatomical and Functional Imaging Methods

Positron emission tomography with 2-[18F]fluor-2-deoxyglucose (FDG-PET) has emerged as a powerful functional imaging tool in HL as well as in most other lymphomas. A major advantage of FDG-PET is its ability to distinguish between viable tumor and necrosis or fibrosis in residual masses after treatment. However, it must be remembered that FDG-PET, like other imaging methods, cannot detect microscopic residual disease.

The widespread use of FDG-PET in the evaluation of HL and other lymphomas prompted an International Harmonization Project to develop recommendations for response criteria that would be used across study groups and for HL and non-Hodgkin lymphomas alike (Cheson et al. 2007). These revised response criteria strongly recommend FDG-PET before treatment for patients with routinely FDG-avid and potentially curable lymphomas such as HL to better delineate the extent of disease, and FDG-PET is considered essential for the posttreatment assessment of HL because a CR is required for a curative outcome. The revised response criteria for use in HL are outlined in Table 12.1. A number of points should be noted:

- The size criteria for normal lymph nodes are identical to those of the original IWG criteria. However, the result of the FDG-PET scan overrides the size criteria with regard to CR in nodal masses.
- For PR, SD and relapse/PD definitions the size criteria are still important, and as in the original IWG criteria they are based on bidimensional measurements. However, the results of the FDG-PET scan must also be included in the evaluation.
- The response category CRu has been eliminated. This is a clear improvement, since there was always considerable uncertainty regarding the precise definition and meaning of this term.
- In some instances microscopic disease will be present in residual masses on CT. As FDG-PET cannot detect microscopic disease there will inevitably be some false-negatives with the new response criteria. Hopefully, the number of false-negatives with the new criteria will be much smaller than the number of false-positives with the old criteria.
- It must be kept in mind that the experience with response assessment with FDG-PET was obtained in patients receiving full conventional treatment, which in many cases in HL meant combined modality treatment. The evaluation of residual masses after chemotherapy only may be more uncertain (Picardi et al. 2007).

Table 12.1 Revised response criteria for Hodgkin lymphoma

Response	Definition	Nodal masses	Spleen, liver	Bone marrow
CR	Disappearance of all evidence of disease	Mass of any size permitted if PET-negative (if PET not available: regression to normal size on CT)	Not palpable, nodules disappeared	Infiltrate cleared on repeat biopsy; if indeterminate by morphology, immunohistochemistry should be negative
PR	Regression of measurable disease and no new sites	≥50% decrease in SPD of up to six largest dominant masses; no increase in size of other nodes; one or more PET-positive at previously involved site (if PET not available: regression on CT)	≥50% decrease in SPD of nodules (for single nodule in greatest transverse diameter); no increase in size of liver of spleen	Irrelevant if positive prior to therapy; cell type should be specified
SD	Failure to attain CR/PR or PD	PET-positive at prior sites of disease and no new sites on CT or PET (if PET not available: no change in size of previous lesions on CT)		
Relapsed disease or PD	Any new lesion or increase by ≥50% of previously involved sites from nadir	Appearance of new lesion(s) >1.5 cm in any axis, ≥50% increase in SPD of more than one node, or ≥50% increase in longest diameter of a previously identified node >1 cm in short axis. Lesions PET-positive.	>50% increase from nadir in SPD of any previous lesions	New or recurrent involvement

CR, complete remission; FDG, 2-[18F]fluor-2-deoxyglucose; PET, positron emission tomography; CT, computed tomography; PR, partial remission; SPD, sum of the products of the diameters; SD, stable disease; PD, progressive disease

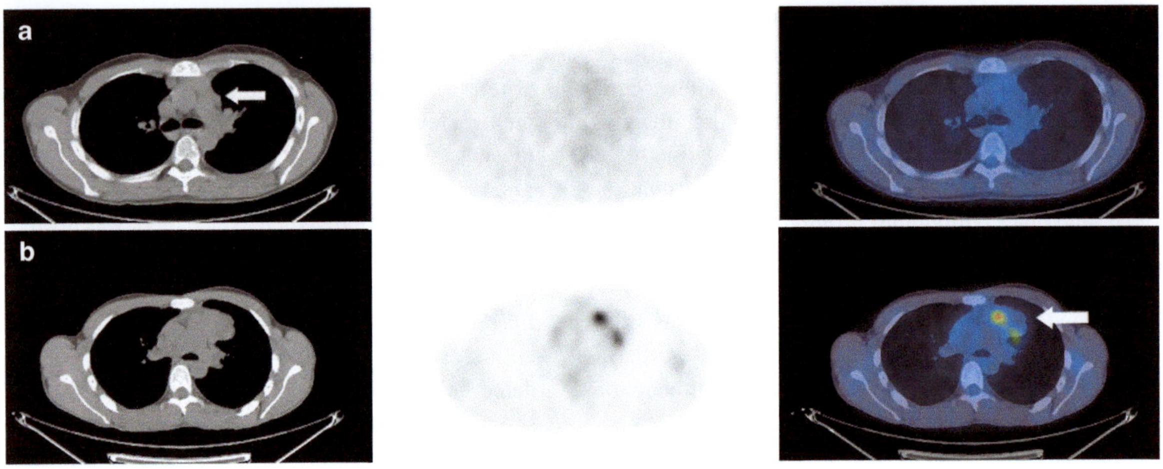

Fig. 12.1 Two HL patients with residual mediastinal masses after treatment. In (**a**) there is no significant FDG uptake. In (**b**) there is focal uptake within the mediastinal mass suggestive of residual tumor. Viable lymphoma cells may be contained within large areas of fibrosis leading to sampling errors at biopsy

The revised IWG criteria were initially based on rather limited clinical data (Juweid et al. 2005), but testing the new criteria in independent data sets of patients with HL seem to confirm that the new criteria provide a more accurate response classification compared with the previous criteria (Brepoels et al. 2007a, 2007b). Figure 12.1 shows examples of residual masses on CT scans after treatment without or with FDG uptake.

12.4 FDG-PET in Response Evaluation of HL

Before including FDG-PET in response evaluation several criteria must be met (Sargent et al. 2009; Shankar et al. 2006). Standardization of the technique and of the interpretation of the images is needed. A subcommittee of the International Harmonization Project developed guidelines for the use of FDG-PET for response assessment of lymphomas intended for use with the revised IWG response criteria (Juweid et al. 2007). They were intended for both HL and non-Hodgkin lymphomas and can be summarized as follows:

- Visual assessment alone is adequate for the interpretation of FDG-PET after completion of therapy.
- Mediastinal blood pool activity is recommended as the reference background activity to define PET positivity for a residual mass larger than 2 cm in greatest transverse diameter, regardless of its location.
- A smaller residual mass or a normal-sized lymph node should be considered positive if its activity is above that of the surrounding background.

These interpretation criteria were based on an expert consensus, but unfortunately they have not been validated in large cohorts of patients nor compared to other interpretation criteria. The authors underline that the criteria are meant for posttreatment assessment only, and they acknowledge that for interim FDG-PET "a dichotomous interpretation based on visual assessment alone may not be sufficiently reliable to distinguish patients with a more favorable from those with less favorable outcome."

Some scans are clearly PET-positive and others are clearly PET-negative. However, there is an intermediate group where the interobserver variability is high if scans are reported *black-and-white* as either positive or negative. Many authors have labeled this group Minimal Residual Uptake (MRU) (Barrington et al. 2009; Hutchings et al. 2005). The evolution has resulted in a widened definition of MRU. As MRU is most commonly counted among the negatives, this has increased the specificity and reduced the number of false-positive interim FDG-PET scans (Gallamini et al. 2009). A recently initiated international collaboration aims to propose simple, reproducible criteria for interim FDG-PET interpretation and to launch international studies to validate these guidelines.

The results of the group's first consensus meeting have been recently published (Meignan et al. 2009b). Briefly, the criteria for interim FDG-PET interpretation in HL were contained in three main points:

- Visual assessment is preferred, but Standardized Uptake Value (SUV) can assist visual assessment in some cases.
- Interim FDG-PET should always be interpreted by comparing the single foci of FDG uptake to the ones recorded in the baseline study.
- The intensity of FDG uptake should be graded according to a five-point scale in which the liver and the mediastinal background are used as references to define different grades of FDG uptake.

The five-point scale allows for different thresholds between negative and positive scans, depending on whether the clinical situations demands an optimal negative predictive value or optimal positive predictive value. Two international validation studies are underway to validate these criteria; one for advanced-stage HL and one for diffuse large B-cell lymphoma. Due to the absence of validated criteria for interim FDG-PET, a central review panel is necessary for PET interpretation in ongoing prospective trials using an interim PET response-adapted strategy (Meignan et al. 2009a).

12.5 Conclusion

Response assessment in patients treated for HL is now carried out according to new revised response criteria including functional imaging with FDG-PET. Recent data seem to indicate that the new criteria provide a more accurate response classification than the previous criteria based solely on the size of lymphoma masses, but more long term follow-up is needed. Standardized and broadly accepted criteria for FDG-PET technique and interpretation for response assessment in HL are being developed.

References

Barrington SF, Qian W, Somer EJ et al (2009) Concordance between four European Centres of PET reporting criteria designed for use in multicentre trials in Hodgkin lymphoma. Eur J Nucl Med Mol Imaging 36(Suppl 2):S252

Brepoels L, Stroobants S, De WW et al (2007a) Hodgkin lymphoma: response assessment by revised International Workshop Criteria. Leuk Lymphoma 48:1539–1547

Brepoels L, Stroobants S, Verhoef G (2007b) PET and PET/CT for response evaluation in lymphoma: current practice and developments. Leuk Lymphoma 48:270–282

Cheson BD, Horning SJ, Coiffier B et al (1999) Report of an international workshop to standardize response criteria for non-Hodgkin's lymphomas. NCI Sponsored International Working Group. J Clin Oncol 17:1244–1253

Cheson BD, Pfistner B, Juweid ME et al (2007) Revised response criteria for malignant lymphoma. J Clin Oncol 25:579–586

Eisenhauer EA, Therasse P, Bogaerts J et al (2009) New response evaluation criteria in solid tumours: revised RECIST guideline (version 1.1). Eur J Cancer 45:228–247

Gallamini A, Fiore F, Sorasio R et al (2009) Interim positron emission tomography scan in Hodgkin lymphoma: definitions, interpretation rules, and clinical validation. Leuk Lymphoma 50:1761–1764

Glazer GM, Gross BH, Quint LE et al (1985) Normal mediastinal lymph nodes: number and size according to American Thoracic Society mapping. AJR Am J Roentgenol 144:261–265

Hutchings M, Mikhaeel NG, Fields PA et al (2005) Prognostic value of interim FDG-PET after two or three cycles of chemotherapy in Hodgkin lymphoma. Ann Oncol 16:1160–1168

Juweid ME, Wiseman GA, Vose JM et al (2005) Response assessment of aggressive non-Hodgkin's lymphoma by integrated International Workshop Criteria and fluorine-18-fluorodeoxyglucose positron emission tomography. J Clin Oncol 23:4652–4661

Juweid ME, Stroobants S, Hoekstra OS et al (2007) Use of positron emission tomography for response assessment of lymphoma: consensus of the Imaging Subcommittee of International Harmonization Project in Lymphoma. J Clin Oncol 25:571–578

Lister TA, Crowther D, Sutcliffe SB et al (1989) Report of a committee convened to discuss the evaluation and staging of patients with Hodgkin's disease: Cotswolds meeting. J Clin Oncol 7:1630–1636

Meignan M, Itti E, Bardet S et al (2009a) Development and application of a real-time on-line blinded independent central review of interim PET scans to determine treatment allocation in lymphoma trials. J Clin Oncol 27:2739–2741

Meignan M, Itti E, Gallamini A et al (2009b) Interim 18F-fluorodeoxyglucose positron emission tomography in diffuse large B-cell lymphoma: qualitative or quantitative interpretation–where do we stand? Leuk Lymphoma 50:1753–1756

Miller AB, Hoogstraten B, Staquet M et al (1981) Reporting results of cancer treatment. Cancer 47:207–214

Picardi M, De Renzo A, Pane F et al (2007) Randomized comparison of consolidation radiation versus observation in bulky Hodgkin's lymphoma with post-chemotherapy negative positron emission tomography scans. Leuk Lymphoma 48:1721–1727

Sargent DJ, Rubinstein L, Schwartz L et al (2009) Validation of novel imaging methodologies for use as cancer clinical trial end-points. Eur J Cancer 45:290–299

Schwartz LH, Bogaerts J, Ford R et al (2009) Evaluation of lymph nodes with RECIST 1.1. Eur J Cancer 45:261–267

Shankar LK, Hoffman JM, Bacharach S et al (2006) Consensus recommendations for the use of 18F-FDG PET as an indicator of therapeutic response in patients in National Cancer Institute Trials. J Nucl Med 47:1059–1066

Therasse P, Arbuck SG, Eisenhauer EA et al (2000) New guidelines to evaluate the response to treatment in solid tumors. European Organization for Research and Treatment of Cancer, National Cancer Institute of the United States, National Cancer Institute of Canada. J Natl Cancer Inst 92:205–216

Vorwerk H, Obenauer S, Schmidberger H et al (2008) The significance of a uniform definition of pathological lymph nodes in Hodgkin lymphoma: impact of different thresholds for positive lymph nodes in CT imaging on staging and therapy. Radiother Oncol 87:74–81

Hodgkin Lymphoma in Special Populations and Rare Localizations

13

Peter Meidahl Petersen

Contents

P.M. Petersen (✉)
Departments of Oncology and Haematology, The Finsen Centre, Rigshospitalet, University of Copenhagen, 9 Blegdamsvej, DK-2100 Copenhagen, Denmark
e-mail: peter.meidahl.petersen@rh.regionh.dk

13.1 Introduction

The presentation of Hodgkin lymphoma (HL) shows special features in certain populations such as the elderly, in pregnant women, and in human immune deficiency virus (HIV)-positive patients. The treatment may also require individualized adjustment for such patients. Rare localizations such as involvement of bone or central nervous system (CNS) may also harbour implications for diagnosis and treatment. The prognosis may differ due to biological differences or differences in treatment feasibilities.

13.2 Hodgkin Lymphoma in Special Patient Populations

13.2.1 Hodgkin Lymphoma in the Elderly

HL is rare in the elderly, the incidence is approximately 2–3/100,000 persons at risk per year in Europe and Northern America in a population aged more than 60 years (Klimm et al. 2007; Proctor et al. 2005). The incidence seems to be stable although more recent studies have shown that the diagnosis in some cases is revised to other B-cell lymphomas if expert panels review the pathology (Jarrett et al. 2003). In population-based studies, 20–30% of the patients are older than 60 (Landgren et al. 2003; Proctor et al. 2005), but only a minor part of patients in clinical studies are over 60, because most studies have an upper age limit for inclusion. Hence, the evidence for the choice of treatment is weaker in elderly than in young patients in many situations. It has been speculated as to whether the biology differs from that of younger patients due to

L. Specht and J. Yahalom (eds.), *Radiotherapy for Hodgkin Lymphoma*,
DOI: 10.1007/978-3-540-78944-4_13, © Springer-Verlag Berlin Heidelberg 2011

the differences in clinical presentation, and because the outcome of treatment seems poorer even after correction from other factors, even in patients who tolerate full-dose chemotherapy (Klimm et al. 2007).

13.2.1.1 Presentation and Staging

The presentation in elderly patients differs from that of younger patients, with more patients presenting with mixed cellularity type, more having B-symptoms, and more having advanced stage disease. Fewer older patients have bulky disease and/or large mediastinal tumours (Engert et al. 2005; Landgren et al. 2003). In general, staging should be done according to the guidelines prescribed for younger patients. However, in many elderly patients the staging may be less extensive compared to younger patients, thus there is a risk of under-staging (Enblad 1994).

13.2.1.2 Comorbidity

With more advanced age, more patients have comorbidity, such as chronic heart or lung disease, which can reduce their tolerance to treatment. A careful assessment of the patient's medical history and a careful workup including assessment of performance status, lung, and heart function is recommended. Also the patient's mental status may be of concern. Collaboration with the patient's general practitioner and home caregivers should be considered to facilitate the treatment (Connors 2008; Enblad 1994; Kennedy 1986; Klimm et al. 2007; Proctor et al. 2005).

13.2.1.3 Treatment

The optimal treatment planning involves assessment of disease stage, prognostic factors according to the international prognostic score (IPS) (Hasenclever and Diehl 1998), the patient's performance status, B-symptoms, and comorbidity (Connors 2005).

13.2.1.4 Chemotherapy

Less intensive chemotherapy in elderly patients clearly results in poorer outcome. Chemotherapy without anthracyclines has shown poorer outcome than anthracycline-containing regimens (Weekes et al. 2002). A complete remission rate of about 90% has been achieved in studies using anthracycline-containing regimens (Levis et al. 2004; Weekes et al. 2002). Use of bleomycin, which is included in the ABVD regimen, is of concern, especially in patients with chronic lung disease (Connors 2005). An alternative may be a regimen with relatively low toxicity, as tested in Canada, containing vincristine, doxorubicin, bleomycin, etoposide, and prednisone (ODBEP) (Macpherson et al. 2002). In patients with cardiac disease, a newer regimen containing another anthracycline, mitoxantrone, instead of doxorubicin, is currently being tested in Europe, containing vinblastine, cyclophosphamide, procarbazine, prednisolone, etoposide, mitoxatrone, and bleomycin (VEPEMB). This regimen seems to show both acceptable outcomes and low toxicity (Levis et al. 2004; Proctor et al. 2005). More intensive regimens like BEACOPP have proven to be not feasible in elderly patients (Ballova et al. 2005). Although more elderly patients showed complete responses, this was counteracted by more toxic deaths. New and less toxic regimens are currently being tested, e.g. prednisone, vinblastine, doxorubicin, gemcitabine (PVAG), and vinblastine, cyclophosphamide, procarbazine, prednisolone, etoposide, mitoxatrone, and bleomycin (VEPEMB) (Levis et al. 2004; Proctor et al. 2005).

Phamacokinetics may differ for elderly patients. They may have a lower distribution volume, as well as lower renal and liver functions than in younger patients, resulting in higher peak concentrations, and slower clearance, therefore resulting in a higher risk of toxicity (Enblad 1994).

13.2.1.5 Radiation Therapy

Localized radiation therapy is usually well tolerated and the concerns of long-term toxicity are less pronounced than in younger patients, therefore, radiation therapy may play a more important role in elderly patients. Radiation therapy does not seem to contribute substantially to pulmonary toxicity (Martin et al. 2005). However, application of larger fields has been shown to worsen outcome in terms of lower overall survival, compared to involved-field treatment in patients treated with chemotherapy followed by radiation therapy (Klimm et al. 2007).

13.2.1.6 Choice of Treatment

Combined modality treatment upfront is the standard treatment whenever possible as elderly patients are in general poor candidates for salvage and thus have limited second-line curative options. The standard treatment in elderly patients with good performance status, with stage I or II HL, should thus be a short course of adriamycin, bleomycin, vinblatsine, dacarbazien (ABVD), ABVD- containing or ABVD-like chemotherapy, followed by involved-node radiotherapy. In more advanced stages, the standard treatment is six series of ABVD or ABVD-like chemotherapy followed by radiation to residual disease (Ballova et al. 2005; Connors 2005; Klimm et al. 2007; Weekes et al. 2002).

We have no evidence to guide us to the choice of treatment if the patient's poor performance status or specific comorbidity precludes standard treatment. The options may vary from radiation alone for localized disease to single-agent chemotherapy with, e.g., vinblastine or gemcitabine, or combination therapy omitting bleomycin in patients with pulmonary insufficiency or antracycline in patients with cardiac disease (Klimm et al. 2007). It is very important that comorbidity is carefully assessed, and the treatment optimized in collaboration with the patient's general practitioner and also that the HL treatment is facilitated by optimal support involving home care nurses and helpers, if needed (Connors 2008; Levis et al. 2004).

In general, treatment response should be assessed exactly the same way as in younger patients (Cheson et al. 2007).

13.2.1.7 Outcome

The fact that the outcome is worse in elderly patients than in younger patients, even if the same staging is done and the patients receive more than 90% of the scheduled dose of chemotherapy, has led to the suggestion that age is an independent poor prognostic factor due to a different biology of the disease than in young patients (Klimm et al. 2007). In fact, age over 45 years is a poor prognostic marker according to the IPS (Bower et al. 2008; Hasenclever and Diehl 1998). However, newer studies have shown CR rates more than 70% and 5-year overall survival/failure-free survival of about 50–80% can be obtained if appropriate anthracycline chemotherapy is given without delay (Ballova et al. 2005; Levis et al. 2004; Weekes et al. 2002). Furthermore, it has been shown that anthracycline-containing combination chemotherapy is needed to obtain such high probability of complete response and survival (Klimm et al. 2007; Weekes et al. 2002). Some clinical studies of different chemotherapy regimens in elderly patients are shown in Table 13.1.

Radiation as a single modality therapy may lead to long-lasting palliation or even in some cases, a cure (Josting et al. 2005). Some investigators find that prognosis is more closely related to comorbidity than age (Specht and Nissen 1989). The fact that prognosis is worse in patients over 70 years of age as opposed to patients who are 60–70 years of age reflects the presence of more comorbidity with increasing age (Landgren et al. 2003). The overall survival is generally lower if less intensive regimens are given, or if the patient cannot tolerate curative intended treatment. This is partly due to the negative selection of patients and partly due to ineffective treatment of the HL (Enblad 1994; Levis et al. 2004).

13.2.2 Hodgkin Lymphoma in Pregnancy

The primary goal of treatment of a pregnant HL patient is to cure the patient; the second goal is to save the life of the child with the fewest possible acute and long-term side effects to the treatment. This paragraph will primarily deal with the issues of diagnosis and treatment of the pregnant patient and the foetus. The aspects of the effects of the mother's treatment on the future life of the child are also discussed.

Pregnancy in HL may have an impact on diagnostic procedures, staging procedures, the treatment options, phamacokinetics of chemotherapy and the options of supportive treatment.

13.2.2.1 Presentation

HL is very rare in pregnant women even though it is one of the most prevalent malignant diseases in pregnancy (1/1,000–1/6,000 pregnancies) (Jacobs et al. 1981; Pavlidis 2002). However, the prevalence seems to vary between different populations (Dilek et al. 2006; Langagergaard et al. 2008).

The risk of HL is not affected by pregnancy and the presentation of the disease concerning stage,

Table 13.1 Clinical studies in elderly patients

Study	Therapeutic regimen	Design	Number of included patients	5 Year outcome (%)
Nebraska Lymphoma Study Group (Weekes et al. 2002	A. 6 × CHIVPP B. 6 × CHLVPP/ABV	Retrospective analysis	31 25Age > 60 years	EFS: 31, OS 39 EFS: 75, OS 87
BC Cancer Agency (Macpherson et al. 2002)	ODBEP	Retrospective analysis	38 Age > 65 years	OS: 42
Intergruppo Italiano Linformi (Levis et al. 2004)	CS I-IIA: 3 × VEPEMB + IFRT CS IIB-IV: 6 × VEPEMB	Prospective phase 2	105 Age > 65 years (66–83 years)	OS: 64, FFS:56
Scotland and Newcastle Group (Proctor et al. 2005)	SHIELD programme VEPEMB	Prospective phase 2	Including	Ongoing
GHSG HD9 Elderly (Ballova et al. 2005)	A. 4 × COPP/ABVD B. 8 × BEACOPP C. 8 × BEACOPP	Randomized Phase 3	26 42 Age > 65 years (66–75 years)	FFTF: 46, OS: 55 HD-FFTF: 55 FFTF: 46, OS: 55 HD-FFTF: 75
GHSG BACOPP (Mueller et al. 2008)	6–8 × BACOPP	Prospective phase 2	60 Age > 60 years (61–75 years)	FFTF: 67, OS: 85 (2 years), final results awaited
GHSG PVAG (Klimm et al. 2005)	6–8 × PVAG	Prospective phase 2	60 Age > 60years (61–75 years)	Results awaited

CHIVPP: chlorambucil 6 mg/m²/day days 1–14, vinblastine 6 mg/m² days 1 and 8, procarbazine 100 mg/m²/day days 1–14, and prednisone 40 mg/day days 1 t- 14. The cycle is repeated after 28 days. CHIVPP/ABV: chlorambucil 6 mg/m²/day days 1–7, vinblastine 6 mg/m² day 1, procarbazine 100 mg/m²/day days 1–7, prednisone 40 mg/day days 1–14, doxorubicin 25 mg/m²day 8, bleomycin 10 mg/m² on day 8 (maximum of 15 mg), and vincristine 1.4 mg/m² on day 8. The cycle is repeated after 28 days. ODBEP, vincrestine 1.2 mg, doxorubicin 50 mg/m² day 1, bleomycin 10 mg/m² on day 8, etoposide 50 mg/m² day 8 and 100 mg/m² days 9–12, prednisone 45 mg/m² p.o. days 1–7 and then every other day days 8–14. Cycle length 28 days. VEPEMB vinblastine 6 mg/m² day 1, cyclophosphamide 500 mg/m² day 1, procarbazine 100 mg/m² p.o. days 1–5, prednisone 30 mg/m² p.o. days 1–5, etoposide 60 mg/m² p.o. days 15–19, mitoxantrone 6 mg/m² day 15, bleomycin 10 mg/m² day 15. Cycle length 28 days. COPP/ABVD: cyclophosphamide 650 mg/m² days 1 and 8, vincristine 1.4 mg/m² days 1 and 8, procarbazine 100 mg/m² p.o. days 1–14, prednisone 40 mg/m² p.o. days 1–14, doxorubicin 25 mg/m² days 29 and 43, bleomycin 10 v mg/m² days 29 and 43, vinblastine 6 mg/m² days 29 and 43, dacarbazine 375 mg/m² days 29 and 43. Cycle length 57 days. BEACOPP: cyclophosphamide 650 mg/m² day 1, doxorubicin 25 mg/m² day 1, etoposide 100 mg/m² days 1–3, procarbazine 100 mg/m² p.o. days 1–7, prednisone 40 mg/m² p.o. days 1–14, bleomycin 10 mg/m² day 8, vincristine 1.4b mg/m² day 8. Cycle length 22 days. BACOPP: bleomycin (10 mg/m²), doxorubicin (50 mg/m²), cyclophosphamide (650 mg/m²), vincristine (1.4 mg/m²), procarbazine 100 mg/m² p.o. days 1–7, prednisone 40 mg/m² p.o days 1–14. Cycle length 22 days. PVAG: Prednisone 40 mg p.p. days 1–5, Vinblastine 6 mg/m² day 1, Doxorubicin 50 mg/m² day 1, Gemcitabine 1,000 mg/m² day 1, Cycle length 21 days

histological subtype, and localization is apparently the same as in non-pregnant HL patients (Pavlidis 2002; Woo et al. 1992). The diagnosis seems not to be delayed due to pregnancy. In one single institution, a series of 750 women with stage I–II HL, 25 (3.5%) were pregnant at diagnosis, seven in first, ten in second, and eight in third trimester. In a study from another institution including 48 women with HL in pregnancy, 70.8% had stage I–II disease and 29.2% had advanced disease, stages III and IV (Pavlidis 2002).

13.2.2.2 General Consideration of Cytotoxic Agents and Radiation to the Foetus

Essentially, all cytotoxic drugs and radiation harbour a risk to the foetus (Cardonick and Iacobucci 2004). The effect of radiation and chemotherapy on the foetus during the first 2 weeks after gestation is primarily cell death leading to early termination of pregnancy. Chemotherapy and radiation during organogenesis (weeks 3–8) harbours a risk of malformation. Later in pregnancy, the treatment implies increased risks of intrauterine foetal death

Table 13.2 Effects and risks after exposure to ionizing radiation in utero, and spontaneous frequency (without exposure) (Adapted from Kal and Struikmans 2005)

Time after conception (weeks)	Effect	Risk per 0.02 GY	Spontaneous frequency of effect
0–2	Prenatal death[a]	0.01–0.001	0.3–0.6
3–8	Malformation[a]	0.005[b]	0.06
8–15	Mental retardation IQ decrease[c]	0.004	0.005
16–25	Mental retardation IQ decrease[d]	0.001	0.005
0–38	Cancer in childhood	0.003–0.004	0.002–0.003

[a]Based on experimental data (UNSCEAR. Sources and effects of ionizing radiation. Annex J, developmental effects of irradiation in utero. New York: United Nations Scientific Committee on the Effects of Atomic Radiation (UNSCEAR), 1977)

[b]Above threshold dose of 0.1–0.2 Gy

[c]Reduction of 21 IQ points per 1 Gy above threshold of about 0·05 Gy; threshold dose for mental retardation about 0·06 Gy

[d]Reduction of 13 IQ points per 0·1 Gy above threshold dose of about 0·05 Gy; 13, 14 threshold dose for mental retardation about 0·25 Gy.15

(IUFD), intrauterine growth retardation (IUGR), mental retardation, and cancer during childhood. From experimental data, a risk of 0.01–0.001 of prenatal deaths per 0.01 Gy to the foetus during the first 2 weeks was calculated. The spontaneous risk is 0.3–0.6. Above the threshold of 0.1 Gy, the risk of malformation during weeks 3–8 is estimated at 0.005 per 0.01 Gy. The spontaneous risk is about 0.06. The risk of mental retardation is 0.001–0.004 per 0.01 Gy above a threshold of 0.06 Gy, with the highest risk early in pregnancy during weeks 8–25. The spontaneous risk is 0.003–0.005 (see Table 13.2) (Kal and Struikmans 2005; Streffer et al. 2003).

13.2.2.3 Diagnosis

A biopsy is always required to obtain the diagnosis of HL. Diagnostic surgery with general anaesthesia is feasible without risk to the mother or child (Cohen-Kerem et al. 2005; Pereg et al. 2007). Optimal staging requires imaging including PET/CT or, less optimally, conventional CT. Foetal exposure to radiation due to a chest X-ray or CT is much lower than the threshold dose for adverse foetal effects. The foetus receives a radiation dose of only about 0.01–0.04 Gy during an abdominal/pelvic CT scan. This dose is still below the threshold dose for severe congenital malformation and should therefore not harm the foetus (Kal and Struikmans 2005). However, the increase in risk of cancers later in life, for which there is no threshold dose, should not be ignored. Iodine-containing contrast agents should be avoided (Chen et al. 2008).

FDG passes the placenta to the foetus, resulting in a higher foetal radiation dose with a PET-CT. PET-CT should therefore be avoided during pregnancy, but a PET-CT should be performed after delivery to assess the actual status and treatment response. In addition, FDG is concentrated in breast milk. Breastfeeding should be discontinued for at least 24 h after injection (Benveniste et al. 2003). Even though the foetal radiation dose from an abdominal/pelvic CT is below the threshold for severe congenital malformations, CT scans should in general be avoided during pregnancy as alternative methods, which cause no radiation dose to the foetus, such as MRI and ultrasound, are available (Benveniste et al. 2003). MRI can be used safely in all trimesters and MRI is in general the recommended imaging method in pregnancy if the required information cannot be obtained by non-ionizing means, e.g. ultrasound, if the information is required and cannot be delayed until after delivery. However, MR contrast agents should *not* be routinely provided to pregnant patients (Kanal et al. 2007).

In summary, a proper histological diagnosis can be obtained, even if a surgical procedure requiring general anaesthesia is needed. Staging can be done with a chest CT scan and abdominal ultrasound or MRI. After delivery a PET-CT scan should be done.

13.2.2.4 Chemotherapy

The knowledge of outcome and toxicity of treatment of HL in pregnancy is based on case reports (see

Table 13.3 Published cases of chemotherapy in pregnancy in HL

Study	Treatment	Phenotype	Age	*n*	Pregnancy complications
	Trimester 1				
(Aviles et al. 1991)	Doxorubicin, vincristine, bleomycin, dacarbazine for all, then melphalan, vincristine, prednisone, procarbazine in one case	Normal	4–14 years	4	–
(Zuazu et al. 1991)	Vincristine, cyclophosphamide, prednisone	Normal	–	1	–
(Nisce et al. 1986)	Vinblastine	Normal	9 years	3	–
(Jacobs et al. 2004)	Chlorambucil	Normal	–	1	–
(Toledo et al. 1971)	Doxorubicin, radiation to abdomen, radiation to pelvis	Absent toes, single coronary artery of pregnancy	–	1	Elective termination
	Trimester 2				
(Peres et al. 2001)	Cytarabine, etoposide, cisplatin	Normal	–	1	Anaemia, jaundice
(Aviles et al. 1991)	Doxorubicin, vincristine, bleomycin, dacarbazine, then melphalan, vincristine, prednisone, procarbazine	Normal	3–16 years	6	–
(Lacher and Geller 1966)	Cyclophosphamide, vinblastine	Normal, normal karyotype	17 months	1	–
	Trimester 3				
(Lacher and Geller 1966)	Vinblastine	Normal	–	2	–

Table 13.3). Based on the fact that the disease in pregnancy has the same clinical picture as in non-pregnant patients, we assume that the optimal treatment is the same as in non-pregnant women with HL. However, it must be considered that phamacokinetics may differ in pregnancy, due to increased volume of distribution (increased plasma volume and amniotic fluid), increased renal clearance and decreased protein-binding capacity. No pharmacokinetic studies have been performed in pregnant women receiving chemotherapy, so the precise implications of these differences of treatments are not known, meaning it is not known whether the dose schedule of chemotherapy should differ to obtain the same outcome and same low toxicity as in non-pregnant HL patients (Cardonick and Iacobucci 2004). The scarce clinical information does not guide us further.

In addition to ensuring the optimal outcome and safety for the mother, the safety of the foetus should be considered. An extensive review of the use of chemotherapy indicates that all cytotoxic drugs and radiation harbours a risk to the foetus (Cardonick and Iacobucci 2004). However, the effects of chemotherapy cannot, in many cases, be distinguished from the effects of the malignant disease itself. Intrauterine growth retardation and foetal death may be due to either the malignant disease or the given chemotherapy. It must also be considered that delay or omission of treatment may put not only the mother, but also the child in danger. In the treatment of pregnant patients, dacarbazine is the least investigated drug of the agents used in the treatment of HL. Doxorubicin seems rather safe even though there might be a small risk of cardiac side effects. Temporary cardiac insufficiency is reported, but long-term follow-up did not show cardiac side effects in a series of 81 children treated in utero (Aviles and Neri 2001). Bleomycin can cause pulmonary long-term effects, but that has never been reported. Vinblastine seems quite safe even though cases of growth retardation and foetal deaths are reported. More than 20 cases of ABVD and ABVD-like treatments in pregnancy have been reported and the treatment seems safe in general during the second and third trimesters.

13.2.2.5 Radiotherapy

The general impact of radiation to the foetus is described above. Clinical studies in lymphomas and solid tumours have shown feasibility of supradiaphragmal radiotherapy in pregnancy (Kal and

Table 13.4 Total dose, fetal dose with shielding and outcome of pregnant patients undergoing radiotherapy (Adapted from Kal and Struikmans 2005

Study	Maternal dose (Gy)	Fetal dose (Gy)	Pregnancy trimester	*n*	Delivery
(Woo et al. 1992)	35–40	0.014–0.055 (6 MV)	1–3	16	Healthy babies
(Nisce et al. 1986)	19	0.09–0.42, head 0.114	3	1	Healthy child at age 8 years
(Mazonakis et al. 2003)	15–20	0.020–0.50	2–3	7	Healthy children at age 6–11 years
(Lishner et al. 1992)				16	Healthy babies
(Cygler et al. 1997)	35	0.1	2	1	Healthy child

Struikmans 2005; Lishner 2003), and it has also been shown that reduction of dose is possible by shielding (Nuyttens et al. 2002). Radiation therapy to mantle fields using 6 MV, which is still the most commonly used radiation energy for the treatment of HL, resulted in an estimated total dose to the mid-foetus below 0.01–0.05 Gy in one study (Woo et al. 1992). Most clinical case reports in HL are from a period when large fields and total doses of about 40 Gy were used (see Table 13.4). However, modern radiotherapy in HL is an integrated part of a combined therapy with chemotherapy using smaller fields and lower doses (Girinsky et al. 2006). This leads to substantially lower doses to the foetus.

13.2.2.6 Treatment Outcome for Mother and Child

The knowledge about the treatment outcome for the mother is based on case reports and small retrospective studies. Most data are old and the diagnostic tools and treatment options have changed considerably since these data were obtained, therefore, it is difficult to interpret the information in the context of modern treatment. The fact that HL in pregnancy shows the same features as in non-pregnant patients, may lead to the assumption that the disease, if possible, shall be treated as in non-pregnant patients.

13.2.2.7 First Trimester Pregnancy

In general, treatment is avoided in the first trimester; therefore, the case studies are few. In a few cases, ABVD has been given without complications to the child but we cannot exclude that the risk of abnormalities is increased. Radiation therapy is often possible without causing any harmful dose to the foetus, and with modern techniques a precise estimate of the dose is possible before the therapy (Woo et al. 1992). Some authors suggest single agent to delay ABVD or more intensive treatment to second or third trimester or even until after delivery even in aggressive disease. Very good results are reported with vinblastine single-agent therapy (Connors 2008).

13.2.2.8 Second and Third Trimester Pregnancy

In the second and third trimesters, ABVD seems to be safe (Anselmo et al. 1999; Aviles et al. 1991). However, an increased risk of IUGR and IUFD cannot be excluded from the present data (Lishner et al. 1996). Radiation therapy has also been shown to be feasible in second and third trimester to supra-diaphragmal disease without complication to mother or child. From case–control studies, it appears that the outcome for the mother is comparable to that of the non-pregnant woman (Langagergaard et al. 2008; Lishner et al. 1996).

13.2.2.9 Supportive Treatment

Most patients get anti-emetics during chemotherapy. Metoclopramide, antihistamines and ondansetron-based anti-emetics are safe in pregnancy. Granulocyte colony-stimulating factor, which is used to prevent neutropenia, is also safe. Antibiotics may be necessary during neutropenia and the choice of antibiotics should be made carefully. Penicillins, cephalosporins and erythromycin are safe and aminoglycosides and metronidazole do not appear to be teratogenic, although the data on these drugs are more limited. Quinolones, which cause arthropathy, tetracyclines, which affect bone and teeth, and sulfonamides, which have been associated with neural tube defects and cardiac malformations should be avoided during pregnancy (Pereg et al. 2007).

13.2.2.10 The Choice of Treatment Strategy

Most authors agree that the treatment should be considered on an individual basis, depending on the clinical situation. Most treatments can be safely delayed to after delivery. About 80% of women had their full staging and treatment safely postponed to after delivery in one experienced centre (Connors 2008).

In the first trimester, induced abortion should be considered in cases with very aggressive disease. If pregnancy is not terminated and if the treatment cannot be delayed to second or third trimester, the treatment options are (1) ABVD,(2) radiation to supra-diaphragmal disease causing severe symptoms, and (3) single agent to delay ABVD or more intensive treatment to second or third trimester or even until after delivery. If more intensive chemotherapy such as BEACOPP is required, it must be delayed until postpartum (Pereg et al. 2007).

In the second and third trimesters, treatment can, in most cases, be delayed to postpartum. Pre-term delivery may be considered in case of aggressive disease (Kal and Struikmans 2005). ABVD is believed to be safe and supra-diaphragmal radiotherapy is also feasible in many cases (Kal and Struikmans 2005). Medical abortion is in general not recommended in second and third trimester (Pereg et al. 2007).

13.2.3 *Hodgkin Lymphoma in HIV*

HL seems to be more frequent in HIV-positive individuals. Even though the assumption of increased incidence among HIV-positive persons is based on few observations, particularly in women, different studies have shown similar estimates of eight to ten times increased risk of HL in HIV-positive individuals. In addition, it has also been suggested that the increased risk of HL is most pronounced in IV drug users. The association between HL and severity of HIV/AIDS, expressed by the CD4 count, is suggested to be more complicated than just showing a higher risk in more affected HIV-positive individuals. In one study, the highest incidence is seen in moderately affected individuals, while individuals with very low CD4 and individuals with higher CD4 counts have a lower risk of developing HL (Biggar et al. 2006). It is unclear how the more widespread use of highly active antiretroviral therapy (HAART) changes the incidence of HL. Some investigators expect a decreased incidence in HIV-positive persons, others an increased risk or an increased number of cases, which is also due to a longer time with a relative immune suppression (Barbaro and Barbarini 2007; Biggar et al. 2006; Spano et al. 2002). The incidence of mixed cellularity type seems to be highest in individuals with very low CD4 counts, while patients with nodular sclerosis type have relatively high CD4 counts. This means that the incidence of mixed cellularity HL may decrease relatively to the incidence of nodular sclerosis type since the development of the use of HAART treatment (Biggar et al. 2006; Grogg et al. 2007).

Table 13.5 Characteristics of HIV patients in two series

Parameter	%	%
Study	(Vaccher et al. 2001b)	(Xicoy et al. 2007)
Histological subtype		
Nodular sclerosis	27	27
Mixed cellularity	53	41
Lymphocyte depletion	18	15
Nodular lymphocytic predominant	4	
Non specified		16
Stage		
I	5	
II	14	
III	28	34
IV	54	66
B-symptoms	80	89
Extranodular involvement	65	
Bone marrow involvement	40	55
Spleen	31	
Liver	19	
Lung	6	

13.2.3.1 Biology/Pathogenesis

More HLs in HIV patients have Epstein-Barr virus (EBV) genome (80%) compared to other groups (<50%) and at least some proteins related to the EBV genome activity are expressed, suggesting that EBV plays a role in the pathogenesis in HIV-related HL. The immunophenotype of HIV-HL, specifically the Reed-Sternberg cells, is similar to that of the morphologic variants of HL in patients without HIV infection (Thompson et al. 2004).

Histology differs in HIV-related HL, with more patients having mixed cellularity subtype (>50%) and lymphocyte depleted (~20%) and fewer having nodular sclerosis than among non-HIV-related HL patients. Another striking feature is that HIV-related HL apparently happens earlier during the HIV infection when the CD 4 count is 200–300/μL or more in most patients, compared to aggressive non-Hodgkin lymphomas in patients with HIV. The explanation for this is unclear.

13.2.3.2 Presentation

The clinical presentation of HIV-related HL differs from non-HIV-related HL by being more disseminated, often having extranodal presentation and more often showing B-symptoms. More than 70% of the patients have B-symptoms, defined as fever more than 38.5°C, weight loss more than 10% of the bodyweight, and/or night sweats. More than 75% have stage III or IV disease (Table 13.5).

In addition, the disease pattern differs in that patients with HIV-related HL may have disease in the liver without lymph node involvement and without spleen involvement, or they may have lung involvement without mediastinal involvement. About (50–60%) have extranodal disease. The most common is involvement of bone marrow (40%), liver (15–40%), and/or spleen (20%) (Table 13.5). There are several case reports about involvement of the central nervous system and other rare locations (Andrieu et al. 1993; Levy et al. 1995; Massarweh et al. 2003; Rubio 1994; Tirelli et al. 1995; Vaccher et al. 2001b; Xicoy et al. 2007).

The diagnosis may be delayed in HIV-related HL, because the patients are more likely to have symptoms such as weight loss and fever due to other reasons. Lymph node swelling is also more prevalent in HIV patients due to other reasons such as chronic infections. Finally, extranodal disease, e.g. in bone or CNS may be more difficult to detect and thus there is a risk of delay of diagnosis.

Staging is more difficult because there is a risk of false-positive findings by physical examination, CT and PET/CT due to lymphadenopathy related to HIV and opportunistic infections. PET/CT is considered to be the standard tool for staging in HL (new response criteria). PET/CT is even more important in HIV-related HL because of the higher risk of extranodal disease. Biopsies should be considered in case of possible false-positive findings, which have impact on the treatment strategy.

The workup in an HIV patient will include a proper assessment of HIV status. In one series, 23% of the patients had AIDS and 20% had an AIDS-related complex. The majority had AIDS due to intravenous drug addiction, which may have implications for the treatment strategy (Tirelli et al. 1995; Vaccher et al. 2001b).

13.2.3.3 Treatment

Treatment strategy in HL is decided based on the extent of the disease – stage and presence of B-symptoms, prognostic factors accordingly to IPS (sex, age > 45, lymphocyte count, leukocyte count, albumin level, haemoglobin level, stage IV, and SR) and patient's characteristics such as performance status, compliance to treatment and comorbidity. This is also true in HIV-related HL (Spina et al. 2002).

The standard treatment in most cases of advanced HL is ABVD or ABVD-like treatment. In phase 2 studies and retrospective series, ABVD has a higher CR rate than MOPP or MOPP-like chemotherapy and a lower rate of opportunistic infections (Vaccher et al. 2001b). Less intensive regimens result in similar rates of opportunistic infections and seem to result in lower CR rates and higher relapse rates (Errante et al. 1994).

ABVD or ABVD-like chemotherapy has become feasible in combination with modern combination antiviral treatments (Bower et al. 2008; Xicoy et al. 2007). However, the risk of haematological toxicity seems higher than in non-HIV-related HL with grade 3/4 neutropenia in about 30–50% (Errante et al. 1994, 1999; Gastaldi et al. 2002; Levine et al. 2000). The outcome of ABVD/ABVD-like chemotherapy has improved substantially after the introduction of HAART (Bower et al. 2008; Hoffmann et al. 2004; Xicoy et al. 2007).

In non-HIV-related HL, more intensive regimens have been introduced to high-risk patients. Randomized studies have shown better overall survival and lower treatment failure rate in patients treated with BEACOOP escalated (Diehl et al. 2003). However, even though standard dose BEACOPP showed better response in elderly patients, this benefit was outweighed by more treatment-related deaths. Thus, more intensive chemotherapy does not improve the outcome in elderly patients. BEACOPP escalated has not been tested in HIV-related HL. More moderate regimens, but still more intensive than the ABVD regimen, such as the standard dose BEACOPP and the Stanford V regimen, have been tested and are shown to be feasible in HIV patients. The haematological and neurological toxicities of these regimens are substantial and the treatment cannot be recommended outside the setting of a clinical trial (Bower et al. 2008; Hartmann et al. 2003; Spina et al. 2002).

In order to reduce the risk of opportunistic infections, prophylaxis to pneumocystis pneumonia (PCP), fungal infections and other diseases, which can be reactivated by chemotherapy-induced relative immune deficiency, e.g. hepatitis C, is initiated before chemotherapy (Bower et al. 2008; Hoffmann et al. 2004). Support with granulocyte colony-stimulating factor is feasible and may reduce haematoxicity (Bower et al. 2008).

Radiotherapy is poorly tested in HIV, primarily because most patients have advanced disease and few patients have bulky disease. In addition, radiation therapy is only used in very few patients even though radiation therapy would have been recommended in similar patients with non-HIV-related HL patients (Bower et al. 2008). However, with modern limited radiation fields and in patients treated with HAART radiotherapy has, in our experience, been well tolerated.

Although different HAART regimens have been used in the different studies, the optimal regimen has not been defined. Complete viral response on HAART is suggested to be associated with higher probability of event-free survival (EFS) and overall survival (OS), but it has yet to be proven as a positive predictor of Hodgkin lymphoma treatment in HIV-related HL (Hoffmann et al. 2004; Xicoy et al. 2007). However, complete immunological response (expressed as CD 4 increasing to > 200/mm^3 and an increase of at least 100/mm^3 on 6 months of HAART) is shown to be a positive predictor of EFS and OS (Xicoy et al. 2007).

The risk of interaction between HAART and chemotherapy should be taken into account when the treatment is planned. Some studies have suggested delaying HAART until after chemotherapy because an increased risk of grade 3–4 side effects was observed when treatments were given concomitantly, while other studies show acceptable toxicity and no differences in haematological toxicity compared to historical controls (Vaccher et al. 2001a).

13.2.3.4 Outcome

Outcome in early series of HIV-linked HL was very poor compared with results in non-HIV-related HL in terms of lower CR rates, lower OS and disease-free survival (DFS) and a higher relapse rate. CR rates were below 45%, median OS as low as below 2 years and relapse rates as high as 38%. High-risk patients with poor-risk HL prognostic factors had a very poor outcome, also due to suboptimal chemotherapy. The OS was highly influenced by the course of HIV and AIDS. Modern combination HAART has changed the course of HIV and AIDS, so OS is less influenced by this disease. In a more recent series of HIV-related HL, only a few patients died of HIV during the first years of follow-up (Xicoy et al. 2007). The proportion of drug addicts in HIV-related HL is high (about 50% in some series) and this group is expected to have a lower life expectancy than the population in general, but the impact of drug addiction on OS is unclear.

Modern HAART has also made more intensive chemotherapy regimens possible resulting in CR as high as more than 80%, the median OS more than 3 years, and a relapse rate of 10% after a medium follow-up of more than 3 years (Xicoy et al. 2007).

In summary, the optimal treatment in HIV-related HL implies the following:

- Combination chemotherapy similar to patients with the same disease characteristics of non-HIV-related HL
- Optimized combination HAART
- Prophylactic treatment of opportunistic infections

13.3 Hodgkin Lymphoma in Rare Locations

Rare location of HL means extranodal disease and HL may be seen in virtually all organs. Most often involvement of extranodal sites is seen concomitantly with involvement of nodal sites, but in rare cases extranodal involvement may be seen as the only involved site. Fourteen per cent of the patients in the GHSG studies had involvement of extranodal involvement (Nogova et al. 2008). The incidence of extranodal HL depends on the methods of staging. Staging including PET-CT scanning contributes to the finding of more extranodal sites (Hutchings et al. 2006).

13.3.1 Bone

Involvement of bone is seen in 9–10% of cases after conventional staging before the PET-CT era (Hutchings et al. 2006). In a report of 495 cases of HL with osseous involvement, only 58 had involvement of bone only. Involvement of bone may often be missed in conventional staging (see Fig. 13.1). Incidences up to 50% have been reported at autopsy in HL patients (Langley et al. 2008). Solitary bone involvement is thus very rare and comprises very few of the cases of malignant bone tumours (Ozdemirli et al. 1996).

13.3.1.1 Presentation

Staging including PET-CT scan may increase the proportion of patients diagnosed with bone involvement (Hutchings et al. 2006). Although bone marrow involvement is not uncommon in later stages of HL, this does not usually produce destructive bone lesions. Bone marrow involvement often causes anaemia, therefore, bone marrow aspiration is recommended in HL patients with anaemia.

HL usually presents as painless adenopathy and may be followed by general symptoms. Presentation with bony lesions may, in addition to these symptoms, cause localized pain (Gebert et al. 2005; Ozdemirli et al. 1996). Spinal cord compression occurs in very rare cases (Cagavi et al. 2006; Citow et al. 2001). Lytic lesions seem to be more common, but also sclerotic or mixed lesions may occur (Ozdemirli et al. 1996). Bony lesions may occur in all histological subtypes of HL.

13.3.1.2 Primary Osseous Hodgkin's Lymphoma

Primary osseous HL (POHL) is a disease entity involving one or multiple foci in patients who have no history of and no evidence of non-osseous foci. Few cases have been reported worldwide (Gebert et al. 2005). In one report of cases, more men than women had POHL and the histology showed the same number of cases with mixed cellularity and nodular sclerosis (Ozdemirli et al. 1996). Most cases have been described before implementation of the current modern imaging modalities in staging of the disease and before the era of modern combination chemotherapy and radiotherapy. Thus, it is likely that POHL is even rarer, and that bone lesions in almost all cases are a part of more advanced disease and should be treated as such.

13.3.1.3 Treatment

In case of localized disease, a combination of chemotherapy and radiation therapy of the involved bone is the optimal treatment. In more widespread disease, combination chemotherapy is recommended (Gebert

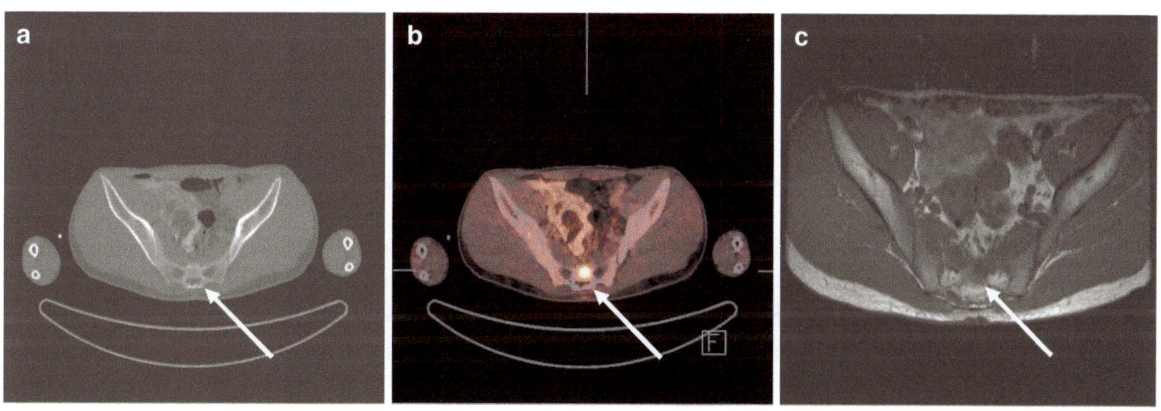

Fig. 13.1 Hodgkin lymphoma in bone (*arrow*): (**a**) CT, (**b**) PET/CT, (**c**) MRI

et al. 2005). We have no data indicating that the choice of chemotherapy should differ from the treatment in patients without bone involvement. Even though we have no evidence, response evaluation done with PET-CT is suggested, because disease involvement in bone cannot be evaluated on CT. Radiation therapy should be considered to solitary bony lesions or to lesions with possible residual disease after chemotherapy.

13.3.1.4 Outcome

The relatively small number of patients makes detailed analyses difficult, but the prognosis in Stage IE seems similar to that of local nodal disease without osseous involvement (Gebert et al. 2005; Kaplan 1980). Extranodal disease could not be shown to be a poor prognostic factor in advanced or more localized HL (Franklin et al. 2000; Hasenclever and Diehl 1998).

13.3.2 *Central Nervous System*

Involvement of the central nervous system (CNS) is very rare in HL. Only 33 cases have been published in the English language medical journals and only a few cases of primary or relapsed CNS HL had no evidence of disease elsewhere. In a series of 2,000 HL patients, none had primary CNS involvement and only 0.5% had involvement at later stage of their disease (Sapozink and Kaplan 1983). The pathogenesis of CNS HL is unknown. Direct invasion from bone, development from meninges and haematological spreading has been suggested (Hirmiz et al. 2004). Epstein Barr virus does not seem to be involved in the pathogenesis of CNS HL.

13.3.2.1 Presentation

Most cases seem to be mixed cellularity, but nodular sclerotic type is also found. Among the limited number of cases, more men than women (1.7/1) are seen and 61% of the patients had disease elsewhere. Symptoms at presentation were mainly cranial nerve palsies (55%), headaches (36%) and paresis (33%) (Cuttner et al. 1979; Hirmiz et al. 2004; Sapozink and Kaplan 1983). Few cases of spinal cord compression have been observed, either caused by invasion from bone or through foramina from nodal disease (Riffaud et al. 2003).

13.3.2.2 Treatment

The treatment has, in most cases, involved combination chemotherapy and whole brain irradiation (Hirmiz et al. 2004; Sapozink and Kaplan 1983). Today ABVD/ABVD-like treatment followed by radiation therapy, in most cases to the whole brain, would be recommended, depending on previous treatment and the presence of poor prognostic factors. The radiation dose used in treated patients has varied from 20 to 40 Gy (Cuttner et al. 1979; Sapozink and Kaplan 1983).

13.3.2.3 Outcome

The prognosis seems poorer than in patients with nodal disease only, with a median interval time from diagnosis of intracranial disease to death of 46 months, with a range from 5 to 168 months (Hirmiz et al. 2004; Sapozink and Kaplan 1983).

13.3.3 *Visceral*

Isolated visceral presentation of HL is very rare, but visceral involvement is not uncommon in advanced HL. For example, in two trials of the EORTC and GELA, 18% and 24% of the patients respectively had lung involvement (Aleman et al. 2007; Ferme et al. 2000). The incidence of visceral involvement is probably higher in patients staged with PET-CT than in patients staged with CT alone (Hutchings et al. 2006).

Visceral presentation in HL has some special implications: (1) Presentation may mimic other diseases and therefore diagnosis might be delayed. (2) The diagnosis may be more difficult because the disease is not visible by conventional X-ray or CT scans, e.g. if the mucosal lining of the gastrointestinal tract is involved.

(3) Evaluation of treatment effect may also be more difficult due to the same reasons.

13.3.3.1 Presentation

Solitary or primary involvement of visceral organs has been reported from the gastrointestinal tract – from the oral cavity to oesophagus, the stomach, duodenum, and bowel. The most common presentations are abdominal pain, nausea, appetite loss and/or weight loss. Gastrointestinal bleeding may also occur (Ogawa et al. 1995). Also, involvement of the respiratory system, trachea and lungs has been reported. Most common symptoms are dry cough, associated with mild chest discomfort. Less common symptoms are dyspnea and hemoptysis (Radin 1990). Some of the cases might be reclassified to non-Hodgkin lymphoma with modern diagnostic techniques available, but some of the cases have clearly been demonstrated to be HL. A higher proportion of mixed cellularity is probably seen in extranodal HL, although the number of patients is limited and does not allow statistical analyses. Thus, HL may arise in most visceral organs, although rarely.

13.3.3.2 Treatment

Even though no solid evidence exists, the optimal treatment of localized visceral disease is assumed to be combined chemotherapy with ABVD, ABVD-like regimen, or BEACOPP and radiation therapy as in localized disease in general. Precise detection of the extent of disease in an organ can be difficult, e.g., the extent of HL in the stomach or bowel. Therefore, treatment of the entire organ or the use of wider margins may be required for radiation therapy in these patients. More advanced disease including visceral organs is treated with ABVD, ABVD-like chemotherapy regimen, or BEACOPP regimens dependent on the extent of the disease and the prognostic factors, as in advanced disease in general. Radiotherapy to the visceral organ is required if residual disease is seen after chemotherapy and may even be indicated if evaluation after chemotherapy is difficult. PET-CT is recommended as a part of the evaluation of treatment because the disease most often is very difficult to assess by CT (Hutchings et al. 2006).

13.3.3.3 Outcome

Outcome is often described as quite poor (Radin 1990). The relatively small number of patients makes detailed analyses difficult, but extranodal involvement has not been identified as an independent poor prognostic factor when other factors, especially the extent of disease, are taken into account (Specht and Hasenclever 2007). In particular, localized extranodal disease, with or without adjacent nodal disease, which can be sensibly contained within a radiation field, does not have a poorer prognosis than other localized presentation, as initially pointed out in the Ann Arbor staging classification (Carbone et al. 1971; Musshoff 1970).

References

Aleman BM, Raemaekers JM, Tomisic R et al (2007) Involved-field radiotherapy for patients in partial remission after chemotherapy for advanced Hodgkin's lymphoma. Int J Radiat Oncol Biol Phys 67:19–30

Andrieu JM, Roithmann S, Tourani JM et al (1993) Hodgkin's disease during HIV1 infection: the French registry experience. French Registry of HIV-associated Tumors. Ann Oncol 4:635–641

Anselmo AP, Cavalieri E, Enrici RM et al (1999) Hodgkin's disease during pregnancy: diagnostic and therapeutic management. Fetal Diagn Ther 14:102–105

Aviles A, Neri N (2001) Hematological malignancies and pregnancy: a final report of 84 children who received chemotherapy in utero. Clin Lymphoma 2:173–177

Aviles A, Diaz-Maqueo JC, Talavera A et al (1991) Growth and development of children of mothers treated with chemotherapy during pregnancy: current status of 43 children. Am J Hematol 36:243–248

Ballova V, Ruffer JU, Haverkamp H et al (2005) A prospectively randomized trial carried out by the German Hodgkin Study Group (GHSG) for elderly patients with advanced Hodgkin's disease comparing BEACOPP baseline and COPP-ABVD (study HD9elderly). Ann Oncol 16:124–131

Barbaro G, Barbarini G (2007) HIV infection and cancer in the era of highly active antiretroviral therapy (Review). Oncol Rep 17:1121–1126

Benveniste H, Fowler JS, Rooney WD et al (2003) Maternal-fetal in vivo imaging: a combined PET and MRI study. J Nucl Med 44:1522–1530

Biggar RJ, Jaffe ES, Goedert JJ et al (2006) Hodgkin lymphoma and immunodeficiency in persons with HIV/AIDS. Blood 108:3786–3791

Bower M, Collins S, Cottrill C et al (2008) British HIV Association guidelines for HIV-associated malignancies 2008. HIV Med 9:336–388

Cagavi F, Kalayci M, Tekin IO et al (2006) Primary spinal extranodal Hodgkin's disease at two levels. Clin Neurol Neurosurg 108:168–173

Carbone PP, Kaplan HS, Musshoff K et al (1971) Report of the Committee on Hodgkin's Disease Staging Classification. Cancer Res 31:1860–1861

Cardonick E, Iacobucci A (2004) Use of chemotherapy during human pregnancy. Lancet Oncol 5:283–291

Chen MM, Coakley FV, Kaimal A et al (2008) Guidelines for computed tomography and magnetic resonance imaging use during pregnancy and lactation. Obstet Gynecol 112:333–340

Cheson BD, Pfistner B, Juweid ME et al (2007) Revised response criteria for malignant lymphoma. J Clin Oncol 25:579–586

Citow JS, Rini B, Wollmann R et al (2001) Isolated, primary extranodal Hodgkin's disease of the spine: case report. Neurosurgery 49:453–456

Cohen-Kerem R, Railton C, Oren D et al (2005) Pregnancy outcome following non-obstetric surgical intervention. Am J Surg 190:467–473

Connors JM (2005) State-of-the-art therapeutics: Hodgkin's lymphoma. J Clin Oncol 23:6400–6408

Connors JM (2008) Challenging problems: coincident pregnancy, HIV infection, and older age. Hematol Am Soc Hematol Educ Prog 2008(1):334–339

Cuttner J, Meyer R, Huang YP (1979) Intracerebral involvement in Hodgkin's disease: a report of 6 cases and review of the literature. Cancer 43:1497–1506

Cygler J, Ding GX, Kendal W et al (1997) Fetal dose for a patient undergoing mantle field irradiation for Hodgkin's disease. Med Dosim 22:135–137

Diehl V, Franklin J, Pfreundschuh M et al (2003) Standard and increased-dose BEACOPP chemotherapy compared with COPP-ABVD for advanced Hodgkin's disease. N Engl J Med 348:2386–2395

Dilek I, Topcu N, Demir C et al (2006) Hematological malignancy and pregnancy: a single-institution experience of 21 cases. Clin Lab Haematol 28:170–176

Enblad G (1994) Hodgkin's disease in young and elderly patients. Clinical and pathological studies. Minireview based on a doctoral thesis. Ups J Med Sci 99:1–38

Engert A, Ballova V, Haverkamp H et al (2005) Hodgkin's lymphoma in elderly patients: a comprehensive retrospective analysis from the German Hodgkin's Study Group. J Clin Oncol 23:5052–5060

Errante D, Zagonel V, Vaccher E et al (1994) Hodgkin's disease in patients with HIV infection and in the general population: comparison of clinicopathological features and survival. Ann Oncol 5(Suppl 2):37–40

Errante D, Gabarre J, Ridolfo AL et al (1999) Hodgkin's disease in 35 patients with HIV infection: an experience with epirubicin, bleomycin, vinblastine and prednisone chemotherapy in combination with antiretroviral therapy and primary use of G-CSF. Ann Oncol 10:189–195

Ferme C, Sebban C, Hennequin C et al (2000) Comparison of chemotherapy to radiotherapy as consolidation of complete or good partial response after six cycles of chemotherapy for patients with advanced Hodgkin's disease: results of the groupe d'etudes des lymphomes de l'Adulte H89 trial. Blood 95:2246–2252

Franklin J, Paulus U, Lieberz D et al (2000) Is the international prognostic score for advanced stage Hodgkin's disease applicable to early stage patients? German Hodgkin Lymphoma Study Group. Ann Oncol 11:617–623

Gastaldi R, Martino P, Gentile G et al (2002) Hodgkin's disease in HIV-infected patients: report of eight cases usefully treated with doxorubicin, bleomycin, vinblastine and dacarbazine (ABVD) plus granulocyte colony- stimulating factor. Ann Oncol 13:1158–1160

Gebert C, Hardes J, Ahrens H et al (2005) Primary multifocal osseous Hodgkin disease: a case report and review of the literature. J Cancer Res Clin Oncol 131:163–168

Girinsky T, van der Maazen R, Specht L et al (2006) Involved-node radiotherapy (INRT) in patients with early Hodgkin lymphoma: concepts and guidelines. Radiother Oncol 79:270–277

Grogg KL, Miller RF, Dogan A (2007) HIV infection and lymphoma. J Clin Pathol 60:1365–1372

Hartmann P, Rehwald U, Salzberger B et al (2003) BEACOPP therapeutic regimen for patients with Hodgkin's disease and HIV infection. Ann Oncol 14:1562–1569

Hasenclever D, Diehl V (1998) A prognostic score for advanced Hodgkin's disease. International Prognostic Factors Project on Advanced Hodgkin's Disease. N Engl J Med 339: 1506–1514

Hirmiz K, Foyle A, Wilke D et al (2004) Intracranial presentation of systemic Hodgkin's disease. Leuk Lymphoma 45: 1667–1671

Hoffmann C, Chow KU, Wolf E et al (2004) Strong impact of highly active antiretroviral therapy on survival in patients with human immunodeficiency virus-associated Hodgkin's disease. Br J Haematol 125:455–462

Hutchings M, Loft A, Hansen M et al (2006) Positron emission tomography with or without computed tomography in the primary staging of Hodgkin's lymphoma. Haematologica 91:482–489

Jacobs C, Donaldson SS, Rosenberg SA et al (1981) Management of the pregnant patient with Hodgkin's disease. Ann Intern Med 95:669–675

Jacobs IA, Chang CK, Salti GI (2004) Coexistence of pregnancy and cancer. Am Surg 70:1025–1029

Jarrett RF, Krajewski AS, Angus B et al (2003) The Scotland and Newcastle epidemiological study of Hodgkin's disease: impact of histopathological review and EBV status on incidence estimates. J Clin Pathol 56:811–816

Josting A, Nogova L, Franklin J et al (2005) Salvage radiotherapy in patients with relapsed and refractory Hodgkin's lymphoma: a retrospective analysis from the German Hodgkin Lymphoma Study Group. J Clin Oncol 23:1522–1529

Kal HB, Struikmans H (2005) Radiotherapy during pregnancy: fact and fiction. Lancet Oncol 6:328–333

Kanal E, Barkovich AJ, Bell C et al (2007) ACR guidance document for safe MR practices: 2007. AJR Am J Roentgenol 188:1447–1474

Kaplan HS (1980) Hodgkin's disease, 2nd edn. Harvard University Press, Cambridge

Kennedy BJ (1986) Leukemia and lymphoma in the elderly. Front Radiat Ther Oncol 20:150–156

Klimm B, Schnell R, Diehl V et al (2005) Current treatment and immunotherapy of Hodgkin's lymphoma. Haematologica 90:1680–1692

Klimm B, Diehl V, Engert A (2007) Hodgkin's lymphoma in the elderly: a different disease in patients over 60. Oncology (Williston Park) 21:982–990

Lacher MJ, Geller W (1966) Cyclophosphamide and vinblastine sulfate in Hodgkin's disease during pregnancy. JAMA 195:486–488

Landgren O, Algernon C, Axdorph U et al (2003) Hodgkin's lymphoma in the elderly with special reference to type and intensity of chemotherapy in relation to prognosis. Haematologica 88:438–444

Langagergaard V, Horvath-Puho E, Norgaard M et al (2008) Hodgkin's disease and birth outcome: a Danish nationwide cohort study. Br J Cancer 98:183–188

Langley CR, Garrett SJ, Urand J et al (2008) Primary multifocal osseous Hodgkin's lymphoma. World J Surg Oncol 6:34

Levine AM, Li P, Cheung T et al (2000) Chemotherapy consisting of doxorubicin, bleomycin, vinblastine, and dacarbazine with granulocyte-colony-stimulating factor in HIV-infected patients with newly diagnosed Hodgkin's disease: a prospective, multi-institutional AIDS clinical trials group study (ACTG 149). J Acquir Immune Defic Syndr 24:444–450

Levis A, Anselmo AP, Ambrosetti A et al (2004) VEPEMB in elderly Hodgkin's lymphoma patients. Results from an Intergruppo Italiano Linfomi (IIL) study. Ann Oncol 15: 123–128

Levy R, Colonna P, Tourani JM et al (1995) Human immunodeficiency virus associated Hodgkin's disease: report of 45 cases from the French Registry of HIV-associated tumors. Leuk Lymphoma 16:451–456

Lishner M (2003) Cancer in pregnancy. Ann Oncol 14(Suppl 3):iii31–iii36

Lishner M, Zemlickis D, Degendorfer P et al (1992) Maternal and foetal outcome following Hodgkin's disease in pregnancy. Br J Cancer 65:114–117

Lishner M, Zemlickis D, Degendorfer P (1996) Maternal and fetal outcome following Hodgkin's disease in pregnancy. In: Koren G, Lishner M, Fell TP (eds) Cancer in pregnancy. Maternal and fetal risks. Cambridge University Press, Cambridge

Macpherson N, Klasa RJ, Gascoyne R et al (2002) Treatment of elderly Hodgkin's lymphoma patients with a novel 5-drug regimen (ODBEP): a phase II study. Leuk Lymphoma 43: 1395–1402

Martin WG, Ristow KM, Habermann TM et al (2005) Bleomycin pulmonary toxicity has a negative impact on the outcome of patients with Hodgkin's lymphoma. J Clin Oncol 23:7614–7620

Massarweh S, Udden MM, Shahab I et al (2003) HIV-related Hodgkin's disease with central nervous system involvement and association with Epstein-Barr virus. Am J Hematol 72: 216–219

Mazonakis M, Varveris H, Fasoulaki M et al (2003) Radiotherapy of Hodgkin's disease in early pregnancy: embryo dose measurements. Radiother Oncol 66:333–339

Mueller H, Nogova L, Eichenauer DA et al (2008) The newly developed modified BEACOPP-regimen (BACOPP) is active and feasible in elderly patients with Hodgkin lymphoma: results of a phase II study of the German Hodgkin Study Group (GHSG). Blood 112:901

Musshoff K (1970) Therapy and prognosis of two different forms of organ involvement in cases of malignant lymphoma (Hodgkin's disease, reticulum sarcoma, lymphosarcoma) as well as a report about stage division in these disease. Klin Wchnschr 48:673–678

Nisce LZ, Tome MA, He S et al (1986) Management of coexisting Hodgkin's disease and pregnancy. Am J Clin Oncol 9:146–151

Nogova L, Reineke T, Brillant C et al (2008) Lymphocyte-predominant and classical Hodgkin's lymphoma: a comprehensive analysis from the German Hodgkin Study Group. J Clin Oncol 26:434–439

Nuyttens JJ, Prado KL, Jenrette JM et al (2002) Fetal dose during radiotherapy: clinical implementation and review of the literature. Cancer Radiother 6:352–357

Ogawa Y, Chung YS, Nakata B et al (1995) A case of primary Hodgkin's disease of the stomach. J Gastroenterol 30: 103–107

Ozdemirli M, Mankin HJ, Aisenberg AC et al (1996) Hodgkin's disease presenting as a solitary bone tumor. A report of four cases and review of the literature. Cancer 77:79–88

Pavlidis NA (2002) Coexistence of pregnancy and malignancy. Oncologist 7:279–287

Pereg D, Koren G, Lishner M (2007) The treatment of Hodgkin's and non-Hodgkin's lymphoma in pregnancy. Haematologica 92:1230–1237

Peres RM, Sanseverino MT, Guimaraes JL et al (2001) Assessment of fetal risk associated with exposure to cancer chemotherapy during pregnancy: a multicenter study. Braz J Med Biol Res 34:1551–1559

Proctor SJ, White J, Jones GL (2005) An international approach to the treatment of Hodgkin's disease in the elderly: launch of the SHIELD study programme. Eur J Haematol 75(Suppl 66):63–67

Radin AI (1990) Primary pulmonary Hodgkin's disease. Cancer 65:550–563

Riffaud L, Adn M, Brassier G et al (2003) Acute cauda equina compression revealing Hodgkin's disease: a case report. Spine (Phila Pa 1976) 28:270–272

Rubio R (1994) Hodgkin's disease associated with human immunodeficiency virus infection. A clinical study of 46 cases. Cooperative Study Group of Malignancies Associated with HIV Infection of Madrid. Cancer 73:2400–2407

Sapozink MD, Kaplan HS (1983) Intracranial Hodgkin's disease. A report of 12 cases and review of the literature. Cancer 52:1301–1307

Spano JP, Atlan D, Breau JL et al (2002) AIDS and non-AIDS-related malignancies: a new vexing challenge in HIV-positive patients. Part I: Kaposi's sarcoma, non-Hodgkin's lymphoma, and Hodgkin's lymphoma. Eur J Intern Med 13: 170–179

Specht L, Hasenclever D (2007) Prognostic factors in Hodgkin lymphoma. In: Hoppe RT, Mauch PM, Armitage JO et al (eds) Hodgkin lymphoma, 2nd edn. Lippincott Williams & Wilkins, Philadelphia

Specht L, Nissen NI (1989) Hodgkin's disease and age. Eur J Haematol 43:127–135

Spina M, Gabarre J, Rossi G et al (2002) Stanford V regimen and concomitant HAART in 59 patients with Hodgkin disease and HIV infection. Blood 100:1984–1988

Streffer C, Shore R, Konermann G et al (2003) Biological effects after prenatal irradiation (embryo and fetus). A report of the International Commission on Radiological Protection. Ann ICRP 33:5–206

Thompson LD, Fisher SI, Chu WS et al (2004) HIV-associated Hodgkin lymphoma: a clinicopathologic and immunophenotypic study of 45 cases. Am J Clin Pathol 121:727–738

Tirelli U, Errante D, Dolcetti R et al (1995) Hodgkin's disease and human immunodeficiency virus infection: clinicopathologic and virologic features of 114 patients from the Italian Cooperative Group on AIDS and Tumors. J Clin Oncol 13:1758–1767

Toledo TM, Harper RC, Moser RH (1971) Fetal effects during cyclophosphamide and irradiation therapy. Ann Intern Med 74:87–91

Vaccher E, Spina M, di Gennaro G et al (2001a) Concomitant cyclophosphamide, doxorubicin, vincristine, and prednisone chemotherapy plus highly active antiretroviral therapy in patients with human immunodeficiency virus-related, non-Hodgkin lymphoma. Cancer 91:155–163

Vaccher E, Spina M, Tirelli U (2001b) Clinical aspects and management of Hodgkin's disease and other tumours in HIV-infected individuals. Eur J Cancer 37:1306–1315

Weekes CD, Vose JM, Lynch JC et al (2002) Hodgkin's disease in the elderly: improved treatment outcome with a doxorubicin-containing regimen. J Clin Oncol 20:1087–1093

Woo SY, Fuller LM, Cundiff JH et al (1992) Radiotherapy during pregnancy for clinical stages IA-IIA Hodgkin's disease. Int J Radiat Oncol Biol Phys 23:407–412

Xicoy B, Ribera JM, Miralles P et al (2007) Results of treatment with doxorubicin, bleomycin, vinblastine and dacarbazine and highly active antiretroviral therapy in advanced stage, human immunodeficiency virus-related Hodgkin's lymphoma. Haematologica 92:191–198

Zuazu J, Julia A, Sierra J et al (1991) Pregnancy outcome in hematologic malignancies. Cancer 67:703–709

Acute and Long-Term Complications of Radiotherapy for Hodgkin Lymphoma

14

Andrea K. Ng and Lois B. Travis

Contents

A.K. Ng (✉)
Department of Radiation Oncology, Brigham & Women's Hospital and Dana-Farber Cancer Institute, Harvard Medical School, 75 Francis St, ASB1-L2, Boston, MA 02115, USA
e-mail: ang@lroc.harvard.edu

L.B. Travis
Philip Rubin Center of Excellence in Cancer Prevention and Survivorship, Wilmot Cancer Center, University of Rochester Medical Center, 601 Elmwood Avenue, Box 647, Rochester, NY 14642, USA
e-mail: lois_travis@URMC.Rochester.edu

14.1 Introduction

Radiation therapy plays a key role as part of curative treatment for Hodgkin lymphoma (HL), especially among patients with early stage disease. The success of radiotherapy for HL, however, is accompanied by untoward sequelae, which are categorized according to latency period. Acute side effects develop during or immediately after treatment, whereas subacute effects become manifest within weeks to months. The late effects of radiation therapy refer to those complications that become apparent several years after treatment has been completed. Table 14.1 summarizes several of the key acute, subacute, and late effects that have been associated with radiation therapy for HL. Most of the acute effects of radiation therapy may temporarily affect a patient's quality of life but tend to be self-limited. On the other hand, a number of the late effects, including second malignancies and cardiovascular disease, may be potentially life-threatening. Raising patient awareness of the various types of late effects of treatment, as well as their timing and associated risk factors, are of particular importance to patients with HL, given the high cure rate, typically young age at diagnosis and resultant long life expectancy. Improved understanding of late effects of treatment can also facilitate the development of follow-up plans, and screening and prevention strategies.

L. Specht and J. Yahalom (eds.), *Radiotherapy for Hodgkin Lymphoma*,
DOI: 10.1007/978-3-540-78944-4_14, © Springer-Verlag Berlin Heidelberg 2011

Table 14.1 Selected, acute, subacute and long-term complications of radiotherapy for HL

Acute and subacute complications	Temporary local alopecia Temporary local skin reaction L'hermitte's syndrome Radiation pneumonitis Xerostomia/dental caries Hypothyroidism Sterility
Long-term complications	Second malignancy Cardiac disease Noncardiac vascular disease

14.2 Acute and Subacute Effects

14.2.1 Temporary Local Alopecia and Skin Reaction

The current standard chemotherapy for most patients with HL is adriamycin, bleomycin, vinblastine, and dacarbazine (ABVD) with or without radiation therapy. Most patients will experience partial or complete alopecia after ABVD treatment. As patients begin consolidative radiation therapy, which typically takes place 3–4 weeks after chemotherapy, they will begin to recover body hair. However, toward the end of radiation treatment, most patients will again experience partial or complete hair loss within the treatment field. Regrowth of hair after radiation therapy typically takes place 3–4 months posttreatment. At the current radiation doses of 30–36 Gy used for the treatment of HL, complete recovery of body hair is expected.

Patients will also likely develop local skin erythema and sensitivity when radiation doses of around 25–30 Gy are reached. The skin reaction may peak 7-10 days after therapy. At the doses that are currently used for the treatment of HL, skin desquamation and chronic skin changes are rarely observed.

14.2.2 Oral Complications: Dysphagia and Xerostomia/Dental Caries

Patients receiving radiation therapy to the neck and mediastinum will likely experience dysphagia 2–3 weeks into treatment, which may persist after the completion of therapy. Most patients, however, experience complete resolution of dysphagia within 1 month after treatment. Depending on the superior extent of the treatment field, if the upper cervical chain is included in the treatment field, patients may also develop temporary taste alteration and decreased salivary output (Bucher et al. 1988). The treatment-related xerostomia may place patients at risk for dental caries as well. It has been demonstrated that the use of supplemental topical fluoride can significantly reduce the risk of dental caries and limit oral concentrations of cariogenic microflora (Keene et al. 1994). At the radiation doses currently used for the treatment of Hodgkin lymphoma, full recovery of taste and salivary gland function is expected, although the recovery time may be longer for older patients.

14.2.3 L'Hermitte's Sign

In patients who receive radiation therapy in which part of the cervical spine was included in the treatment field, L'hermitte's sign has been reported in about 5%. It has also been described in patients who have received radiation therapy for primary head and neck cancers (Lewanski et al. 2000). The symptoms typically manifest themselves 3 months following radiation therapy and gradually disappear within 6 months (Carmel and Kaplan 1976). Patients typically complain of electric shock-like sensation down the extremities, precipitated by neck flexion. The syndrome is thought to be related to transient demyelination of sensory fibers in the cervical spine (Esik et al. 2003a, b). It is typically self-limiting and is not associated with any permanent neurological sequelae.

14.2.4 Radiation Pneumonitis

Radiation pneumonitis is an acute-phase response to radiation therapy. The risk of radiation pneumonitis after mantle radiation therapy alone for HL has been estimated to be less than 5% (Tarbell et al. 1990). Typical symptoms include dry cough, dyspnea, and shortness of breath, all of which occur several weeks posttreatment. In most cases, these symptoms are self-limited and do not require treatment, although in more severe cases, nonsteroidal anti-inflammatory agents or steroid treatments may be required. The risk is higher for patients treated with whole lung irradiation, an approach, which is now almost never used, and in patients who received chemotherapy in conjunction with radiation (Hirsch et al. 1996; Horning et al. 1994; Tarbell et al. 1990). In the setting of modern radiation therapy utilizing smaller fields and lower doses, the prevalence of radiation pneumonitis is well under 5% even when chemotherapy is used (Koh et al. 2006). In the era of three-dimensional radiation therapy, data are also emerging on the relationship between radiation dosimetric parameters in the treatment of HL and pulmonary toxicity. In a study conducted at Princess Margaret Hospital, which included 64 HL patients treated with mediastinal radiation therapy using three-dimensional radiation planning (Koh et al. 2006), the median mean lung dose (MLD) was 12.2 Gy for the entire cohort, and in the two patients who developed radiation pneumonitis, the MLD was 16.4 and 17.6 Gy, respectively.

14.2.5 Thyroid Abnormalities

The most common thyroid abnormality after radiation therapy for HL is hypothyroidism. In a landmark study from Stanford University, the actuarial risk of hypothyroidism 26 years after radiation therapy for HL was 47% (Hancock et al. 1991). Other less common thyroid abnormalities included Graves' disease, thyroiditis, thyrotoxicosis, thyroid nodules, and thyroid malignancies. Most of the data on the effect of radiation dose to treat HL on the risk of thyroid dysfunction have been derived from the pediatric population. In a study of HL patients by Constine et al., only 17% of children developed thyroid abnormalities at doses of 26 Gy or lower, as compared with 78% of children who received 26 Gy or higher (Constine et al. 1984). Results in the Childhood Cancer Survivor Study showed that survivors of HL demonstrated a 17-fold increased risk of hypothyroidism compared to a sibling cohort (Sklar et al. 2000). The risk of hypothyroidism increased significantly with increasing dose, and at 45 Gy or higher the actuarial risk of hypothyroidism at 20 years was 50%. In a study from the University of Minnesota, which included 89 children and young adults treated for HL, the median time to the development of hypothyroidism was 6 years (Bhatia et al. 1996). The estimated actuarial risk of developing hypothyroidism was 60% at 11 years. In addition, the relative risk of hypothyroidism was estimated to increase by 1.02/Gy. Age, gender, chemotherapy, and prior lymphangiography were not significantly associated with development of hypothyroidism.

14.2.6 Sterility

14.2.6.1 Reproductive Function After Chemotherapy

Both chemotherapy and radiotherapy may induce gonadal failure. For patients with HL, however, most of the accrued data have focused on chemotherapy-related sterility. In a recent cohort study of 518 female survivors of HL (De Bruin et al. 2008), after a median follow-up of 9.4 years, chemotherapy was associated with a 12.3-fold increased risk of premature menopause compared with radiotherapy alone. A significant dose–response relationship was demonstrated with exposure to alkylating chemotherapy, most notably, procarbazine and cyclophosphamide. In a separate study of male survivors of HL, it was reported that 80–90% developed azoospermia after six to eight cycles of mechlorethamine, vincristine, procarbazine, and prednisone (MOPP) chemotherapy (Anselmo et al. 1990). In a cohort study of male patients treated on the European Organisation for Research and Treatment of Cancer (EORTC) protocols for HL, exposure to alkylating chemotherapy was associated with a significantly higher risk of gonadal dysfunction and longer recovery time of gonadal function (van der Kaaij et al. 2007). It has been shown, however, that most male patients with HL have poor sperm quality even before treatment. Adriamycin, bleomycin, vinblastine, and dacarbazine (ABVD), the current standard systemic therapy for HL does not appear to affect fertility (van der Kaaij et al. 2007). In a case–control study of female HL survivors treated with ABVD, no significant evidence for subfertility was found (Hodgson et al. 2007b). In male survivors of HL, transient azoospermia was observed in about one third of those given ABVD, but the majority of patients showed recovery of spermatogenesis following completion of treatment (Anselmo et al. 1990; Viviani et al. 1985). The bleomycin, etoposide, doxorubicin, cyclophosphamide, vincristine, procarbazine, and prednisone (BEACOPP) regimen, developed by the German Hodgkin Study Group (GHSG) for patients with advanced-stage or unfavorable HL, has been shown to result in significantly higher overall survival (OS) than standard dose cyclophosphamide, vincristine, procarbazine, and prednisone alternating with doxorubicin, bleomycin, vinblastine, and dacarbazine (COPP-ABVD) (Diehl et al. 2003). However, an increased risk of sterility is associated with BEACOPP. Behringer et al. described that more than 50% of women who received eight cycles of BEACOPP for HL had continuous amenorrhea (Behringer et al. 2005). In a more recent study from the GHSG which evaluated the fertility status of 38 male patients with advanced-stage HL treated with BEACOPP, 77% patients had dysspermia at baseline. After treatment, 89% patients had azoospermia and 11% had other types of dysspermia; in no patients was normozoospermia observed (Sieniawski et al. 2008).

14.2.6.2 Reproductive Function After Radiation Therapy

In general, the gonadal toxicity of radiation therapy is well established (Lushbaugh and Casarett 1976; Ogilvy-Stuart and Shalet 1993; Sklar et al. 2006; Wallace et al. 1989, 2005). However, in the HL population, radiation-induced sterility is of relevance mainly in those patients given pelvic radiation therapy for infradiaphragmatic involvement, which is rarely observed among those patients presenting with early stage disease. For women, ionizing radiation can cause direct DNA damage to ovarian follicles, leading to follicular atrophy and decreased follicular reserve within the ovary. This injury can subsequently hasten the natural decline of follicle numbers, leading to impaired ovarian hormone production, uterine dysfunction due to inadequate estrogen exposure, and early menopause (Wallace et al. 1989). An ovarian dose of 4 Gy may cause a 30% incidence of sterility in young women, but is associated with 100% sterility in women over 40 years of age (Ogilvy-Stuart and Shalet 1993). The radiosensitivity of the oocyte is thought to vary during the growth phase, with primordial follicles being more radioresistent than maturing follicles. In a mathematical model developed by Wallace et al. (2005), based on the known radiosensitivity of the human oocyte according to age at exposure, the effective sterilizing dose (ESD), or dose of fractionated radiotherapy at which premature ovarian failure occurs immediately after treatment in 97.5% of patients was estimated. The estimated ESD at birth was found to be 20.3 Gy; at 10 years of age, 18.4 Gy; at 20 years of age 16.5 Gy; and at 30 years of age, 14.3 Gy. These doses are well within the dose ranges used in the treatment of HL. This mathematical model can allow physicians to counsel women on their reproductive potential following radiation therapy. In female patients receiving pelvic irradiation, oophoropexy, which can be achieved laparoscopically, can substantially reduce the dose delivered to the ovaries and thereby preserve fertility (Williams et al. 1999; Williams and Mendenhall 1992)

For male patients, radiation therapy can induce germinal epithelium depletion in a dose-related manner (Clifton and Bremner 1983; Lushbaugh and Casarett 1976; Meistrich 1993; Ogilvy-Stuart and Shalet 1993). Decrease in sperm counts can be observed after doses as low as 0.15 Gy. A one-time dose of 0.35 Gy or higher can cause transient azoospermia. The recovery time increases with increasing dose, and doses of 2 Gy or higher to the germinal epithelium can result in permanent azoospermia. At doses of 15 Gy or higher, Leydig cell function can be affected, with the potential need for testosterone replacement therapy. In men who receive pelvic radiation therapy, cryopreservation of semen prior to initiation of therapy should be strongly considered. Adequate testicular shielding can also reduce the risk of permanent azoospermia.

14.3 Late Effects

14.3.1 Second Malignancies

Several studies have shown significantly increased risks of mortality due to late effects in long-term survivors of HL, with second malignancies comprising the leading cause of death (Aleman et al. 2003; Ng et al. 2002a). Ample data exist, largely in the form of single-institutional retrospective cohort or case–control studies, as well as population-based studies, characterizing second malignancies after HL. It is important to recognize that in addition to radiation therapy, other factors also contribute to the increased risks of second malignancies. Chemotherapy, in particular, alkylator-containing regimens of the past, is associated with increased risks of both leukemia and lung cancer.

However, long-term data on second malignancy risks among patients given modern chemotherapy alone is sparse. The increased risk of selected second malignancies observed among HL survivors can also be related to other nontreatment-related factors, including underlying genetic predisposition, compromised immune function, tobacco use, and heightened surveillance.

Historically, second malignancies after HL were divided into three main categories: leukemia, non-Hodgkin's lymphoma, and solid tumors. However, recent studies have focused on the more common subtypes of second malignancies, most notably, breast cancer and lung cancer (Aleman et al. 2003; Swerdlow et al. 2001; Travis et al. 2002, 2003; Travis 2002; van Leeuwen et al. 2003). Given the magnitude of the problem, efforts to reduce the negative impact of second malignancies on the survival of patients with HL have been increasingly emphasized. These include prevention and screening strategies in survivors, and treatment modifications in newly diagnosed patients (Friedman and Constine 2006; Mauch et al. 2005).

14.3.1.1 Leukemia

An increased risk of leukemia in patients treated for HL was first described in the early 1970s (Arseneau et al. 1972), with the largest excesses observed within the first 10 years after treatment. It later became apparent that the risk was largely related to the use of alkylating chemotherapy in a dose-related manner (Kaldor et al. 1990; van Leeuwen et al. 1994). In a case–control study conducted by van Leeuwen et al., among HL patients who received chemotherapy alone, the relative risk of developing leukemia was 44.6, compared to patients who were treated with radiation therapy alone (van Leeuwen et al. 1994). A significant dose–response relationship was also demonstrated. Using patients who received radiation therapy alone as a reference group, patients given more than six cycles of alkylating chemotherapy had a relative risk of leukemia of 57.1 compared with 12.9 for those treated with one to six cycles.

The use of large-field radiation therapy has also been implicated as a contributing factor to leukemia excesses in HL. In the study by van Leeuwen et al., overall, the addition of radiation therapy to chemotherapy did not significantly increase the risk of leukemia (relative risks of chemotherapy alone versus combined modality therapy: 44.6 vs 20.9. $p = 0.16$) (van Leeuwen et al. 1994). However, total-nodal irradiation given with combination chemotherapy was associated with a 2.5-fold increased risk of leukemia compared with patients treated with chemotherapy alone, although the increase was not statistically significant ($p = 0.39$).

Several studies have suggested that a history of splenectomy is associated with an increased risk of leukemia after HL (Tura et al. 1993; van Leeuwen et al. 1987). A postulated biological mechanism for the increased second leukemia risk is the reduced tumoral immunosurveillance capabilities in asplenic patients. However, similarly elevated risks of leukemia have not been observed in patients who were splenectomized for other reasons, e.g., trauma, implying that cancer risk after a splenectomy may be influenced by a patient's baseline immune status. In the case–control study by van Leeuwen et al., a fivefold elevated leukemia risk was found in patients with persistent thrombocytenia after treatment (van Leeuwen et al. 1994). This finding may reflect the association between treatment-related marrow damage and leukemia risk.

The prognosis of leukemia after HL is extremely poor, with a median survival of less than 1 year (Ng et al. 2002b). With the replacement of MOPP by ABVD, the risk of leukemia has been substantially reduced. In a recent large, international population-based study by Schonfeld et al. (2006), a significant reduction in absolute excess risk of acute myeloid leukemia was found in HL patients who were treated after 1985, an observation, which is likely explained by changes in chemotherapy over time.

Leukemogenic agents, however, are still often used in the setting of salvage therapy for HL, and are present in some of the newer regimens, including BEACOPP and Stanford V, which consists of mechlorethamine, doxorubicin, vinblastine, vincristine, bleomycin, etoposide, and prednisone. In the updated 10-year results of the GHSG HD 9 trial, a total of 14 cases of acute myelogenous leukemia were documented among the 466 patients randomized to receive eight cycles of dose-escalated BEACOPP (Engert et al. 2009). However, the leukemia risk was only 0.9% in the succeeding study that also employed dose-escalated BEACOPP, at a median follow-up of 4 years. In a recent report from Stanford, among the group of patients who received mostly Stanford V chemotherapy (Advani et al. 2006), the incidence of acute myelogenous leukemia/myelodysplasia was only 0.3%, which likely reflects lower cumulative doses of alkylating chemotherapy.

14.3.1.2 Non-Hodgkin's Lymphoma

An increased risk of non-Hodgkin's lymphoma after HL has also been observed (Ng et al. 2002b; Swerdlow et al. 2000; van Leeuwen et al. 2000). The timing of these excesses and the relationship with prior therapy, however, is unclear. The lack of a consistent pattern of factors associated with the development of non-Hodgkin's lymphoma can be attributed to a number of influences. First, the discrepant results may partly reflect pathologic misclassification in some of the studies, or differences in diagnostic criteria for HL and non-Hodgkin's lymphoma. Development of non-Hodgkin's lymphoma after HL may be treatment induced, or may represent the natural course of selected subtypes of HL, such as the lymphocyte predominant group. The excessive risk could also reflect in part the immunosuppressed status of HL patients, similar to the increased risk of non-Hodgkin's lymphoma observed in other groups of immunocompromised patients such as transplant recipients.

In a detailed analysis of 52 cases of non-Hodgkin's lymphoma that developed after HL, which was conducted by the GHSG, the most common histology was diffuse large B-cell lymphoma (Rueffer et al. 2001). With a median follow-up of 26 months, the actuarial 2-year freedom from treatment failure (FFTF) was 24%, and the actuarial 2-year overall survival (OS) was 30%. For patients with diffuse large-cell lymphoma treated with a doxorubicin-containing regimen, the 2-year FFTF and OS were 50% and 54%, respectively. Patients who developed non-Hodgkin's lymphoma within 3 months after completion of HL therapy had a significantly worse prognosis than patients who developed non-Hodgkin's lymphoma beyond 12 months (2-year OS, 20% vs 42%). The age-adjusted International Prognostic Score also significantly predicted for treatment outcome.

14.3.1.3 Solid Tumors

As the number of long-term survivors of HL has increased, solid tumors have emerged as the major subtype of second malignancy, accounting for up to 75–80% of all cases (Behringer et al. 2004; Hodgson et al. 2007a; Ng et al. 2002b; Swerdlow et al. 2000; van Leeuwen et al. 2000). Solid tumors typically develop after a long latency period following initial treatment of HL. In addition, the excess risk appears to persist as long as 30 years. The most common solid tumors observed in long-term survivors of HL include cancers of breast, lung, and gastrointestinal tract (Behringer et al. 2004; Dores et al. 2002; Hodgson et al. 2007a; Ng et al. 2002b).

The contribution of radiation therapy to the development of solid tumors after HL is supported by the observation that the majority of these tumors arise within or at the edges of prior radiation treatment fields. In addition, several recent studies have shown a significant radiation dose–response relationship in the development of specific types of solid tumors after HL (Travis et al. 2002, 2003; van Leeuwen et al. 2003).

Two case–control studies, which overlapped in patient populations, examined in detail the relationship between radiation dose and the risk of breast cancer after HL therapy (Travis et al. 2003; van Leeuwen et al. 2003). In both studies, the radiation dose at the site of the breast cancer was estimated in the case patients and compared to the dose to a comparable location in the control subjects. In the study by van Leeuwen et al., which consisted of 48 cases of breast cancer and 175 matched controls, the breast cancer risk was significantly increased only after a radiation dose of 38.5 Gy or higher, but not at lower doses (van Leeuwen et al. 2003). Forty of the 48 cases were also included in the study by Travis et al. (2003). The significant dose–response relationship observed by van Leeuwen et al. (2003) was limited to women who received radiation therapy alone and was not observed among women who received both chemotherapy and radiation therapy, which is likely due to the effect of chemotherapy on ovarian function. In the large, international case–control study by Travis et al. (2003), which consisted of 105 breast cancer cases and 266 matched controls, a radiation dose of >4 Gy to the breast was associated with a 3.2-fold breast cancer risk compared with women who received lower doses of radiation and no alkylating chemotherapy. The risk increased to eightfold for women who received >40 Gy to the breast (p trend < 0.001).

A significant radiation dose–response relationship has similarly been shown for the development of lung cancer after HL. Travis et al. conducted a case–control study of 222 cases of lung cancer and 444 matched controls among patients who had been treated for HL (Travis et al. 2002). Using patients who received <5 Gy to the area of the lung in which cancer developed as the reference group, the lung cancer risk increased with increasing dose to the lung (p trend < .001), although the increased risk was statistically significantly only after exposure to doses of 30 Gy or higher.

It is important to recognize that the data on solid tumors after radiation therapy for HL were based on patients treated in an era in which large treatment fields and higher radiation doses were routinely used. The radiation treatment field is significantly smaller with the current standard of involved-field radiation therapy given as part of combined modality therapy. In a study by Koh et al., organ-specific cancer risks after mantle-field radiation therapy versus involved-field radiation therapy were calculated using a dosimetric risk-modeling approach (Koh et al. 2007). It was estimated that the excess relative risks for female breast and lung cancer were reduced by approximately 65%, and for male lung cancer, by approximately 35%, when an involved-field instead of a mantle field was used. A recent meta-analysis showed that the risk of breast cancer is significantly higher after extended-field than involved-field radiation therapy (OR, 3.25, $p = 0.04$), which is likely related to the reduced amount of breast tissue in a more limited treatment field (e.g. exclusion of the axillae) (Franklin et al. 2006). More recently, there has been a movement toward the use of involved-node radiation therapy, which will further reduce the exposure of normal tissue to radiation (Girinsky et al. 2006b).

Clinical trials which further explore reductions in the dose of radiation therapy used to treat HL are ongoing, and it is likely that these results will have important implications, given the known dose–response relationships for some of the more common secondary cancers. With these modifications, it is expected that HL patients given radiation therapy in the modern era will face a lower risk of second malignancy.

There is a paucity of long-term data on HL patients treated with chemotherapy alone because of the historically prominent role of radiation therapy in the cure of this disease. Most studies do not have large enough numbers of patients given chemotherapy alone with sufficient follow-up time to meaningfully examine the long-term risk of solid tumors. In a collaborative British cohort study, which included 1,693 patients treated with chemotherapy alone, the relative risk of lung cancer after chemotherapy alone was found to be significantly increased at 3.3 (95% CI, 2.2–4.7) (Swerdlow et al. 2000). This increased risk was of comparable magnitude to the patients who received radiation therapy alone (RR, 2.9, 95% CI, 1.9–4.1) or the patients who received combined modality therapy (RR, 4.3, 95% CI, 2.9–6.2). The majority of patients in this study were treated with alkylating-agent-based chemotherapy. Also, because tobacco history was not available for the majority of patients, the analyses were not controlled for tobacco use. The significance of alkylating agent in subsequent lung cancer development after HL was confirmed in a case–control study by the same group (Swerdlow et al. 2001), and in the case–control study by Travis et al. (2002), with both studies showing a significant dose–response relationship between cumulative doses of alkylating-agent chemotherapy and lung cancer risk. All analyses in this case–control study by Travis and colleagues were controlled for tobacco use (Travis et al. 2002).

Several other factors have been identified to influence the risk of treatment-related second malignancy after HL. Young age at mantle irradiation has been consistently shown to be associated with significantly increased risks of breast cancer in women (Hodgson et al. 2007a; Ng et al. 2002b; van Leeuwen et al. 2000). In a recent population-based cohort study by Hodgson et al., the absolute risks of breast cancer in women diagnosed with HL at ages 15–25 were 34–47 per 10,000 person years at 10 years, which were higher than the absolute risks of women in the general population of ages between 50 and 54 years, a typical age when mammography screening is recommended (Hodgson et al. 2007a).

Hormonal exposures appear to play an important role in the development of breast cancer after HL. Treatment exposure to alkylating chemotherapy and pelvic irradiation had been shown to confer a protective effect against breast cancer in a dose-related manner, as documented in the two case–control studies described above (Travis et al. 2003; van Leeuwen et al. 2003). This reduction in risk appears related to treatment-induced premature menopause. These findings may have implications on recommendations for the use of hormone replacement therapy, and the role of chemopreventive agents in female survivors of HL.

The modifying effect of other known cancer risk factors on treatment-induced malignancies after HL has also been explored. In the case–control study by van Leeuwen et al., the effect of several traditional breast cancer risk factors, including family history, on breast cancer risks among HL survivors were evaluated (van Leeuwen et al. 2003). None of the factors were found to have a significant influence, although the negative findings may be due to the small number of cases. In a larger, case–control study by Hill et al., the authors showed that radiation therapy did not further increase the risk of breast cancer in women with a family history of breast cancer (Hill et al. 2005). Among women with a positive family history, the addition of radiation therapy was associated with a relative risk of breast cancer of 0.8. It was postulated that women with a family history of breast or ovarian cancer may have an altered response to radiation, and that in mutation carriers, unrepaired damaged cells might undergo cell death rather than serve as cancer-initiating cells.

The role of tobacco use in the etiology of lung cancer is well established. The modifying effect of smoking history on treatment-related lung cancer in HL survivors was explored in a case–control study by Travis et al. Using patients who had minimal radiation or alkylating chemotherapy exposure and who were nonsmokers as the reference group, exposure to >5 Gy of radiation therapy and/or alkylating-agent chemotherapy was associated with a 4.3- to 7.2-fold increased risk of lung cancer (Travis et al. 2002). The relative risk increased to 16.8–20.2 in patients who had either one of the treatment exposures and a positive smoking history, and the relative risk further increased to 49.1 in patients who had >5 Gy of radiation therapy, received alkylating chemotherapy and had a history of smoking, consistent with a multiplicative effect of tobacco use on the risk of treatment-related lung cancer.

14.3.1.4 Follow-Up Strategies for Second Malignancies

Given the significantly increased risk of second malignancies in survivors of HL, strategies need to be developed to minimize the impact of this serious late effect on patient survival. For a number of second malignancies after HL, data on their temporal trend and associated risk factors are well established. These data may allow us to ascertain the appropriate follow-up tests, optimal timing and frequency, as well as assist in identifying high-risk survivors for closer follow-up. Specific examples include mammographic screening in women who received chest irradiation at a young age, to start around 8–10 years after treatment completion. In the most recent American Cancer Society Guidelines, which are based on expert consensus, breast MRI as an adjunct to mammography is also recommended for these patients (Saslow et al. 2007). Other potential screening studies to consider in selected survivors of HL include low-dose chest CT screening for lung cancer among patients given chest irradiation and/or alkylating chemotherapy and who have a history of tobacco use, and colonoscopy among patients given infradiaphragmatic irradiation (Das et al. 2006; Hodgson et al. 2007a). In the follow-up of long-term survivors, counseling on lifestyle changes, including smoking cessation and sun-safety practices, will serve to lower risks of selected second cancers. Extrapolating data from other high-risk population, chemoprevention may also have a role in selected HL survivors. For instance, selective estrogen-receptor modulators might be considered in women who are deemed at high risk based on their treatment history. Trials designed to test the efficacies of these interventions are an important part of survivorship research.

14.3.2 Cardiovascular Disease

Cardiovascular disease is the second leading cause of death in long-term survivors of HL. A number of studies have shown that patients who have been cured of HL are at significantly increased risk of death from cardiac disease compared with the normal population (Eriksson et al. 2000; Hancock et al. 1993a, b; Henry-Amar et al. 1990; Ng et al. 2002a; Swerdlow et al. 2007; van Rijswijk et al. 1987). The estimated relative risks of cardiac mortality range from 2.2 to 7, and the absolute excess risks range from 9.3 to 28/10,000 person years (Eriksson et al. 2000; Hancock et al. 1993b; Hoppe 1997; Ng et al. 2002a). A wide spectrum of cardiac complications have been reported in long-term survivors of HL (Adams et al. 2004; Aviles et al. 2005; Heidenreich et al. 2003, 2005; Hull et al. 2003). These include pericardial disease, valvular disorders, conduction abnormalities, ventricular dysfunction, and coronary disease. Among these cardiac abnormalities, coronary artery disease is the major contributor to the excess risk of cardiac mortality, accounting for two thirds of all cases of fatal cardiac events in survivors of HL.

14.3.2.1 Cardiovascular Disease After Mediastinal Irradiation

Earlier reports focused largely on the relationship between mediastinal irradiation for HL and the risk of fatal cardiovascular complications, predominantly in the form of acute myocardial infarctions (MI) (Boivin et al. 1992; Cosset et al. 1991; Hancock et al. 1993a, b). The cardiac complications after radiation therapy are thought to be due to radiation-induced inflammation and fibrosis of individual cardiac structures, with signs and symptoms typically becoming manifest 5–10 years after completion of treatment. Boivin et al. showed that compared with patients who did not receive mediastinal irradiation, the relative risk of death from MI in patients given mediastinal irradiation was significantly increased at 2.6 (Boivin et al. 1992). Cosset et al. reported a 10-year cumulative incidence of acute MI of 3.9% in patients who underwent radiation treatment to the mediastinum, although no cases were observed in patients who did not receive radiation therapy (Cosset et al. 1991). Hancock et al. demonstrated a dose–response relationship in that cardiac mortality was significantly increased in patients who received more than 30 Gy to the mediastinum, but the increase was not significant in patients who received 30 Gy or less (Hancock et al. 1993b). In a study from Switzerland that included 352 patients treated with radiation therapy alone (Glanzmann et al. 1998), the relative risks of fatal MI was significantly elevated at 4.2 at a mean follow-up of 11.2 years. Because of the narrow range of radiotherapy doses used, the relationship between amount of radiation and risk of fatal MI could not be evaluated.

In addition to cardiac mortality, cardiac morbidity after treatment for HL has also been described. In a retrospective study from the University of Florida on 415 patients with history of HL (Hull et al. 2003), 10.4% patients developed coronary artery disease (defined as history of documented MI, coronary artery bypass graft surgery, percutaneous coronary intervention, and >75% diameter stenosis on coronary angiography or autopsy) at a median follow-up of 9 years posttreatment. On multivariable analysis, the only treatment-related risk factor significantly associated with the risk of coronary artery disease was the use of a matched mantle and para-aortic field as compared with mantle alone or subdiaphragmatic treatment alone. Aleman et al. from the Netherlands reviewed 1,474 survivors of HL younger than 41 years at treatment (Aleman et al. 2007). At a median follow-up of 18.7 years, the relative risks of MI and congestive heart failure were significantly increased at 3.6 and 4.9, respectively, and the absolute excess risks were 35.7 and 25.6 per 10,000 person years of follow-up, respectively. The relative risk of MI became significantly elevated after 10 years, and remained significantly elevated for at least 25 years after treatment. On multivariable analysis, mediastinal radiotherapy was associated with significantly increased risks of valvular disorders, coronary heart disease, and congestive heart failure.

Most of the data on radiation-related cardiac complications were derived from HL patients treated with outdated techniques and doses. There are ongoing efforts to reduce treatment especially among patients with early stage HL. Over the past few decades, the radiation field sizes have decreased from extended-field to involved-field (Bonadonna et al. 2004; Engert et al. 2003; Ferme et al. 2007), and more recently there is increasing interest in the concept of involved-node radiation therapy (Girinsky et al. 2006b), as mentioned above. Other recent advances in radiation therapy techniques include intensity-modulated radiation therapy (IMRT), which can allow specification of dose constraints to individual normal structures while delivering the full prescribed dose to the tumor target (Ghalibafian et al. 2008; Girinsky et al. 2006a). In addition, the use of respiratory gating, which is especially important for mediastinal structures, can further improve targeting of tumor tissue (Girinsky and Ghalibafian 2005). Radiation doses to individual cardiac structures as well as the risk of cardiac complications with these newer radiation therapy approaches need to be verified.

14.3.2.2 Cardiovascular Disease After Chemotherapy

In recent years, additional data have been generated on the relationship between chemotherapy for HL and risk of cardiac complications. Aviles et al. reviewed 399 HL patients who achieved a complete remission after chemotherapy alone (163 with ABVD, 71 patients with MBVD [mitoxantrone instead of doxorubicin], and 165 with EBVD [epirubicin instead of doxorubicin]) (Aviles et al. 2005). Cardiac examination and testing were performed every 4 months for 2 years, every 6 months for 2 years and then yearly. At a median follow-up of 11.5 years, 20 patients developed congestive heart failure and 19 patients developed MI. A total of 21 cardiac deaths were reported, and the relative risks of cardiac mortality compared to the matched normal population after MBVD, ABVD, and EBVD were 67.8, 46.4, and 19.4, respectively.

A British study also demonstrated the independent effect of chemotherapy on risk of cardiac mortality, although the relative risks were elevated to a considerably lesser extent. Swerdlow et al. reported on 7,033 patients with HL treated from 1967 to 2000 (Swerdlow et al. 2007). At a mean follow-up of 11.1 years, a total of 166 MI deaths were observed. The risk of cardiac mortality was separately analyzed for patients who received chemotherapy with and without mediastinal irradiation. Among patients who were treated with ABVD and mediastinal irradiation, the relative risk of cardiac mortality was significantly elevated at 12.1 ($p = 0.004$). However, patients who received ABVD without mediastinal irradiation were also found to have a significantly elevated relative risk of cardiac mortality of 7.8 ($p = 0.01$). Similarly, the relative risk of cardiac mortality after treatment with any adriamycin-based chemotherapy with and without mediastinal irradiation was 2.4 ($p = 0.05$) and 3.2 ($p < 0.001$), respectively.

14.3.2.3 Screening for Cardiovascular Disease

Because of the well-documented increased risks of cardiac complications in HL survivors, investigators have described the use of cardiac screening tools in asymptomatic patients. In a prospective study conducted at Stanford University, 294 asymptomatic patients treated with mediastinal irradiation for HL underwent electrocardiography and echocardiography screening (Heidenreich et al. 2003). The median time following initial treatment was 15 years. The prevalence of valvular abnormalities increased significantly with increasing follow-up time. For those patients for whom more than 20 years had elapsed since treatment, mild to severe aortic regurgitation was detected by echocardiography in 60%, which was significantly higher than the expected prevalence of 4% in an age- and gender-matched sample from the Framingham cohort ($p < 0.0001$). It was further noted that aortic regurgitation was rarely picked up on auscultation. A diastolic murmur was detected in only 6.3% of the patients who were found to have valvular disease on echocardiogram. These results support the use of routine screening echocardiogram in identifying patients with valvular disease who would benefit from endocarditis prophylaxis. In addition to valvular disease, patients were also found to be significantly more likely than expected to have depressed left ventricular fractional shortening, regional wall motion abnormality, decreased left ventricular mass, and pericardial thickening, all of which also increased with increasing time from initial irradiation. The finding of increasing prevalence of asymptomatic cardiac structural abnormalities requiring interventions with increasing follow-up time led to the authors' conclusion that screening echocardiography may be beneficial, particularly in those who have survived 10 years following mediastinal irradiation. The same group subsequently separately reported on the diastolic function of the screened patients (Heidenreich et al. 2005). A high prevalence of diastolic dysfunction was found, with increased incidence related to older age, presence of hypertension, diabetes, wall motion abnormalities, and those with a longer latency period from radiation treatment to screening. For patients who were 11–20 years and longer than 20 years out from radiation treatment, 15% and 23%, respectively, had mild to moderate diastolic dysfunction. Diastolic dysfunction was sevenfold more common in this population than in community-based data from Rochester, Minnesota. Moreover, on stress echocardiography, coronary artery disease was found to be significantly more common in patients with diastolic dysfunction than in patients with normal function (10% vs 2%; $p = 0.005$). Deaths or events due to coronary artery disease were significantly more common in patients with diastolic dysfunction compared with patients with normal function (25% vs 8%; $p = 0.002$). Sixty-three patients (21.4%) had abnormal ventricular images at rest, suggesting prior myocardial injury. In the most recent report from the Stanford group, the focus was on coronary disease among 294 participants of the screening trial (Heidenreich et al. 2007). During stress testing, 40 patients (14%) developed perfusion defects, impaired wall motion, or both abnormalities. Based on the imaging results, these 40 patients underwent coronary angiography. The angiography showed >50%, <50%, and no stenosis in 55%, 22.5%, and 22.5% of patients, respectively. As a result of the screening, seven of these asymptomatic patients (2.4%) underwent bypass graft surgery. In addition, 23 patients (8%) subsequently developed coronary events during a median of 6.5 years of follow-up, including ten cases of acute myocardial infarction. Of note, the median dose to the mediastinum among patients included in the Stanford screening study was 44 Gy (range, 35–54.6 Gy), which is considerably higher than those used in current practice.

In a prospective cardiac screening study by Adams et al. (2004), the incidence of asymptomatic cardiac disease in 48 survivors of childhood HL was reported. The median age of the study population at the time of initial therapy was 16.5 years, and the median dose received was 40 Gy. The median follow time was 14.3 years. On echocardiogram, 42% were found to have significant valve defects, 75% had conduction defects, and 22% had echocardiographic changes suggestive of restrictive cardiomyopathy. Aortic regurgitation was found to be associated with a decreased physical component score (PCS) on the SF-36 ($r = -.371$, $p = .011$). A decreased peak myocardial oxygen uptake during exercise (VO2max), a predictor of mortality in heart failure, was associated with increased fatigue ($r = -.35$, $p = .02$), increased shortness of breath ($r = -.35$, $p = .02$) and decreased PCS ($r = .554$, $p = .00017$). These findings suggest that the late effects of treatment can contribute to the increased fatigue level seen in long-term HL survivors. In addition, in survivors with symptoms of fatigue, evaluation for underlying cardiac disease should be considered.

14.3.2.4 Modifying Effect of Traditional Cardiac Risk Factors

Several studies have addressed the contribution of traditional cardiac risk factors to the subsequent risk of cardiac disease after HL therapy. In the study by Hull et al. (2003), all patients who developed coronary artery disease had at least one traditional cardiac risk factor. In addition, both hypertension and hypercholesterolemia were significantly associated with the risk of coronary artery disease. Similarly, in the Swiss study by Glanzmann et al. (1998), the relative risk of ischemic cardiac disease in patients with known cardiac risk factors was significantly elevated at 2.36, whereas in patients without risk factors, the relative risk was only 0.96. The study from the Netherlands identified a history of recent smoking and hypercholesterolemia as both independent factors for myocardial infarction (Aleman et al. 2007). These findings emphasize the importance of minimizing underlying cardiac risk factors (e.g., lipid screening, controlling hyperlipidemia and hypertension, smoking cessation, weight control, enhanced physical activity, and diet modification) in HL survivors, and also help identify high-risk patients for screening and intervention.

14.3.2.5 Cardiac Follow-Up Guidelines

Currently, expert opinion- and consensus-based guidelines for cardiac follow-up are available for cancer survivors at increased risk for cardiac complications. The Children's Oncology Group (COG) guidelines recommend baseline and periodic screening with echocardiogram and MUGA scans after exposure to anthracyclines (Children's Oncology Group 2008). For patients treated with chest irradiation, the COG guidelines recommend fasting blood glucose, a lipid profile every 3–5 years, as well as baseline and periodic echocardiograms. For survivors of HL, the National Comprehensive Cancer Network (NCCN) recommends annual blood pressure, serum glucose, and lipid screening, and suggests that baseline stress test/echocardiogram should be considered at 10 years of follow-up (National Comprehensive Cancer Network 2009).

14.3.3 Noncoronary Vascular Complications

Emerging data describe the risk of noncoronary vascular disease as a late complication after HL therapy. In a retrospective review of 415 HL patients who were at least 2 years out from treatment, Hull et al. reported an actuarial incidence of noncoronary atherosclerotic disease (including stroke, transient ischemic attack, carotid artery stenosis, and subclavian artery stenosis) of 2% at 5 years, 3% at 10 years, and 7% at 20 years, respectively (Hull et al. 2003). A significant radiation dose–response was observed. The median dose to the low neck was significantly higher in patients who developed subclavian artery stenosis than those who did not (44 and 36 Gy, respectively, $p = 0.002$). Similarly, the median dose to the low neck was 38 Gy among patients who developed carotid artery stenosis and 36 Gy in patients in whom this endpoint was not detected (p = 0.05). In addition, both hypertension (p = 0.003) and diabetes mellitus (p = 0.001) were significant independent factors associated with noncoronary atherosclerotic disease in this population. A report from the Childhood Cancer Survivor Study examined the incidence of stroke in survivors of pediatric HL (Bowers et al. 2005). Compared with siblings, there was a 5.6-fold higher risk of stroke in survivors of HL who received mantle radiation therapy. The median dose to the mantle field in survivors who developed a stroke was 40 Gy. Unlike the study by Hull et al., hypertension and diabetes mellitus did not significantly increase the risk of stroke, but a history of smoking was a significant predictor of stroke (OR = 3.37, p = 0.026). It is important to note, however, that modern approaches to HL therapy employ lower radiation doses, smaller fields, and planning techniques that limit dose inhomogeneity and hot spots commonly seen in the neck area with older techniques. It is therefore anticipated that noncoronary vascular complications will be less of a concern in more recently treated patients.

References

Adams MJ, Lipsitz SR, Colan SD et al (2004) Cardiovascular status in long-term survivors of Hodgkin's disease treated with chest radiotherapy. J Clin Oncol 22:3139–3148

Advani R, Hoppe R, Rosenberg SA et al (2006) Incidence of secondary leukemia/myelodysplasia (AML/MDS) in Hodgkin's disease (HD) with three generations of therapy at Stanford University. J Clin Oncol 24:426

Aleman BM, van den Belt-Dusebout AW, Klokman WJ et al (2003) Long-term cause-specific mortality of patients treated for Hodgkin's disease. J Clin Oncol 21:3431–3439

Aleman BM, van den Belt-Dusebout AW, De Bruin ML et al (2007) Late cardiotoxicity after treatment for Hodgkin lymphoma. Blood 109:1878–1886

Anselmo AP, Cartoni C, Bellantuono P et al (1990) Risk of infertility in patients with Hodgkin's disease treated with ABVD vs MOPP vs ABVD/MOPP. Haematologica 75:155–158

Arseneau JC, Sponzo RW, Levin DL et al (1972) Nonlymphomatous malignant tumors complicating Hodgkin's disease. Possible association with intensive therapy. N Engl J Med 287:1119–1122

Aviles A, Neri N, Nambo JM et al (2005) Late cardiac toxicity secondary to treatment in Hodgkin's disease. A study comparing doxorubicin, epirubicin and mitoxantrone in combined therapy. Leuk Lymphoma 46:1023–1028

Behringer K, Josting A, Schiller P et al (2004) Solid tumors in patients treated for Hodgkin's disease: a report from the German Hodgkin Lymphoma Study Group. Ann Oncol 15:1079–1085

Behringer K, Breuer K, Reineke T et al (2005) Secondary amenorrhea after Hodgkin's lymphoma is influenced by age at treatment, stage of disease, chemotherapy regimen, and the use of oral contraceptives during therapy: a report from the German Hodgkin's Lymphoma Study Group. J Clin Oncol 23:7555–7564

Bhatia S, Ramsay NK, Bantle JP et al (1996) Thyroid abnormalities after therapy for Hodgkin's disease in childhood. Oncologist 1:62–67

Boivin JF, Hutchison GB, Lubin JH et al (1992) Coronary artery disease mortality in patients treated for Hodgkin's disease. Cancer 69:1241–1247

Bonadonna G, Bonfante V, Viviani S et al (2004) ABVD plus subtotal nodal versus involved-field radiotherapy in early-stage Hodgkin's disease: long-term results. J Clin Oncol 22:2835–2841

Bowers DC, McNeil DE, Liu Y et al (2005) Stroke as a late treatment effect of Hodgkin's Disease: a report from the Childhood Cancer Survivor Study. J Clin Oncol 23:6508–6515

Bucher JA, Fleming TJ, Fuller LM et al (1988) Preliminary observations on the effect of mantle field radiotherapy on salivary flow rates in patients with Hodgkin's disease. J Dent Res 67:518–521

Carmel RJ, Kaplan HS (1976) Mantle irradiation in Hodgkin's disease. An analysis of technique, tumor eradication, and complications. Cancer 37:2813–2825

Children's Oncology Group (2008) Long-Term Follow-Up Guidelines for Survivors of Childhood, Adolescent, and Young Adult Cancers Version 3.0. www.survivorshipguidelines.org

Clifton DK, Bremner WJ (1983) The effect of testicular x-irradiation on spermatogenesis in man. A comparison with the mouse. J Androl 4:387–392

Constine LS, Donaldson SS, McDougall IR et al (1984) Thyroid dysfunction after radiotherapy in children with Hodgkin's disease. Cancer 53:878–883

Cosset JM, Henry-Amar M, Pellae-Cosset B et al (1991) Pericarditis and myocardial infarctions after Hodgkin's disease therapy. Int J Radiat Oncol Biol Phys 21:447–449

Das P, Ng AK, Earle CC et al (2006) Computed tomography screening for lung cancer in Hodgkin's lymphoma survivors: decision analysis and cost-effectiveness analysis. Ann Oncol 17:785–793

De Bruin ML, Huisbrink J, Hauptmann M et al (2008) Treatment-related risk factors for premature menopause following Hodgkin lymphoma. Blood 111:101–108

Diehl V, Franklin J, Pfreundschuh M et al (2003) Standard and increased-dose BEACOPP chemotherapy compared with COPP-ABVD for advanced Hodgkin's disease. N Engl J Med 348:2386–2395

Dores GM, Metayer C, Curtis RE et al (2002) Second malignant neoplasms among long-term survivors of Hodgkin's disease: A population-based evaluation over 25 years. J Clin Oncol 20:3484–3494

Engert A, Schiller P, Josting A et al (2003) Involved-field radiotherapy is equally effective and less toxic compared with extended-field radiotherapy after four cycles of chemotherapy in patients with early-stage unfavorable Hodgkin's lymphoma: results of the HD8 trial of the German Hodgkin's Lymphoma Study Group. J Clin Oncol 21:3601–3608

Engert A, Diehl V, Franklin J et al (2009) Escalated-dose BEACOPP in the treatment of patients with advanced-stage Hodgkin's lymphoma: 10 years of follow-up of the GHSG HD9 study. J Clin Oncol 27:4548–4554

Eriksson F, Gagliardi G, Liedberg A et al (2000) Long-term cardiac mortality following radiation therapy for Hodgkin's disease: analysis with the relative seriality model. Radiother Oncol 55:153–162

Esik O, Csere T, Stefanits K et al (2003a) A review on radiogenic Lhermitte's sign. Pathol Oncol Res 9:115–120

Esik O, Csere T, Stefanits K et al (2003b) Increased metabolic activity in the spinal cord of patients with long-standing Lhermitte's sign. Strahlenther Onkol 179:690–693

Ferme C, Eghbali H, Meerwaldt JH et al (2007) Chemotherapy plus involved-field radiation in early-stage Hodgkin's disease. N Engl J Med 357:1916–1927

Franklin J, Pluetschow A, Paus M et al (2006) Second malignancy risk associated with treatment of Hodgkin's lymphoma: meta-analysis of the randomised trials. Ann Oncol 17:1749–1760

Friedman DL, Constine LS (2006) Late effects of treatment for Hodgkin lymphoma. J Natl Compr Canc Netw 4:249–257

Ghalibafian M, Beaudre A, Girinsky T (2008) Heart and coronary artery protection in patients with mediastinal Hodgkin lymphoma treated with intensity-modulated radiotherapy: dose constraints to virtual volumes or to organs at risk? Radiother Oncol 87:82–88

Girinsky T, Ghalibafian M (2005) Radiation treatment in non Hodgkin's lymphomas: present and future directions. Cancer Radiother 9:422–426

Girinsky T, Pichenot C, Beaudre A et al (2006a) Is intensity-modulated radiotherapy better than conventional radiation treatment and three-dimensional conformal radiotherapy for mediastinal masses in patients with Hodgkin's disease, and is there a role for beam orientation optimization and dose constraints assigned to virtual volumes? Int J Radiat Oncol Biol Phys 64:218–226

Girinsky T, van der Maazen R, Specht L et al (2006b) Involved-node radiotherapy (INRT) in patients with early Hodgkin lymphoma: concepts and guidelines. Radiother Oncol 79:270–277

Glanzmann C, Kaufmann P, Jenni R et al (1998) Cardiac risk after mediastinal irradiation for Hodgkin's disease. Radiother Oncol 46:51–62

Hancock SL, Cox RS, McDougall IR (1991) Thyroid diseases after treatment of Hodgkin's disease. N Engl J Med 325:599–605

Hancock SL, Donaldson SS, Hoppe RT (1993a) Cardiac disease following treatment of Hodgkin's disease in children and adolescents. J Clin Oncol 11:1208–1215

Hancock SL, Tucker MA, Hoppe RT (1993b) Factors affecting late mortality from heart disease after treatment of Hodgkin's disease. JAMA 270:1949–1955

Heidenreich PA, Hancock SL, Lee BK et al (2003) Asymptomatic cardiac disease following mediastinal irradiation. J Am Coll Cardiol 42:743–749

Heidenreich PA, Hancock SL, Vagelos RH et al (2005) Diastolic dysfunction after mediastinal irradiation. Am Heart J 150:977–982

Heidenreich PA, Schnittger I, Strauss HW et al (2007) Screening for coronary artery disease after mediastinal irradiation for Hodgkin's disease. J Clin Oncol 25:43–49

Henry-Amar M, Hayat M, Meerwaldt JH et al (1990) Causes of death after therapy for early stage Hodgkin's disease entered on EORTC protocols. EORTC Lymphoma Cooperative Group. Int J Radiat Oncol Biol Phys 19:1155–1157

Hill DA, Gilbert E, Dores GM et al (2005) Breast cancer risk following radiotherapy for Hodgkin lymphoma: modification by other risk factors. Blood 106:3358–3365

Hirsch A, Vander EN, Straus DJ et al (1996) Effect of ABVD chemotherapy with and without mantle or mediastinal irradiation on pulmonary function and symptoms in early-stage Hodgkin's disease. J Clin Oncol 14:1297–1305

Hodgson DC, Gilbert ES, Dores GM et al (2007a) Long-term solid cancer risk among 5-year survivors of Hodgkin's lymphoma. J Clin Oncol 25:1489–1497

Hodgson DC, Pintilie M, Gitterman L et al (2007b) Fertility among female hodgkin lymphoma survivors attempting pregnancy following ABVD chemotherapy. Hematol Oncol 25:11–15

Hoppe RT (1997) Hodgkin's disease: complications of therapy and excess mortality. Ann Oncol 8(Suppl 1):115–118

Horning SJ, Adhikari A, Rizk N et al (1994) Effect of treatment for Hodgkin's disease on pulmonary function: results of a prospective study. J Clin Oncol 12:297–305

Hull MC, Morris CG, Pepine CJ et al (2003) Valvular dysfunction and carotid, subclavian, and coronary artery disease in survivors of hodgkin lymphoma treated with radiation therapy. JAMA 290:2831–2837

Kaldor JM, Day NE, Clarke EA et al (1990) Leukemia following Hodgkin's disease. N Engl J Med 322:7–13

Keene HJ, Fleming TJ, Toth BB (1994) Cariogenic microflora in patients with Hodgkin's disease before and after mantle field radiotherapy. Oral Surg Oral Med Oral Pathol 78:577–582

Koh ES, Sun A, Tran TH et al (2006) Clinical dose-volume histogram analysis in predicting radiation pneumonitis in Hodgkin's lymphoma. Int J Radiat Oncol Biol Phys 66:223–228

Koh ES, Tran TH, Heydarian M et al (2007) A comparison of mantle versus involved-field radiotherapy for Hodgkin's lymphoma: reduction in normal tissue dose and second cancer risk. Radiat Oncol 2:13

Lewanski CR, Sinclair JA, Stewart JS (2000) Lhermitte's sign following head and neck radiotherapy. Clin Oncol (R Coll Radiol) 12:98–103

Lushbaugh CC, Casarett GW (1976) The effects of gonadal irradiation in clinical radiation therapy: a review. Cancer 37:1111–1125

Mauch P, Ng A, Aleman B et al (2005) Report from the Rockefellar Foundation Sponsored International Workshop on reducing mortality and improving quality of life in long-term survivors of Hodgkin's disease: July 9–16, 2003, Bellagio, Italy. Eur J Haematol Suppl 75:68–76

Meistrich ML (1993) Effects of chemotherapy and radiotherapy on spermatogenesis. Eur Urol 23:136–141

National Comprehensive Cancer Network (2009) Clinical Practice Guidelines in Oncology. www.nccn.org

Ng AK, Bernardo MP, Weller E et al (2002a) Long-term survival and competing causes of death in patients with early-stage Hodgkin's disease treated at age 50 or younger. J Clin Oncol 20:2101–2108

Ng AK, Bernardo MVP, Weller E et al (2002b) Second malignancy after Hodgkin disease treated with radiation therapy with or without chemotherapy: long-term risks and risk factors. Blood 100:1989–1996

Ogilvy-Stuart AL, Shalet SM (1993) Effect of radiation on the human reproductive system. Environ Health Perspect 101(Suppl 2):109–116

Rueffer U, Josting A, Franklin J et al (2001) Non-Hodgkin's lymphoma after primary Hodgkin's disease in the German Hodgkin's Lymphoma Study Group: incidence, treatment, and prognosis. J Clin Oncol 19:2026–2032

Saslow D, Boetes C, Burke W et al (2007) American Cancer Society guidelines for breast screening with MRI as an adjunct to mammography. CA Cancer J Clin 57:75–89

Schonfeld SJ, Gilbert ES, Dores GM et al (2006) Acute myeloid leukemia following Hodgkin lymphoma: a population-based study of 35, 511 patients. J Natl Cancer Inst 98:215–218

Sieniawski M, Reineke T, Nogova L et al (2008) Fertility in male patients with advanced Hodgkin lymphoma treated with BEACOPP: a report of the German Hodgkin Study Group (GHSG). Blood 111:71–76

Sklar C, Whitton J, Mertens A et al (2000) Abnormalities of the thyroid in survivors of Hodgkin's disease: data from the Childhood Cancer Survivor Study. J Clin Endocrinol Metab 85:3227–3232

Sklar CA, Mertens AC, Mitby P et al (2006) Premature menopause in survivors of childhood cancer: a report from the childhood cancer survivor study. J Natl Cancer Inst 98:890–896

Swerdlow AJ, Barber JA, Hudson GV et al (2000) Risk of second malignancy after Hodgkin's disease in a collaborative British cohort: the relation to age at treatment. J Clin Oncol 18:498–509

Swerdlow AJ, Schoemaker MJ, Allerton R et al (2001) Lung cancer after Hodgkin's disease: a nested case-control study of the relation to treatment. J Clin Oncol 19:1610–1618

Swerdlow AJ, Higgins CD, Smith P et al (2007) Myocardial infarction mortality risk after treatment for Hodgkin disease: a collaborative British cohort study. J Natl Cancer Inst 99:206–214

Tarbell NJ, Thompson L, Mauch P (1990) Thoracic irradiation in Hodgkin's disease: disease control and long-term complications. Int J Radiat Oncol Biol Phys 18:275–281

Travis LB (2002) Therapy-associated solid tumors. Acta Oncol 41:323–333

Travis LB, Gospodarowicz M, Curtis RE et al (2002) Lung cancer following chemotherapy and radiotherapy for Hodgkin's disease. J Natl Cancer Inst 94:182–192

Travis LB, Hill DA, Dores GM et al (2003) Breast cancer following radiotherapy and chemotherapy among young women with Hodgkin disease. JAMA – J Am Med Assoc 290:465–475

Tura S, Fiacchini M, Zinzani PL et al (1993) Splenectomy and the increasing risk of secondary acute leukemia in Hodgkin's disease. J Clin Oncol 11:925–930

van der Kaaij MA, Heutte N, Le SN et al (2007) Gonadal function in males after chemotherapy for early-stage Hodgkin's lymphoma treated in four subsequent trials by the European Organisation for Research and Treatment of Cancer: EORTC Lymphoma Group and the Groupe d'Etude des Lymphomes de l'Adulte. J Clin Oncol 25:2825–2832

van Leeuwen FE, Somers R, Hart AA (1987) Splenectomy in Hodgkin's disease and second leukaemias. Lancet 2:210–211

van Leeuwen FE, Chorus AM, Belt-Dusebout AW et al (1994) Leukemia risk following Hodgkin's disease: relation to cumulative dose of alkylating agents, treatment with teniposide combinations, number of episodes of chemotherapy, and bone marrow damage. J Clin Oncol 12:1063–1073

van Leeuwen FE, Klokman WJ, Veer MB et al (2000) Long-term risk of second malignancy in survivors of Hodgkin's disease treated during adolescence or young adulthood. J Clin Oncol 18:487–497

van Leeuwen FE, Klokman WJ, Stovall M et al (2003) Roles of radiation dose, chemotherapy, and hormonal factors in breast cancer following Hodgkin's disease. J Natl Cancer Inst 95:971–980

van Rijswijk RE, Verbeek J, Haanen C et al (1987) Major complications and causes of death in patients treated for Hodgkin's disease. J Clin Oncol 5:1624–1633

Viviani S, Santoro A, Ragni G et al (1985) Gonadal toxicity after combination chemotherapy for Hodgkin's disease. Comparative results of MOPP vs ABVD. Eur J Cancer Clin Oncol 21:601–605

Wallace WH, Shalet SM, Hendry JH et al (1989) Ovarian failure following abdominal irradiation in childhood: the radiosensitivity of the human oocyte. Br J Radiol 62:995–998

Wallace WH, Thomson AB, Saran F et al (2005) Predicting age of ovarian failure after radiation to a field that includes the ovaries. Int J Radiat Oncol Biol Phys 62:738–744

Williams RS, Mendenhall N (1992) Laparoscopic oophoropexy for preservation of ovarian function before pelvic node irradiation. Obstet Gynecol 80:541–543

Williams RS, Littell RD, Mendenhall' NP (1999) Laparoscopic oophoropexy and ovarian function in the treatment of Hodgkin disease. Cancer 86:2138–2142

15 Proton Therapy for Hodgkin Lymphoma

Bradford Hoppe, Roelf Slopsema, and Lena Specht

Contents

B. Hoppe (✉) and R. Slopsema
University of Florida Proton Therapy Institute, 2015 N. Jefferson St, Jacksonville, FL 32206, USA
e-mail: bhoppe@floridaproton.org; slopsema@ufl.edu

L. Specht
Departments of Oncology and Haematology, The Finsen Centre, Rigshospitalet, University of Copenhagen, 9 Blegdamsvej, 2100 Copenhagen, Denmark
e-mail: specht@dadlnet.dk

15.1 Introduction to Proton Therapy

Even though proton therapy has been used in clinical medicine since the late 1950s and early 1960s, its use has been significantly restricted due to the limited number of proton facilities around the world. Before 1990, there were about 10 facilities in the world treating patients, but currently there are more than 30 either in operation or under construction worldwide (including five operational in the USA with more than five under construction). This growth in proton therapy facilities has developed out of an interest to safely escalate radiation doses while reducing toxicity and improving cure rates in some cancers as well as reducing the amount of normal tissue irradiated in cancers with high cure rates where the late toxicities from treatment may present a problem.

Proton therapy is an exciting treatment approach in radiation oncology. Although the relative biologic effectiveness (RBE), oxygen enhancement ratio (OER), and linear transfer energy (LET) of protons (RBE = 1.1, OER = 2.5–3) are similar to 250 kV X-rays, the proton's unique properties produce a depth–dose curve that is distinctly different from that of a photon. Due to the proton's large mass (about 1,800 times the electron mass) and positive charge, the dose deposited by a monoenergetic proton beam remains quite flat until it gets close to the end of its range at which point the dose increases steeply, peaks, and then ends abruptly. The high-dose peak over which the majority of the dose is dispersed is referred to as the Bragg peak. The ≥90% isodose width of the Bragg peak is typically 4–7 mm, depending on the energy of the proton beam.

The limited width of the Bragg peak, in and of itself, is not very useful, unless the tumor is just a few

L. Specht and J. Yahalom (eds.), *Radiotherapy for Hodgkin Lymphoma*,
DOI: 10.1007/978-3-540-78944-4_15, © Springer-Verlag Berlin Heidelberg 2011

millimeter in length; however, by adding peaks of different energy physicists can produce a "spread-out Bragg peak" (SOBP) with a uniform dose extending over a larger region. Each of the peaks is shifted in depth (typically 6–8 mm) and given a "weight" (number of protons) so that the sum of all peaks produces a flat dose distribution. By adding more or less peaks the extent of the uniform region ("modulation width") can be adjusted depending on the target length. As a result, a typical proton beam disperses a low dose of radiation as it enters the patient, increases the dose distribution just proximal to the tumor where the SOBP is calculated to begin, and continues to distribute the dose throughout the length of the tumor until just distal to the tumor where the SOBP is calculated to stop and from which no further dose passes through the medium (i.e., the patient's body). This type of treatment which leads to virtually no exit dose of radiotherapy can be strategically utilized to significantly reduce the dose to non-targeted tissue and lessen both the acute and late side effects of treatment. Figure 15.1a shows the depth–dose curve in water for a 147 MeV proton beam with the Bragg peak at 15 cm. Figure 15.1b shows the creation of an SOBP by addition of five Bragg peaks with decreasing energy and weight. The resulting uniform-dose region extends about 4 cm in depth.

Proton beams with energy between 70 and 230 MeV, which correspond to a range in water of 4–33 cm, are of

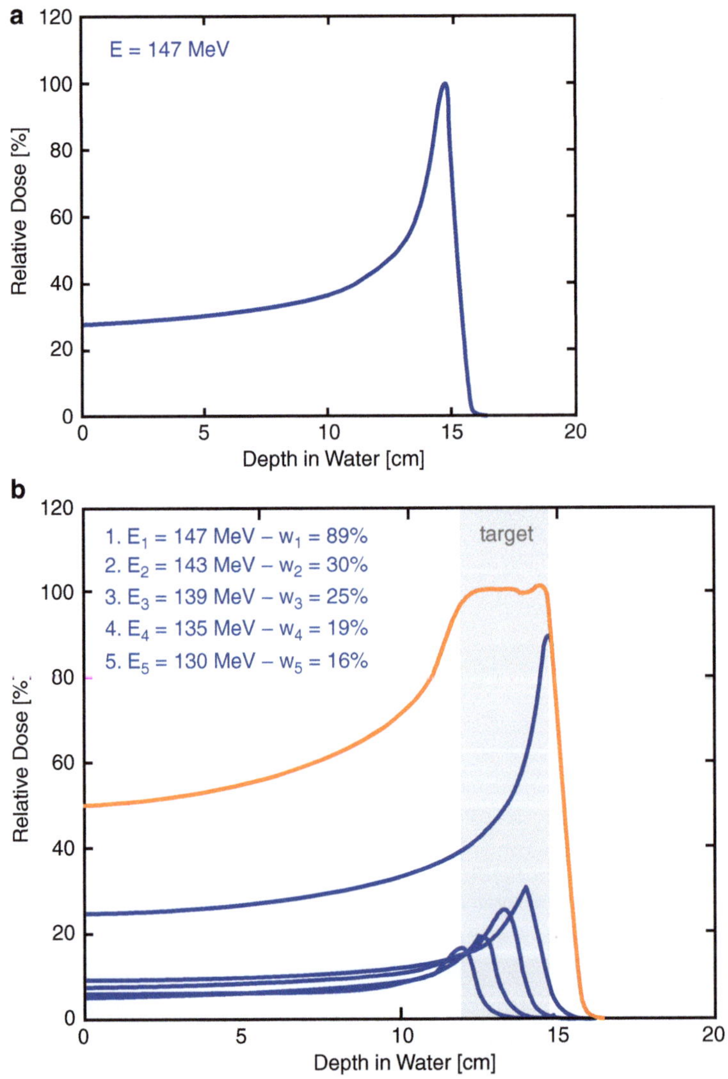

Fig. 15.1 (**a**) Percentage depth–dose curve for a 147MeV proton beam in water. This 'Bragg peak' has a range of 15cm. (**b**) Generation of a spread-out Bragg peak (SOBP) by summation of five Bragg peaks, sequentially shifted 6 mm in depth and decreased in weight. The resulting uniform-dose region covers about 3.5 cm in depth

particular interest to clinical radiation oncology. The protons are accelerated either by a cyclotron or a synchrotron and directed into one of the gantry or fixed-beam rooms (one accelerator may deliver protons in up to five separate rooms) for patient treatment. Once the beam has entered the room, the small diameter of the beam is spread out laterally through a "scattering" technique or by way of a "scanning" technique. A lengthy description of these various techniques is beyond the scope of this chapter, however, it suffices to point out that there are pro's and con's to each technique. The scattering technique utilizes a target (typically lead) to scatter the proton beam to a large-enough area to be useful for treatment. Following the scattering of the beam a field-specific brass aperture gives the beam its final shape before entering the patient. A field-specific range compensator (made of Lucite or wax) degrades the beam energy as function of lateral position, conforming the dose to the distal end of the target. An unfortunate consequence of the "scattering" technique is that neutrons are produced in the scattering elements of the treatment head as well as in the brass aperture. Neutrons are concerning because of their large RBE, which raises concerns of risks of late toxicities in patients, specifically, secondary malignancies. The amount of neutrons produced is still in debate and further investigation is needed before final conclusions can be drawn. Scanning beam technique utilizes magnets to shape the field. A small "pencil beam" is scanned over the target, eliminating the need of a beam scattering target and the brass aperture,[1] therefore significantly reducing the amount of neutrons produced. In addition, no range compensator is required, since the beam can be conformed to the target at different depths. The proton fluence can be optimized both as function of lateral position and energy which enables the delivery of intensity-modulated proton therapy (IMPT). IMPT optimizes the dose to the target using multiple fields and can deliver a more conformal dose distribution even to concave structures. Unfortunately, this technique is still in its infancy and requires further investigation, due to sensitivities to tumor movement (especially during respiration), which can lead to much higher dose uncertainties compared with the scattering technique.

[1] A simpler scanning technique (uniform scanning) scans the beam into a rectangular uniform dose distribution and still requires an aperture and range compensator to conform the dose to the target.

15.2 Rationale for Proton Therapy in Hodgkin Lymphoma

Due to the young age at diagnosis and excellent outcomes for patients with HL treated with a combined-modality approach, the major focus for researchers has been in identifying treatment-related late toxicities and finding ways of reducing them. One of the largest studies analyzing this issue was the Childhood Cancer Survivor Study by Oeffinger et al., which looked at the outcome of 10,397 survivors of childhood cancer (18% with HL) and compared them with over 3,000 siblings (Oeffinger et al. 2006). In this study, they found that survivors of HL were one of the three groups at the greatest risk of severe or life-threatening chronic health conditions and specifically were at the highest risk of developing a second cancer and heart disease. Additionally, associated with standard treatment of irradiation of the chest with either bleomycin or an anthracycline, they were at the highest risk of developing a Grade 3 or 4 chronic toxicity (relative risk = 13).

Researchers have evaluated how to minimize these often devastating toxicities by modifying the treatment techniques in patients with HL by changing the chemotherapy and reducing the radiation dose or field size, while maintaining high levels of disease control and survival. Constine et al. and Leeuwen et al. reported that lower radiation doses were associated with a lower risk of developing secondary cancers without compromising disease control (Constine et al. 2008; van Leeuwen et al. 2003). Additionally, Hancock et al. revealed that decreasing the dose to the heart by adding a heart block decreased "non-myocardial infarction" cardiac deaths (Hancock et al. 1993). Ng et al. and Behringer et al., on the other hand, showed a reduction in secondary malignancies when the field size decreased from an extended field to an involved field (Behringer et al. 2004; Ng et al. 2002). Radiobiological modeling studies predict very substantial reductions in the risk of secondary malignancies from reductions in radiation volumes and doses (Hodgson et al. 2007). The risk of cardiovascular disease also increases significantly with the radiation dose and the irradiated heart volume (Adams et al. 2003). Recently, Campbell et al. reported the disease-specific outcomes of field reduction from extended field to involved field to involved node all following standard chemotherapy, and showed that control rates and survival rates were equivalent regardless of field size, although longer follow-up is still required to determine whether the field reductions translate into fewer late toxicities (Campbell et al. 2008).

Another treatment strategy that has been proposed for reducing radiation-related toxicities uses more complex radiation-field designs and respiratory gating to try and minimize the radiation dose to normal tissues while maintaining appropriate nodal coverage. Researchers have shown in selected patients that the dose to the lungs, esophagus, heart, and coronary arteries could be reduced by using more conformal methods like intensity-modulated radiation therapy (IMRT) (Girinsky et al. 2006; Goodman et al. 2005; Loo and Hoppe 2005; Nieder et al. 2007a). Unfortunately, IMRT comes at the price of spreading out the low-dose region, encompassing a large volume of normal tissue (the integral dose), which could place the patients at a higher risk of secondary malignancies (Nieder et al. 2007b; Schneider et al. 2000; Sigurdson et al. 2005). In fact, studies have shown that doses as low as 4 Gy can be associated with an increased risk of secondary solid tumors in Hodgkin lymphoma survivors (Nieder et al. 2007b; Schneider et al. 2000; Sigurdson et al. 2005; Travis et al. 2002; Travis et al. 2003). A possible solution to this problem is proton therapy.

15.3 Dosimetry for Supradiaphragmatic Hodgkin Lymphoma

The supradiaphragmatic region is the most common site for HL to present. This region includes many critical structures, such as the salivary glands, thyroid gland, esophagus, heart, lungs, spinal cord, breasts, as well as critical arteries and veins, that have traditionally been affected both by acute and late side effects from treatment. In a conventional involved-field radiotherapy AP/PA plan, large portions of these critical normal structures are needlessly irradiated by photons as they exit the tumor and pass through distal structures before exiting the body. For example, to cover an anterior pericardial lymph node, the beam may need to exit through the entire heart (including the coronary vessels), part of the lung, esophagus, vertebral body (bone marrow storage), and the spinal cord. However, with the use of protons, a more limited beam can be used that stops just past the targeted region, sparing the spinal cord, esophagus, aorta, lung, and the posterior aspects of the heart and pericardium. The dosimetric benefit with proton therapy has been explored and reported for mantle-field irradiation as well as in supradiaphragmantic involved-nodal-field design.

Schneider et al. performed a study comparing the dosimetric outcomes of a conventional AP/PA photon plan, 9-field IMRT plan, 1-field proton plan, and a 9-field IMPT plan (Schneider et al. 2000). Furthermore, the investigators attempted to predict the secondary cancer rate based on the dosimetry of the various plans and yielded a result favoring the proton plans. Specifically, with 100% PTV coverage, the two proton plans had the lowest mean dose to the total body, liver, breasts, spinal cord, lung, and vertebral body compared to either the IMRT or AP/PA photon plans. They also saw lower mean doses to the heart, thyroid gland, and esophagus with the proton plan compared with the AP/PA photon plan. The subsequent calculated secondary cancer risk was reduced by 50% as a result of using protons compared with photons in this study. More specifically, the one-field proton plan alone could potentially reduce the breast cancer incidence by a factor of 10 compared to the AP/PA photon plan.

In a recent dosimetric study by Chera et al., nine consecutive patients who were treated at the University of Florida with a conventional AP/PA photon plan were replanned to be treated with either involved-nodal radiotherapy with conventional AP/PA photons, IMRT, or 3D-conformal protons with 100% of the prescription dose covering 95% of the planning target volume (PTV; Fig. 15.2a–c) (Chera et al. 2009).

A pairwise comparison of the conventional AP/PA photon plan with the 3D-conformal proton plan revealed a significant reduction in the volume of the body receiving ≥4, ≥10, ≥16, ≥24, and ≥30 Gy as well as the mean total body dose when treated with protons. In the comparison of IMRT with proton therapy, the volume of the body receiving ≥4 Gy as well as the mean total body dose was significantly reduced with proton therapy. When evaluating the percentage of the lung exposed to various radiation doses, protons significantly reduced the amount of lung receiving ≥4, ≥10, and ≥16 Gy as well as the mean lung dose compared with the conventional AP/PA photon plans. When compared with IMRT, the proton plan significantly reduced the mean lung dose as well as the percent of lung receiving ≥4 and ≥10 Gy. Furthermore, when evaluating breast dose, the proton plan

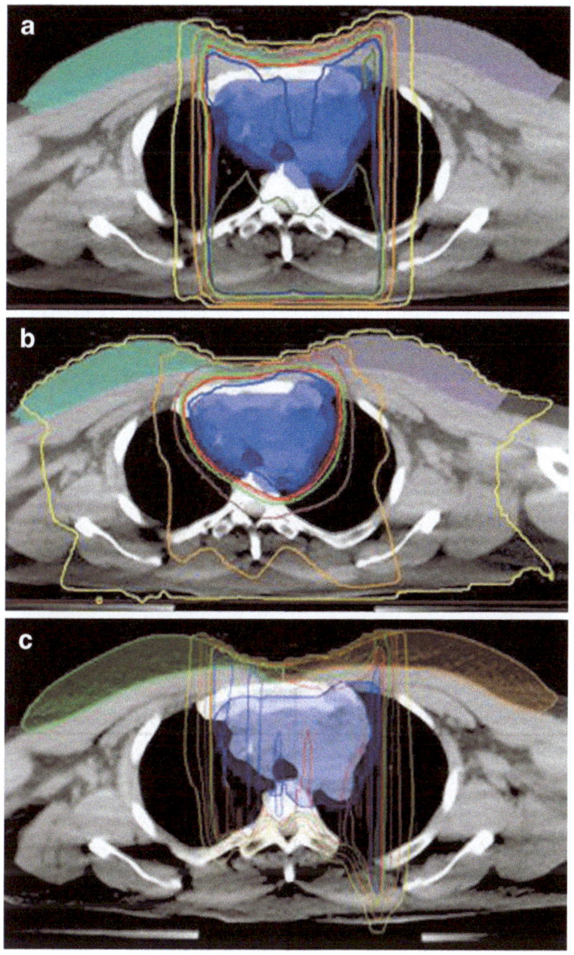

Fig. 15.2 (**a**–**c**) CT axial images through the middle of the planning target volume (*shaded blue*) in the mediastinum demonstrating isodose distribution for conventional photon radiotherapy (RT), intensity-modulated radiotherapy (IMRT), and three-dimensional proton therapy plans. (**a**–**c**) Isodose lines include: blue (105%), red (100%), green (95%), brown (80%), orange (50%), and yellow (10%) (Reprinted with permission from Chera et al. 2009)

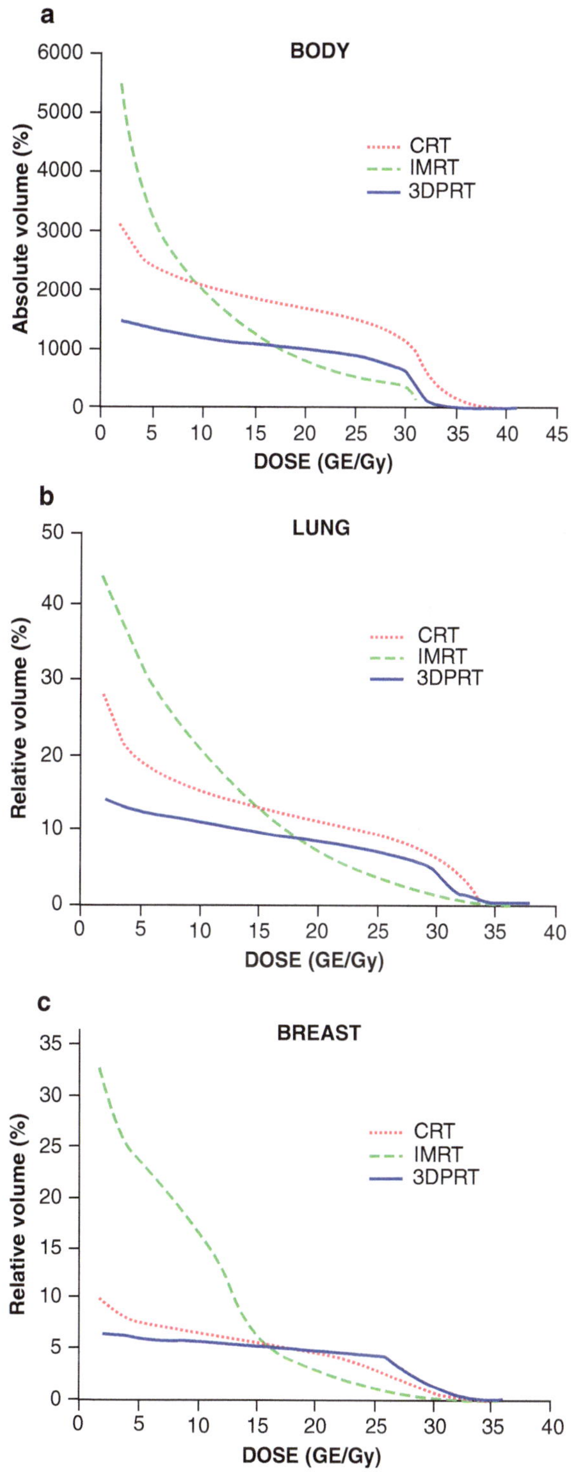

Fig. 15.3 (**a**–**c**) Dose volume histograms of total body (**a**), lung (**b**), and breast (**c**) for conventional radiotherapy (*red dotted line*), intensity-modulated radiotherapy (*green dashed line*), and three-dimensional proton therapy (*blue solid line*) (Reprinted with permission from Chera et al. 2009)

significantly reduced the mean breast dose compared with either the conventional AP/PA photon plan or the IMRT plan. Figure 15.3 shows the comparison of DVHs or the different modalities for total body (a), lung (b), and breast (c).

Based on this retrospective dosimetry study, the University of Florida now has a prospective dosimetric/clinical study open for stage IA–IIIB classical HL with mediastinal involvement, where, depending on the final treatment plans, the patient will be treated accordingly (AP/PA photon plan, IMRT, or 3D-PRT plan) and followed for disease-specific outcomes and treatment toxicities. The primary objective of the study is to evaluate whether protons can reduce the amount of normal tissue exposed to carcinogenic doses of radiation (>4 Gy), although other dosimetric outcomes will be evaluated as secondary objectives.

15.4 Dosimetry for Infradiaphragmatic Hodgkin Lymphoma

The infradiaphragmatic region also includes a number of important critical organs, although the dosimetric benefits with protons for sparing these organs have not been as thoroughly explored. This lack of research may be somewhat due to the unpredictable movement of bowel and gastric distention, which could dramatically affect the range of an anterior proton field. A posterior proton field approach, however, might be utilized and, while it would not spare the bone marrow or cord, could potentially spare the anterior structures in the abdomen and pelvis, such as the stomach, duodenum, small and large intestines, pancreas, liver, uterus, or ovaries. In fact, Kirsch et al. reported on a case of a 14-year-old girl with stage IVA HL involving the sacrum who received chemotherapy and then received consolidation proton therapy to the sacrum to reduce the amount of normal tissue exposed to radiation (Fig. 15.4) (Kirsch et al. 2005)

15.5 Dosimetry for Total Nodal Irradiation

Although the popularity of total nodal irradiation (TNI) for definitive management of HL has faded with the improved outcomes and lower toxicities observed with combined-modality approaches that include involved-field radiotherapy techniques, there are still some circumstances that warrant TNI. As a result, it is worth discussing what may have been one of the first papers to explore the role of proton therapy in HL patients from Archambeau et al. published in 1974 (Archambeau et al. 1974). In this study, a dosimetric comparison of a conventional X-ray TNI plan is compared with a proton plan. With the use of an anterior beam for the thorax, the group reports being able to spare the bone marrow within the thoracic spine, while encompassing the mediastinal disease. In the abdomen, the posterior beam allowed sparing of the bowel anterior to the involved lymph node groups. They concluded that proton therapy allows a threefold reduction in the irradiated volume of normal tissue while achieving appropriate coverage of the region at interest. Furthermore, through the sparing of bone marrow and reduction of side effects from treatment, it was hypothesized that the typical split course of treatment for TNI (treatment of a mantle field followed by a short break followed by treatment of the inverted Y) could be eliminated and that patients could tolerate a full-course treatment all at once.

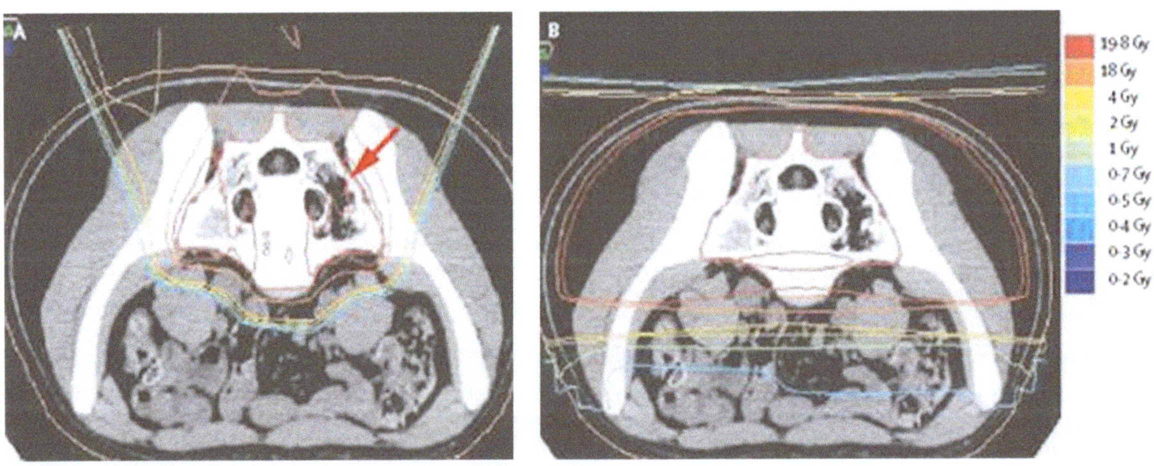

Fig. 15.4 CT axial images through the sacrum demonstrating isodose distribution for three-dimensional proton therapy (*left*) and conventional photon radiotherapy (*right*). (Reprinted with permission from Kirsch et al. 2005)

15.6 Conclusion

Proton therapy is an exciting treatment approach that may considerably benefit HL survivors, who have traditionally suffered from the late effects of cancer treatments like cardiotoxic chemotherapy and radiotherapy. Research shows that compared to other recent treatment innovations, proton therapy may help further reduce the amount of normal tissue exposed to radiotherapy and thereby lessen the number of complications that occur in this patient population years later.

References

Adams MJ, Hardenbergh PH, Constine LS et al (2003) Radiation-associated cardiovascular disease. Crit Rev Oncol Hematol 45:55–75

Archambeau JO, Bennett GW, Chen ST (1974) Potential of proton beams for total nodal irradiation. Acta Radiol Ther Phys Biol 13:393–401

Behringer K, Josting A, Schiller P et al (2004) Solid tumors in patients treated for Hodgkin's disease: a report from the German Hodgkin Lymphoma Study Group. Ann Oncol 15:1079–1085

Campbell BA, Voss N, Pickles T et al (2008) Involved-nodal radiation therapy as a component of combination therapy for limited-stage Hodgkin's lymphoma: a question of field size. J Clin Oncol 26:5170–5174

Chera BS, Rodriguez C, Morris CG et al (2009) Dosimetric comparison of three different involved nodal irradiation techniques for stage II Hodgkin's lymphoma patients: conventional radiotherapy, intensity-modulated radiotherapy, and three-dimensional proton radiotherapy. Int J Radiat Oncol Biol Phys 75:1173–1180

Constine LS, Tarbell N, Hudson MM et al (2008) Subsequent malignancies in children treated for Hodgkin's disease: associations with gender and radiation dose. Int J Radiat Oncol Biol Phys 72:24–33

Girinsky T, Pichenot C, Beaudre A et al (2006) Is intensity-modulated radiotherapy better than conventional radiation treatment and three-dimensional conformal radiotherapy for mediastinal masses in patients with Hodgkin's disease, and is there a role for beam orientation optimization and dose constraints assigned to virtual volumes? Int J Radiat Oncol Biol Phys 64:218–226

Goodman KA, Toner S, Hunt M et al (2005) Intensity-modulated radiotherapy for lymphoma involving the mediastinum. Int J Radiat Oncol Biol Phys 62:198–206

Hancock SL, Tucker MA, Hoppe RT (1993) Factors affecting late mortality from heart disease after treatment of Hodgkin's disease. JAMA 270:1949–1955

Hodgson DC, Koh ES, Tran TH et al (2007) Individualized estimates of second cancer risks after contemporary radiation therapy for Hodgkin lymphoma. Cancer 110:2576–2586

Kirsch DG, Ebb DH, Hernandez AH et al (2005) Proton radiotherapy for Hodgkin's disease in the sacrum. Lancet Oncol 6:532–533

Loo BW, Hoppe RT (2005) Hodgkin's disease: case study. In: Mundt AJ, Roeske JC (eds) Intensity modulated radiation therapy – a clinical perspective, 1st edn. BC Decker, Hamilton, Ontario

Ng AK, Bernardo MVP, Weller E et al (2002) Second malignancy after Hodgkin disease treated with radiation therapy with or without chemotherapy: long-term risks and risk factors. Blood 100:1989–1996

Nieder C, Schill S, Kneschaurek P et al (2007a) Comparison of three different mediastinal radiotherapy techniques in female patients: Impact on heart sparing and dose to the breasts. Radiother Oncol 82:301–307

Nieder C, Schill S, Kneschaurek P et al (2007b) Influence of different treatment techniques on radiation dose to the LAD coronary artery. Radiat Oncol 2:20-

Oeffinger KC, Mertens AC, Sklar CA et al (2006) Chronic health conditions in adult survivors of childhood cancer. N Engl J Med 355:1572–1582

Schneider U, Lomax A, Lombriser N (2000) Comparative risk assessment of secondary cancer incidence after treatment of Hodgkin's disease with photon and proton radiation. Radiat Res 154:382–388

Sigurdson AJ, Ronckers CM, Mertens AC et al (2005) Primary thyroid cancer after a first tumour in childhood (the Childhood Cancer Survivor Study): a nested case-control study. Lancet 365:2014–2023

Travis LB, Gospodarowicz M, Curtis RE et al (2002) Lung cancer following chemotherapy and radiotherapy for Hodgkin's disease. J Natl Cancer Inst 94:182–192

Travis LB, Hill DA, Dores GM et al (2003) Breast cancer following radiotherapy and chemotherapy among young women with Hodgkin disease. JAMA 290:465–475

van Leeuwen FE, Klokman WJ, Stovall M et al (2003) Roles of radiation dose, chemotherapy, and hormonal factors in breast cancer following Hodgkin's disease. J Natl Cancer Inst 95:971–980

Future Prospects for Radiotherapy for Hodgkin Lymphoma

16

Lena Specht and Joachim Yahalom

Contents

L. Specht (✉)
Departments of Oncology and Haematology, Finsen Centre, Rigshospitalet, The University of Copenhagen, 9 Blegdamsvej, 2100 Copenhagen, Denmark
e-mail: specht@dadlnet.dk

J. Yahalom
Department of Radiation Oncology, Memorial Sloan-Kettering Cancer Center, 1275 York Ave, New York, NY 10021-6094, USA
e-mail: yahalomj@mskcc.org

16.1 Introduction

Radiotherapy remains the single most effective modality for the treatment of Hodgkin lymphoma (HL). The challenge for the future is to implement radiotherapy in the most rational and intelligent way possible, in order to maximize the benefit while keeping the total burden of long-term complications from the entire treatment program, including all treatment modalities, as low as possible. Research in long-term complications from all treatment modalities, including different chemotherapy regimens and possible future biological therapies, is needed. Quantitative data are required in order to allow the development of mathematical models that can predict with some accuracy the different types of long-term complications from different treatments. This should enable us to choose the optimal treatment strategy in different clinical settings and in different patients. A number of issues are still unresolved.

16.2 Staging

The Ann Arbor staging system was created in a different era, with limited information from imaging studies. It was meant to divide patients into groups with different prognosis depending on the anatomic extent of disease. It mostly reflected radiation-alone treatment results and was influenced by the extended field approach early experience. The limitations of the Ann Arbor system have been recognized for a long time. The regions defined in the Ann Arbor system are quite arbitrary, based mainly on bony landmarks visible on conventional X-ray images, and they were never meant for guidance of radiotherapy planning. Measures

L. Specht and J. Yahalom (eds.), *Radiotherapy for Hodgkin Lymphoma*,
DOI: 10.1007/978-3-540-78944-4_16, © Springer-Verlag Berlin Heidelberg 2011

giving a more accurate reflection of the total lymphoma burden have been introduced (Specht 1996). Today, positron emission tomography with 2-[18F]fluor-2-deoxyglucose (FDG-PET) and CT is used for staging of patients with HL in most centers, usually as a combined PET/CT-scan. It gives a more accurate definition of the localization and volume of lymphoma, and the volume of metabolically active tissue has been shown to be prognostically important (Grow et al. 2005; Hutchings et al. 2005). A staging system taking advantage of modern imaging techniques and incorporating an anatomical description reflecting the continuous distribution of the lymphatic system in the body, would be more helpful in the management of HL in the modern era. Incorporating biological characteristics, e.g., new immunohistochemistry information, into the prognostic evaluation might also yield additional valuable information (Steidl et al. 2010).

In recent years, most study groups that designed prospective studies for HL or developed national guidelines for staging and treatment of HL categorized patients into three groups. The two early-stage (stages I–II) groups favorable and unfavorable are based on the total absence or presence of at least one adverse prognostic factor, respectively. This distinction by the presence of an adverse factor is supported by results of recent trials and allows the reduction of both chemotherapy and radiotherapy in the favorable group and helped the optimization of treatment in unfavorable early-stage ("intermediate group"). While all groups accept bulky disease, presence of B symptoms, and elevated sedimentation rate as adverse prognostic markers in early stage, there is no complete agreement on other adverse factors; for example, the German Hodgkin Study Group (GHSG) considers involvement of three or more nodal sites (based on the aging Ann Arbor map of nodal sites) as a qualifier for an unfavorable group, while the other groups such as the EORTC/GELA will allow a favorable patient to have involvement of three sites. While this difference may sound subtle, it applies to many patients with early-stage disease. With the expected wide acceptance of the recent excellent data of the GHSG HD10 as a standard of care that allows reduction of the recommended treatment for favorable patients to only two cycles of ABVD followed by IFRT of only 20 Gy, patient allocation will be even more important (Engert et al. 2009). Extranodal involvement (GHSG) and age over 50 years (EORTC/GELA) as adverse prognosis qualifiers also differ among study groups and require consensus building. We will need to harmonize these categories for extracting the most benefit from future studies.

The advanced-stage category lumps together patients with stage III and patients with stage IV. While this approach may be appropriate for identifying optimal chemotherapy regimens, it is probably suboptimal for evaluating the benefit of consolidation with radiotherapy.

The international prognostic score (IPS) for advanced-stage disease is also becoming outdated and of limited use. New biological markers such as the number of tumor-associated macrophages that can be identified in formalin-fixed material by using staining for CD68 may correlate well with prognosis of advanced- and early-stage patients (Steidl et al. 2010). In one recent study a high proportion of CD68+ cells in the tumor specimen outperformed the IPS in identifying shortened progression-free survival. Validation of this study results is obviously still required in order to incorporate its parameters into a prognostic system that may influence the management algorithm of HL.

16.3 Radiotherapy as Single Modality: Lymphocyte Predominant HL

Localized lymphocyte predominant HL (LPHL) is the only subgroup of patients still treated upfront with radiotherapy alone. The course of the disease is indolent, and it has been questioned if watchful waiting after complete resection is a safe option (Mauz-Korholz et al. 2007; Murphy et al. 2003). In general, there is agreement that standard treatment for localized disease is radiotherapy, but the dose and volume have not been determined in randomized trials. For patients with advanced disease, the optimal chemotherapy regimen, the role of rituximab, and the role of additional radiotherapy are still unclear.

16.4 Radiotherapy in the Combined Modality Setting

Except for LPHL, radiotherapy will practically always be used as part of combined modality therapy in HL, both in the primary setting and in the recurrent situation.

16.4.1 Radiotherapy in the Primary Treatment

16.4.1.1 Target Volume

The target volume in the combined modality setting includes only the initially involved lymphoma volume. However, systemic treatment is given first, and radiotherapy is given after shrinkage of lymphoma tissue has occurred. The issue of using pre-chemotherapy imaging for the planning of post-chemotherapy radiotherapy poses challenges both with regard to technique and organization.

With regard to technique, some form of co-registration of the pre- and post-chemotherapy images is needed. In its crudest form, this consists in the radiation oncologist drawing the initial lymphoma volume on the post-chemotherapy planning CT-scan based on the visual analysis of the pre-chemotherapy images. However, this is a quite inaccurate method, especially if the patient's position differed significantly, making large margins for uncertainty necessary. Some form of mathematical co-registration is faster and potentially also more accurate. At present only rigid co-registration, mostly based on bony landmarks, is widely implemented. This technique is hampered by differences in position of the patients before and after chemotherapy, and by changes in patient anatomy during treatment due to tumor shrinkage and to weight loss etc. Deformable co-registration is now being developed (Gu et al. 2010; Yang et al. 2010), but the technique still suffers from major problems when the difference between the images to be co-registered are substantial, as they may well be in the pre- and post-chemotherapy situations.

Organizational problems may be an impediment to the optimal use of radiotherapy in HL. Ideally, all information needed for radiotherapy should be collected for each individual patient before the start of chemotherapy by the radiation oncologist responsible for the subsequent radiotherapy planning. Specifically, imaging (typically PET/CT) should be acquired in the right patient position and with techniques suitable for later co-registration. If these requirements are not fulfilled the only way the radiation oncologist can compensate is by increasing the irradiated volume in order to accommodate the uncertainties caused by the suboptimal technical conditions. However, the best should not be the enemy of the good, and some form of reasonable compromise will have to be developed which will allow the use of radiotherapy in the best possible way even in situations where the ideal conditions cannot be fulfilled. Moreover, with the dissemination of the information of the technical possibilities of modern radiotherapy in a wider circle than just radiation oncologists, hopefully, the implementation of the pre-chemotherapy imaging techniques required for optimal radiotherapy planning can be implemented also by hematologists and medical oncologists treating HL.

A caveat to the universal acceptance of the involved node radiation therapy (INRT) is the absence of randomized studies comparing it to the widely adopted involved field radiation therapy (IFRT) and the paucity of documented experience of using INRT. Thus far, only one retrospective study that compared reduced IFRT field that has some similarities to the new INRT field documented the safety of the reduced IFRT (quasi INRT) in terms of in-field and margin control (Campbell et al. 2008). A randomized study of INRT versus IFRT is planned by the GHSG in the HD17 trial (Eich et al. 2008). The current ongoing prospective study conducted by the EORTC, GELA, and IIL groups H10, is using well-outlined INRT and is expected to finish accruing over 1,400 patients this year. Although, the radiation field extent is not the trial question, it will likely provide important information regarding the efficacy of using INRT following chemotherapy.

16.4.1.2 Dose

Radiation dose in early-stage disease is at present being modified, and the prescribed dose in the combined modality setting will most likely be reduced further from 30 to 20 Gy for patients with favorable characteristics. The recent results of the GHSG HD10 have documented the safety of this dose reduction following only two cycles of ABVD (Engert et al. 2009). For patients with unfavorable disease there is randomized evidence to show that 30 Gy is as effective as 40 Gy. Further reduction to the 20 Gy range may be dependent on the choice of chemotherapy. In the randomized GHSG study of unfavorable patients (HD11) (Borchmann et al. 2009), the groups that received standard BEACOPP × 4 had similar excellent disease control and OS whether they received 30 Gy of IFRT or only 20 Gy. Unfavorable early-stage patients that received ABVD × 4 followed by IFRT of 30 Gy did equally well to the BEACOPP groups, but ABVD × 4 followed by IFRT of 20 Gy yielded slightly inferior results. For patients with advanced disease treated for residual and/or bulky disease the optimal dose level has not been determined in randomized trials.

16.4.2 *Radiotherapy in Salvage Treatment*

Radiotherapy as the only treatment of relapse is probably indicated in a highly selected group of patients. However, the precise definition of this group, the volume to be irradiated, and the radiation dose have not determined.

The role of radiation therapy as a component of a high-dose salvage program that includes autologous stem cell transplantation has not been studied in a randomized trial and clear guidelines for incorporation of radiotherapy are not available. Thus, many groups often take patients who failed chemotherapy alone and either remained refractory or relapsed in only single site through stem cell transplantation without considering the benefit of radiation therapy. Multiple retrospective studies and pattern of failure analyses suggested an important role for radiotherapy in salvage programs. The timing of radiotherapy, before the transplant or after the transplant, remains unclear and is discussed in the relevant chapter. Several reports have shown the efficacy and safety of the high-dose chemo-radiotherapy salvage approach (Yahalom et al. 1993). Patient selection criteria, the timing of radiotherapy, the extent of the field, and dose have not been clearly defined and thus may need to be determined by the multidisciplinary transplant team. Still, an important challenge remains – raising the awareness of transplantation teams to the benefits of radiotherapy in this critical stage of a second attempt to obtain cure after failure of standard chemotherapy alone or a combined modality treatment. Unfortunately, too often, a patient is referred to radiation oncology for the first time only after he/she had already failed a chemotherapy-only-based stem cell transplantation.

16.5 FDG-PET Response and the Need for Radiotherapy

In an effort to reduce the exposure of patients to radiation, some have speculated that a negative FDG-PET obtained at the end of a chemotherapy course or at the completion of only two cycles of chemotherapy will serve as an indicator of the safety of eliminating radiotherapy without compromising progression-free survival rate. In one published prospective randomized trial that included mostly advanced-stage bulky (>5 cm) patients who after chemotherapy converted into a negative PET status, the idea of avoiding radiation did not work too well (Picardi et al. 2007). PET-negative patients that were randomized to observation alone had significantly more relapses than patients that received IFRT of 32 Gy.

Three large studies with interesting different designs are currently looking into the same question – is chemotherapy alone as effective as combined modality therapy in those patients who achieved a PET-negative status after chemotherapy? The EORTC/GELA/IIL H10 study in early-stage HL (protocol 20015) is assessing PET response after two cycles of ABVD in all patients. Patients with favorable disease that were originally randomized to the "standard arm" receive three cycles of ABVD followed by INRT of 30 Gy, independent of the interim PET results. Unfavorable "standard arm" patients receive four cycles of ABVD followed by INRT of 30 Gy. On the "experimental arm," favorable patients that became PET-negative after only two cycles receive two additional cycles of ABVD and no radiotherapy (more chemotherapy is given to substitute for radiotherapy); unfavorable patients on the "experimental arm" receive a total of six cycles of ABVD and no radiotherapy. Patients that remained with a positive PET on the experimental arm are switched to escalated BEACOPP × 2 followed by INRT of 30 Gy. This study will have the power to show if in PET-negative patients more chemotherapy can safely substitute for INRT.

As this book was going into print, an interim analysis of the H10 study disclosed that a statistically significant higher number of patients with either favorable or unfavorable early-stage who obtained a PET-negative status after 2 cycles of ABVD and thus received additional chemotherapy but no RT consolidation on the experimental arm relapsed compared to those that received RT consolidation (and less ABVD) on the standard arm. Following the interim analysis, the study monitoring committee closed the no-RT arms to both favorable and unfavorable patients. The study is still inconclusive with regard to the best chemotherapy approach in patients that remain PET-positive after 2 cycles of ABVD. They all receive consolidation RT after wither additional ABVD (standard arm) or escalated BEACOPP (experimental arm).

Another ongoing randomized study in patients with non-bulky early-stage HL is being conducted in Great Britain. Responding patients that achieved a PET-negative status after three cycles of ABVD are randomized to either IFRT or observation alone. The other study is conducted by GHSG (study HD16) in patients with favorable early-stage HL. It is based on the excellent results of the HD10 trial that showed that even without the benefit of an interim PET, only two cycles of ABVD followed by IFRT of 20 Gy yielded an excellent outcome (5-year freedom from treatment failure greater than 90%). In HD16, the "standard arm" patients will receive ABVD × 2+IFRT 20 Gy independent of their PET response prior to radiotherapy. Those randomized to the "experimental arm" and have achieved a PET-negative status receive no further treatment, those that are still PET-positive proceed to receive only IFRT of 20 Gy, but no further chemotherapy.

We are eagerly awaiting the results of these prospective randomized trials. They will clarify the role of radiotherapy in PET-negative patients and may help to optimize treatment in those who remained PET-positive after a relatively short course of chemotherapy.

It is concerning, however, that while the HL community is waiting for the completion and analysis of these interesting studies, some have already decided that a PET-negative status is already a permit to eliminate radiotherapy from the combined modality approach in favorable and unfavorable early-stage patients.

16.6 Conclusion

Radiotherapy is a highly efficient treatment for HL. Present and future refinements in radiation and imaging technology should be used to their full capacity to benefit patients with HL, keeping the cure rate, both from primary and salvage treatment, as high as possible while at the same time reducing radiation doses to normal tissues to an absolute minimum, thus reducing the risk of long-term complications from radiotherapy. Further research is needed with regard to radiation dose and volume in different clinical situations. Data on the risk of long-term complications from all treatment modalities are needed, and mathematical modeling and risk calculations should be developed in order to enable the rational choice of combinations of the different modalities for the optimal outcome in the individual patient.

References

Borchmann P, Diehl V, Goergen H et al (2009) Combined modality treatment with intensified chemotherapy and dose-reduced involved field radiotherapy in patients with early unfavourable Hodgkin lymphoma (HL): final analysis of the German Hodgkin Study Group (GHSG) HD11 trial. Blood 114: 717

Campbell BA, Voss N, Pickles T et al (2008) Involved-nodal radiation therapy as a component of combination therapy for limited-stage Hodgkin's lymphoma: a question of field size. J Clin Oncol 26:5170–5174

Eich HT, Muller RP, Engenhart-Cabillic R et al (2008) Involved-node radiotherapy in early-stage Hodgkin's lymphoma. Definition and guidelines of the German Hodgkin Study Group (GHSG). Strahlenther Onkol 184:406–410

Engert A, Diehl V, Pluetschow A et al (2009) Two cycles of ABVD followed by involved field radiotherapy with 20 Gray (Gy) is the new standard of care in the treatment of patients with early-stage Hodgkin lymphoma: final analysis of the randomized German Hodgkin Study Group (GHSG) HD10. Study supported by the Deutsche Krebshilfe and in part by the Competence Network Malignant Lymphoma. Blood 114(22): Abstract 716

Grow A, Quon A, Graves EE et al (2005) Metabolic tumor volume as an independent prognostic factor in lymphoma. J Clin Oncol 23 (Suppl.):583S

Gu X, Pan H, Liang Y et al (2010) Implementation and evaluation of various demons deformable image registration algorithms on a GPU. Phys Med Biol 55:207–219

Hutchings M, Berthelsen AK, Jakobsen AL et al (2005) Volume of abnormal tumour tissue on FDG-PET - a predictor of progression-free survival in Hodgkin lymphoma? Int J Radiat Oncol Biol Phys 63:S45

Mauz-Korholz C, Gorde-Grosjean S, Hasenclever D et al (2007) Resection alone in 58 children with limited stage, lymphocyte-predominant Hodgkin lymphoma-experience from the European network group on pediatric Hodgkin lymphoma. Cancer 110:179–185

Murphy SB, Morgan ER, Katzenstein HM et al (2003) Results of little or no treatment for lymphocyte-predominant Hodgkin disease in children and adolescents. J Pediatr Hematol Oncol 25:684–687

Picardi M, De Renzo A, Pane F et al (2007) Randomized comparison of consolidation radiation versus observation in bulky Hodgkin's lymphoma with post-chemotherapy negative positron emission tomography scans. Leuk Lymphoma 48:1721–1727

Specht L (1996) Prognostic factors in Hodgkin's disease. Semin Radiat Oncol 6:146–161

Steidl C, Lee T, Shah SP et al (2010) Tumor-associated macrophages and survival in classic Hodgkin's lymphoma. N Engl J Med 362:875–885

Yahalom J, Gulati SC, Toia M et al (1993) Accelerated hyperfractionated total-lymphoid irradiation, high-dose chemotherapy, and autologous bone marrow transplantation for refractory and relapsing patients with Hodgkin's disease. J Clin Oncol 11:1062–1070

Yang D, Goddu SM, Lu W et al (2010) Technical note: deformable image registration on partially matched images for radiotherapy applications. Med Phys 37:141–145

Index